2Cd Navelbine

Pam Curry

THE
Oncology
WORD
BOOK

mental health team

DeB

79,

Nancy 74, 209l

D0808439

THE
Oncology
WORD
BOOK

Krista
6321

Helen E. Littrell, CMT
Private Practice
Klamath Falls, Oregon

 F. A. DAVIS COMPANY • Philadelphia

F. A. Davis Company
1915 Arch Street
Philadelphia, PA 19103

Printed in the United States of America

Last digit indicates print number: 10 9 8 7 6 5 4 3 2 1

Editor: *Lynn Borders Caldwell*
Production Editor: *Jody E. Gould*
Cover Design By: *Donald B. Freggens, Jr.*

As new scientific information becomes available through basic and clinical research, recommended treatments and drug therapies undergo changes. The author(s) and publisher have done everything possible to make this book accurate, up to date, and in accord with accepted standards at the time of publication. The authors, editors, and publisher are not responsible for errors or omissions or for consequences from application of the book, and make no warranty, expressed or implied, in regard to the contents of the book. Any practice described in this book should be applied by the reader in accordance with professional standards of care used in regard to the contents of the book. Any practice described in this book should be applied by the reader in accordance with professional standards of care used in regard to the unique circumstances that may apply in each situation. The reader is advised always to check product information (package inserts) for changes and new information regarding dose and contraindications before administering any drug. Caution is especially urged when using new or infrequently ordered drugs.

Library of Congress Cataloging-in-Publication Data

Littrell, Helen E.
    The oncology word book / Helen E. Littrell.
      p. cm.
    ISBN 0-8036-5649-1 (pbk. : alk. paper)
    1. Oncology—Terminology. I. Title.
    [DNLM: 1. Medical Oncology—terminology. QZ 15 L7820 1993]
RC254.5.L58 1993
616.99′2′0014—dc20
DNLM/DLC
for Library of Congress
                          93-18230
                              CIP

To the memory of my daughter
Sharon Mae Simpson,
whose lifelong dedication to
helping those less fortunate
did make a difference.

Acknowledgments

I wish to thank Jean-François Vilain and Lynn Borders Caldwell for their confidence in me, as well as their encouragement and assistance throughout this project.

To the reviewers listed below goes a most special thanks for many tedious hours spent in careful reading and researching the manuscript, and for the very constructive comments and suggestions that helped so much in finalizing the book.

Sarah Lu Mitchell-Hatton, CMT
Author, *The Davis Book of Medical Abbreviations*
Private Practice
Sacramento, California

Mimi Phillips, CMT
Hospital Transcriptionist
Nehalem, Oregon

Jeanne M. Schneider, CMT
Hospital Transcriptionist
Eugene, Oregon

Lois A. Thistle, CMT
Private Practice
Stockton, California

Introduction

The Oncology Word Book was written for use primarily by medical transcriptionists at hospitals, clinics, and transcription services, as well as those at the university research level. Others in the allied health field including radiation therapy technicians, medical records personnel, coders, tumor board personnel, billing clerks, hospice workers, nurses, educators, authors, and students will find this book the most comprehensive and timely reference source available.

Some AIDS terms are included as well as many terms applicable to the specialties of immunology, microbiology, immunogenetics, hematology, virology, epidemiology, cellular biology, molecular biology, molecular genetics, and cancer genetics, because all of these are incorporated into oncology. In all, over 33,000 entries are included in the text. An extensive listing of anticancer and chemotherapy protocols is included under *protocol.*

Because new discoveries in the various fields of research are constantly being made, *The Oncology Word Book* will be updated at regular intervals in order to provide current information. I welcome all suggestions and contributions of new terms to be included in upcoming revisions.

Please send your suggestions to:

Helen E. Littrell, CMT
c/o Lynn Borders Caldwell
Editor, Allied Health
F.A. Davis Company
1915 Arch Street
Philadelphia, PA 19103

References

Literally hundreds of hours were spent researching and compiling the information contained in *The Oncology Word Book*. Hospital libraries, textbooks, reference books, and journals were primary sources for much of the data. Fred Hutchinson Cancer Research Center, Dana-Farber Cancer Institute, Memorial Sloan-Kettering Cancer Center, and Baylor-Charles A. Hammons Cancer Center responded overwhelmingly to my request for information and have enabled me to present the newest drugs, protocols, procedures, and therapies in this book.

How To Use This Book

The format is strictly alphabetical with extensive cross-referencing employed for maximum ease and speed in finding a desired term. Many entries appear as both primary entries and subentries under the appropriate cross-reference category. Examples of this are *anemia, biopsy, leukemia, radiation, tumor,* and *cancer.*

When an entry is modified by several other terms, as in the case of the different kinds of cancer, the subentries are indented and punctuated as follows:

> *cancer* (main entry)
> > *atrophicans, c.* (when main entry comes before subentry)
>
> *colorectal c.* (when main entry comes after subentry)

Immediately following the list of various types of cancer are phrases in which the word *cancer* comes first. For example:

> *cancer cachexia*
> *cancer chemotherapy*

This is a streamlined format used throughout the book to provide maximum clarity, especially in the case of main entries such as *cell, gene, tumor, anemia,* and so on, which have many subentries listing the various types of each in addition to numerous phrases in which the main entry is the first word.

In the case of anticancer drug–chemotherapy drug combinations, generic or chemical names are used wherever possible, but it is sometimes necessary to use the trade name in order to fit the initialism. Generic, trade, chemical, National Formulary, U.S.P., British Approved Names, United States Adopted Names, and so on, may be used interchangeably in various combinations, according to the preference of the individual physician, institution, or writer. For example:

> *CAP (Cytoxan, Adriamycin, Platinol)*—using trade names to fit initialism
> *CAP (cyclophosphamide, doxorubicin, cisplatin)*—using generic names
> *CAP (Neosar, doxorubicin, DDP)*—using a combination of generic and trade names

Over 550 chemotherapy drug combinations are listed under the main heading of *protocol,* as well as in their respective alphabetical positions.

Plurals of Latin or Greek origin are shown in parentheses following the root word. For example:

> *carcinoma (pl. carcinomata)*
> *carcinomata (pl. of carcinoma)* is also listed alphabetically

Abbreviations used interchangeably with the full entry are shown as:

> *PSA (prostate-specific antigen)*
> *prostate-specific antigen (PSA)* is also listed alphabetically

Where an abbreviation has more than one meaning, a separate entry is made for each, and each is cross-referenced; however, cross-referencing is not done in the case of chemotherapy drug combinations such as *MOPP.*

In accordance with standards approved by the American Association for Medical Transcription (AAMT), the possessive form is not used with eponyms in this book. For example:

> *Lindau's tumor* is shown as
> *Lindau tumor*

Many genes and oncogenes have names that appear to be abbreviations but are not. For example:

> *kit* gene

Entries beginning with a number are listed by the first letter following the number. For example:

> *11-deoxycorticosterone (DOC)*

A A-2371
A-8103
A antigen
A cell
A factor
AA (ara-C, Adriamycin)
AA (arachidonic acid)
AAA (adenosine-adenosine-adenosine)
AAAF (albumin autoagglutinating factor)
AAF (2-acetylaminofluorene)
AAS (atomic absorption spectrophotometry)
Aase syndrome
AAT (alpha1-antitrypsin)
AAV (adeno-associated virus)
Aavala lung biopsy needle
Ab (antibody)
AB-100
AB-132
Abbe
    condenser, A.
    flap, A.Abbé
Abbé
    condenser, A.
Abbe-Estlander flap
Abbé-Zeiss
    apparatus, A.
    counting cell hemocytometer, A.
    counting chamber, A.
Abbott
    AFP-EIA monoclonal, A.
    anti-delta EIA, A
    CEA-EIA monoclonal, A.
    CMV total AB EIA, A.
    -HB EIA, A.
    -HBe test, A.
    HTLV III antigen EIA, A.
    IgE EIA, A.
    PAP-EIA, A.
    TdT EIA, A.
    Toxo-G EIA, A.
    Toxo-M EIA, A.
Abbott-Rawson tube
ABC (Adriamycin, BCNU, cyclophosphamide)
ABC (American Blood Commission)
ABC (antigen-binding capacity)
ABC (aspiration biopsy cytology)
ABCD (Adriamycin, bleomycin, CCNU, dacarbazine)
ABCD (amphotericin B colloid dispersion)

ABCDs (asymmetry, border, color, diameter) of melanoma
ABCM (Adriamycin, bleomycin, cyclophosphamide, mitomycin-C)
ABCX (Adriamycin, bleomycin, cisplatin, radiation therapy)
ABD (Adriamycin, bleomycin, DTIC)
Abderhalden dialysis
ABDIC (Adriamycin, bleomycin, dacarbazine, CCNU, prednisone)
abdominopelvic
abdominoperineal resection (APR)
abdominosacral resection
abducens nerve
ABDV (Adriamycin, bleomycin, DTIC, vinblastine)
Abelson
    murine leukemia virus, A.
    oncogene, A.
Abercrombie syndrome
Abernethy sarcoma
aberrant
aberration
    chromosome a.
abetalipoproteinemia
abevacuation
ABGs (arterial blood gases)
ABH blood group
    antigen, A.
Abitrexate
abl oncogene
ablate
ablation
    pituitary a.
    radioiodine a.
ablation dose
ablation therapy
ablative
    hormonal therapy, a.
    laser therapy, a.
ABLC (amphotericin B lipid complex)
ABMA (antibasement membrane antibody)
ABMT (autologous bone marrow transplant)
abnormally banding region
ABO (blood groups A, AB, B, and O)
    antigen, A.
    blood group system, A.
    compatibility, A.
    erythroblastosis, A.
    hemolytic disease, A.
    incompatibility, A.

ADDITIONAL TERMS

above-knee amputation (AKA)
ABP (Adriamycin, bleomycin,
 prednisone)
ABP (arterial blood pressure)
ABPP (bropirimine)
Abrami disease
Abrams biopsy needle
Abrikosov tumor
Abrikossoff tumor
abscess
abscise
abscissa
abscission
abscopal
Absidia
 corymbifera, A.
 ramosa, A.
absolute
 basophil count, a.
 eosinophil count, a.
 ethanol, a.
 leukocytosis, a.
 lymphocyte count, a.
 neutrophil count, a. (ANC)
 reticulocyte count, a.
 zero, a.
absorb
absorbable
 carrier, a.
absorbance
absorbed
 dose, a. (AD)
absorber
absorbifacient
absorptiometry
absorption
 agglutinin, a.
 atelectasis, a.
 cell, a.
 coefficient, a.
 dose, a.
 equivalent thickness, a. (AET)
 peak, a.
 spectrophotometer, a.
 spectrum, a.
absorptive
absorptivity
abstinence
abstinent
ABV (actinomycin-D, bleomycin,
 vincristine)
ABVD (Adriamycin, bleomycin,
 vinblastine, dacarbazine)

ABVE (Adriamycin, bleomycin,
 vincristine, etoposide)
Ac (actinium)
AC (Adriamycin, carmustine)
AC (Adriamycin, CCNU)
AC (Adriamycin, cisplatin)
5-AC (azacitidine)
acanthamebiasis
Acanthamoeba
 astronyxis, A.
 castellani, A.
 culbertsoni, A.
 hartmannella, A.
 polyphaga, A.
acanthocyte
acanthocytosis
acanthoma
 adenoides cysticum, a.
 basal cell a.
acanthosis
 glycogenic a.
 nigricans, a.
acanthotic
ACAT (automated computerized axial
 tomography)
acatalasemia
acatamathesia
acataphasia
ACBE (air contrast barium enema)
accelerated
 fractionation, a.
 myeloproliferative phase, a.
 treatment, a.
accelerator
 betatron a.
 bevatron a.
 C3b inactivator a.
 charge-exchange a.
 electron a.
 electrostatic a.
 induction a.
 linear a.
 microwave linear a.
 positive-ion a.
 proton beam a.
 serum prothrombin conversion a.
 (SPCA)
 serum thrombotic a.
accelerator factor
accelerator globulin (AcG)
accelerin
accessory
 cells, a.

ADDITIONAL TERMS

spleen, a.
thyroid gland, a.
accrementition
accretion
Accu-Chek II Freedom
Accucore II core biopsy needle
accumulated dose equivalent
Accutane (isotretinoin)
ACD (acid citrate dextrose)
ACD (annihilation coincidence detection)
AC-DC (bisexual)
ACe (Adriamycin, cyclophosphamide)
ACE (adrenocortical extract)
ACE (Adriamycin, cyclophosphamide,
  etoposide)
    -II, A. (Adriamycin,
      cyclophosphamide, etoposide in
      high-dose infusion)
ACE (angiotensin-converting enzyme)
ACEH (acid cholesteryol ester
  hydrolase)
acellular
acemannan (Carrisyn)
acervuline
acervuloma
acervulus
acestoma
acetabulectomy
acetabulum
acetic acid
acetoacetic acid
acetone
    -insoluble antigen, a.
acetonemia
acetrizoate
acetrizoic acid
acetylaminofluorene
acetylcholine (ACh)
    receptor antibody, a. (AChRab)
acetylcholinesterase
acetyl-CoA
    acetyltransferase, a.
    carboxylase, a.
acetylcysteine
N-acetylgalactosamine-4-sulfatase
acetylphenylhydrazine
N-acetyltransferase
ACFUCY (actinomycin D, 5-fluorouracil,
  cyclophosphamide)
AcG (acclerator globulin)
ACh (acetylcholine)
achaete-scute protein
achalasia

AChRab (acetylcholine receptor
  antibody)
achrestic anemia
achroacytosis
achromasia
achromatin
achromic
Achromobacter
achromocyte
achylanemia
achylia
achylic anemia
acid
    aerosol, a.
    agglutination, a.
    -base, a.
    cholesterol ester hydrolase, a.
      (ACEH)
    citrate dextrose, a. (ACD)
    -elution test, a.
    fallout, a.
    -fast, a.
    -fast bacilli, a. (AFB)
    helix-turn activator motif, a.
    hemolysis test, a.
    -labile alpha interferon, a.
    lability test, a.
    lipase deficiency, a.
    maltase deficiency, a.
    phosphatase, a. (AP)
    rain, a.
    Schiff stain, a.
ACID (Adriamycin, cyclophosphamide,
  imidazole, dactinomycin)
Acidaminococcus
acidemia
acidic
acidified serum test
acidocyte
acidocytopenia
acidocytosis
acidophilic
    adenoma, a.
acidophilism
acidophilus
acidosis
    lactic a.
    metabolic a.
acidotic
Acidulin
aciduria
acinar
    cell, a.

ADDITIONAL TERMS

acinar —*Continued*
   cell carcinoma, a.
   cell tumor, a.
Acinetobacter
   anitratus, A.
   calcoaceticus, A.
   lwoffi, A.
   parapertussis, A.
acinic
   cell carcinoma, a.
   cell tumor, a.
acinose
acinous
acinus
   liver a.
acivicin
Ackerman biopsy needle
aclacinomycin A
acladiosis
aclarubicin
ACM (Adriamycin, cyclophosphamide,
   methotrexate)
acne
   fulminans, a.
acneiform
acnemia
ACNU (nimustine)
ACOAP (Adriamycin,
   cyclophosphamide, Oncovin, cytosine
   arabinoside, prednisone)
acodazole hydrochloride
acomia
aconitase
ACOP (Adriamycin, cyclophosphamide,
   Oncovin, prednisone)
ACOPP (Adriamycin,
   cyclophosphamide, Oncovin,
   prednisone, procarbazine)
Acosta classification
acoustic
   neurilemoma, a.
   neurinoma, a.
   neuroma, a.
   schwannoma, a.
   tumor, a.
acoustical shadowing
acquired
   agammaglobulinemia, a.
   hemolytic anemia, a. (AHA)
   immune hemolytic disease, a.
      (AIHD)
   immunity, a.

immunodeficiency syndrome, a.
   (AIDS or AIS)
red cell aplasia, a. (ARCA)
sideroblastic anemia, a.
siderochrestic anemia, a.
acral lentiginous melanoma
acraturesis
Acremoniella
acridine orange
acridinyl
   anisidide, a. (amsacrine or AMSA)
acridinylamino
   -carbamate derivative, a.
acridone
acriflavine
acrokeratosis
acrolein
acronine
acronycine
ACS (American Cancer Society)
ACT (actinomycin)
ACT (activated clotting time)
ACT (activated coagulation time)
ACT-C (actinomycin-C)
ACT-D (actinomycin-D)
ACT-FU-Cy (actinomycin-D, 5-FU,
   cyclophosphamide)
ACTG (AIDS Clinical Trials Group)
ACTH (adrenocorticotropic hormone)
   -Cushing syndrome, A.
   -producing tumors, A.
   -RF, A. (adrenocorticotropic
      hormone-releasing factor)
   stimulation test, A.
   tumor marker, A.
Acthar
Actimmune
actin
   F (fiber) a.
   G (globular) a.
actinic
   burn, a.
   elastosis, a.
   keratosis, a.
   light rays, a.
   radiation, a.
actinicity
actiniform
actinism
actinium (Ac)
   emanation, a.
Actinobacillus

ADDITIONAL TERMS

actinomycetemcomitans, A.
actinocutitis
actinodermatitis
Actinomadura
   madurae, A.
   pelletierii, A.
actinometer
actinometry
Actinomyces
   asteroides, A.
   bovis, A.
   eppingeri, A.
   eriksonii, A.
   gonidiaformis, A.
   israelii, A.
   naeslundii, A.
   necrophorus, A.
   odontolyticus, A.
   pseudonecrophorus, A.
   viscosus, A.
actinomycetoma
actinomycin (ACT)
   C, a. (ACT-C)
   D, a. (ACT-D or dactinomycin)
actinomycoma
actinomycosis
actinomycotic
actinon
actinopraxis
actinoquinol sodium
actinotherapy
Activase
activated
   clotting time, a. (ACT)
   partial thromboplastin time, a.
    (APTT)
   prothrombin complex concentrates,
    a. (APCC)
   T-cells, a.
activation
   lymphocyte a.
activation factor
activator
   plasminogen a.
   polyclonal a.
   tissue plasminogen a. (t-PA)
Active Life ostomy pouch
activities of daily living (ADL)
activity
   leukemia-associated inhibitory a.
   tumor a.
actoquinol sodium

ACTP (adrenocorticotropic polypeptide)
acupoint
acupressure
acupuncture
acusection
acusector
acute
   cerebellar ataxia, a.
   disseminated histiocytosis X, a.
   encephalopathy, a.
   febrile leukemia, a.
   fulminating toxoplasmosis, a.
   granulocytic leukemia, a. (AGL)
   intermittent porphyria, a. (AIP)
   leukemia, a.
   lymphoblastic leukemia, a. (ALL)
   lymphocytic leukemia, a. (ALL)
   monoblastic leukemia, a. (AMOL)
   monocytic leukemia, a. (AML)
   monomyelocytic leukemia, a.
    (AMML)
   myeloblastic leukemia, a. (AML)
   myelogenous leukemia, a. (AML)
   myeloid leukemia, a.
   myelomonoblastic leukemia, a.
    (AMML)
   myelomonocytic leukemia, a.
   nonlymphocytic leukemia, a.
    (ANLL)
   nonlymphoid leukemia, a. (ANLL)
   promyelocytic leumemia, a. (APL)
   radiation syndrome, a. (ARS)
   renal failure, a. (ARF)
   transforming retrovirus, a.
   tubular necrosis, a. (ATN)
   tumor lysis, a. (ATL)
   undifferentiated leukemia, a. (AUL)
   viral hepatitis, a.
ACV (acyclovir)
acycloguanosine
acyclovir (ACV)
AD (absorbed dose)
AD (ara-C, daunorubicin)
AD (diphenylchlorarsine or Clark I)
A+D (ara-C, daunorubicin)
ADA (adenosine deaminase)
   deficiency, A.
   -deficient, A.
ADA gene
ADAC EXL-22 DP accelerator
Adagen
adamantine

ADDITIONAL TERMS

adamantine—*Continued*
  epithelioma, a.
adamantinoblastoma
adamantinocarcinoma
adamantinoma
  long bones, a. of
  pituitary a.
  polycysticum, a.
adamantoblast
adamantoblastoma
adamantoma
Adam's apple
adaptogen
ADBC (Adriamycin, DTIC, bleomycin, CCNU)
ADC (AIDS dementia complex)
  staging, A. (stages 0 through 4)
ADCC (antibody-dependent cell-mediated cytolysis)
ADCC (antibody-dependent cell-mediated cytotoxicity)
Addis count
Addison
  anemia, A.
  disease, A.
  melanoderma, A.
  syndrome, A.
Addison-Biermer anemia
addisonian
  anemia, a.
  crisis, a.
  syndrome, a.
addisonism
ADE (ara-C, daunorubicin, etoposide)
adenectomy
adenine
  arabinoside, a.
  deaminase, a.
  diphosphate, a.
  hypoxanthine, a.
  nucleotide, a.
  phosphoribosyltransferase, a. (APRT)
  sulfate, a.
  triphosphate, a.
adenitis
adenoacanthoma
adenoameloblastoma
adenoangiosarcoma
adenoassociated virus (AAV)
adenoblast
adeno-CA (adenocarcinoma)
adenocancroid

adenocarcinoma
  acinar a.
  acinous a.
  alveolar a.
  anaplastic a.
  axillary lymph node a.
  clear cell a.
  colloid a.
  ductal a.
  follicular a.
  gelatinous a.
  Gleason II a.
  hilar a.
  Hurthle cell a.
  kidney, a. of
  metastatic prostatic a.
  mucinous a.
  papillary a.
  polypoid a.
  prostatic a.
  salivary gland a.
  signet ring a.
  undifferentiated a.
adenocele
adenocellulitis
adenochondroma
adenochondrosarcoma
adenocyst
adenocystic
adenocystoma
  papillary a.
  lymphomatosum, a.
adenocyte
adenoepithelioma
adenofibroma
  edematodes, a.
adenofibrosis
adenogenous
adenography
adenohypophysectomy
adenohypophysial
adenohypophysis
adenoid
  cystic carcinoma, a.
adenoleiomyofibroma
adenolipoma
adenolipomatosis
adenolymphitis
adenolymphocele
adenolymphoma
adenoma (pl. adenomata)
  acidophilic a.
  adamantinum, a.

ADDITIONAL TERMS

alveolare, a.
apocrine a.
basophil a.
basophilic a.
benign a.
bronchial a's
carcinoid a. of bronchus
ceruminous a.
chief cell a.
chromophile a.
chromophobe a.
chromophobic a.
colloid a.
cortical a's
destruens, a.
embryonal a.
endometrioides ovarii, a.
eosinophil a.
fetal a.
fibroid a.
fibrosum, a.
follicular a.
gelatinosum, a.
hidradenoides, a.
Hurthle cell a.
islet a.
langerhansian a.
macrofollicular a.
malignant a.
microfollicular a.
mucinous a.
mucous gland a.
oncocytic a.
ovarian tubular a.
ovarii testiculare, a.
oxyphil a.
oxyphilic granular cell a.
papillary cystic a.
Pick tubular a.
pituitary a.
pituitary basophil a.
pleomorphic a.
polypoid a.
racemose a.
sebaceous a.
sebaceum, a.
sudoriparum, a.
testicular tubular a.
thyroid a.
tubular a.
tubulare testiculare ovarii, a.
villous a.
adenomalacia

adenomata (pl. of adenoma)
adenomatoid
adenomatosis
fibrosing a.
multiple endocrine a.
oris, a.
pluriglandular a.
polyendocrine a.
pulmonary a.
adenomatous
goiter, a.
hyperplasia, a.
polyp, a.
polyposis coli, a.
tumor, a.
adenomegaly
adenomeloblastoma
adenomere
adenomyoepithelioma
stomach, a. of
adenomyofibroma
adenomyoma
psammopapillare, a.
adenomyomatosis
adenomyomatous
adenomyometritis
adenomyosarcoma
embryonal a.
adenomyosis
externa, a.
stromal a.
subbasalis, a.
tubae, a.
uteri, a.
adenomyxoma
adenomyxosarcoma
adenoncus
adenopathy
hilar a.
mediastinal a.
adenorhabdomyosarcoma
adenosarcoma
embryonal a.
mullerian a.
adenosclerosis
adenosclerotic
adenosine
analogue, a.
arabinoside, a.
cyclic a. monophosphate (5'-AMP or cAMP)
3',5'-cyclic a. phosphate
deaminase, a. (ADA)

ADDITIONAL TERMS

adenosine—*Continued*
  diphosphate, a. (ADP)
  kinase, a.
  monophosphate, a. (AMP)
  phosphate, a.
  3'-phosphate, a.
  5'-phosphate, a.
  triphosphatase, a. (ATPase)
  triphosphate, a. (ATP)
adenosinetriphosphatase
adenosis
  blunt duct a.
  vaginae, a.
adenosquamous
  carcinoma, a.
adenosylcobalamin
S-adenosylmethionine
  carcinoma, a.
  deficiency, a.
adenous
adenoviral
adenovirus
  avian a.
  bovine a.
  canine a.
  human a.
  murine a.
  simian a.
adenyl cyclase
  pathway, a.
adenylate
  cyclase, a.
  deaminase, a.
  kinase, a.
adenylic acid
adenylosuccinate lyase
adenylyltransferase
ADH (antidiuretic hormone)
adherence
  immune a.
adhesiolysis
adhesiveness
  platelet a.
adiactinic
ADIC (Adriamycin, DTIC)
adipocyte
  P2 gene, a.
adipofibroma
adipogenesis
adipohepatic
adipoma
adiponecrosis
adipsin

adjunct
adjunctive
  therapy, a. (AT)
adjusted survival rate
adjuvant
  Freund complete a.
  Freund incomplete a.
  mycobacterial a.
adjuvant chemotherapy
adjuvant radiotherapy
adjuvant therapy
adjuvanticity
ADL (activities of daily living)
ADM (Adriamycin)
adnexa
adnexectomy
AdOAP (Adriamycin, Oncovin, ara-C,
  prednisone)
AdOP (Adriamycin, Oncovin,
  prednisone)
adoptive
  immunity, a.
  immunotherapy, a.
adozelesin
ADP (adenosine diphosphate)
ADR (Adriamycin or doxorubicin)
ADR-529
adrenal
  adenoma, a.
  cortex, a.
  corticosteroid, a.
  failure, a.
  feminizing syndrome, a.
  gland, a.
  insufficiency, a.
  medullary hyperplasia, a.
  metastases, a.
  suppression, a.
  virilism, a.
  virilizing syndrome, a.
adrenalectomize
adrenalectomy
Adrenalin
adrenaline
adrenalitis
adrenalopathy
adrenergic
  blocking agent, a.
adrenoceptor
adrenocortical
  carcinoma, a.
  extract, a. (ACE)
  hormone, a.

ADDITIONAL TERMS

insufficiency, a.
adrenocorticohyperplasia
adrenocorticomimetic
adrenocorticosteroids
adrenocorticotropic
 hormone, a. (ACTH)
 polypeptide, a. (ACTP)
adrenocorticotropin
adrenodoxin
adrenogenic
adrenogenous
adrenoglomerulotropin
adrenogram
adrenokinetic
adrenoleukodystrophy
adrenolytic
adrenomegaly
adrenomimetic
adrenoprival
adrenoreceptive
adrenoreceptor
adrenostatic
adrenotoxin
adrenotropic
adrenotropin
Adria + BCNU (Adriamycin, BCNU)
Adria-L-PAM (Adriamycin, melphalan)
Adriamycin (doxorubicin)
 flare, A.
 toxicity, A.
Adroyd (oxymetholone)
Adrucil (fluorouracil)
ADS (antibody deficiency syndrome)
ADS (antidiuretic substance)
adsorb
adsorption
 agglutinin a.
adult
 acute lymphocytic leukemia, a.
 cystic teratoma, a.
 respiratory distress syndrome, a.
 (ARDS)
 T-cell leukemia, a. (ATL)
 T-cell lymphoma, a. (ATL)
adumbration
adventitia
adventitial
adventitious cyst
AECL
 Brachytron afterloader, A.
 Therac 25 accelerator, A.
AEF (allogeneic effect factor)
Aerobacter

aerobe
 facultative a.
 obligate a.
aerobic
aerocele
aerocystography
aerocystoscopy
aerogram
Aeropent
Aeroseb-Dex
aerosol
 pentamidine isethionate, a.
aerosolization
aerosolized pentamidine
Aerosporin
aerotonometer
aesthetically
aesthetics
AET (absorption-equivalent thickness)
AEV (avian erythroblastosis virus)
AF 1890 (lonidamine)
AFB (acid-fast bacilli)
afferent
afferentia
affinity
 chromatography, a.
 labeling, a.
afibrinogenemia
afibrogenemia
 congenital a.
aflatoxin
 B1, a.
AFM (Adriamycin, 5-fluorouracil,
 methotrexate)
AFP (alpha-fetoprotein)
African
 AIDS, A.
 anemia, A.
 Burkitt lymphoma, A.
 green monkey, A.
 green monkey kidney, A. (AGMK)
 Kaposi sarcoma, A.
 lymphoma, A.
 sleeping sickness, A.
 trypanosome, A.
afterload applicator
afterloading (AL)
 applicator, a.
 colpostat, a.
 Heyman applicator, a.
 tandem, a.
 technique, a.
Ag (antigen)

ADDITIONAL TERMS

A/G (albumin/globulin) ratio
agammaglobulinemia
    acquired a.
    Bruton a.
    common variable a.
    congenital a.
    lymphopenic a.
    nonsecretory a.
    Swiss type a.
    X-linked a.
    X-linked infantile a.
agar
Agar-IF (immunofixation in agar)
agarose gel electrophoresis (AGE)
AGE (agarose gel electrophoresis)
age spots
agenesis
Agent Orange
AGEPC (acetyl glyceryl ether
  phosphoryl choline)
agger nasi cells
agglutinable
agglutinant
agglutination
    bacteriogenic a.
    cold a.
    cross a.
    group a.
    intravascular a.
    macroscopic a.
    microscopic a.
    passive a.
    platelet a.
    Vi a.
agglutinative
agglutinator
agglutinin
    anti-Rh a.
    atypical a.
    chief a.
    cold a.
    complete a.
    cross a.
    cross-reacting a.
    febrile a.
    flagellar a.
    group a.
    H a.
    immune a.
    incomplete a.
    leukocyte a.
    major a.
    MG a.

    minor a.
    nonspecific a.
    O a.
    partial a.
    platelet a.
    saline a.
    somatic a.
    T a.
    warm a.
agglutinogen
    A and B a's
    M and N a's
    Rh a.
agglutinogenic
agglutinoid
agglutometer
aggregate
aggregated
    human IgG, a. (AHuG)
    lymphatic nodules, a.
    radiopharmaceutical, a.
aggregation
    platelet a.
aggregen
aggregometer
aggressin
aggressive
    disease, a.
    treatment, a.
AGL (acute granulocytic leukemia)
AGL (aminoglutethimide)
aglycemia
aglycon
aglycone
AGM-1470
agminated
AGMK (African green monkey kidney)
agnocobalamin
agnogenic
    myeloid metaplasia, a. (AMM)
AgNOR (silver-staining nucleolar
  organizer region)
agonal respiration
agonist
    opioid a.
agranulocyte
agranulocytosis
    infantile genetic a.
    Kostmann infantile a.
agranuloplastic
agranulosis
AGT (antiglobulin test)
AHA (acquired hemolytic anemia)

ADDITIONAL TERMS

AHA (autoimmune hemolytic anemia)
ahaptoglobin
ahaptoglobinemia
AHF (antihemophilic factor)
AHG (antihemophilic globulin)
AHLS (antihuman lymphocyte serum)
AHuG (aggregated human IgG)
AID (Adriamycin, ifosfamide,
dacarbazine, mesna)
AIDS (acquired immunodeficiency
syndrome)
    arthritis, A.
    dementia complex, A. (ADC)
    drugs, A.
    enteritis, A.
    enteropathy, A.
    psychosis, A.
    -related complex, A. (ARC)
    -related disease, A. (ARD)
    -related syndrome, A. (ARS)
    -related virus, A. (ARV)
    vaccine, A.
    virus, A.
    wasting, A.
AIHA (autoimmune hemolytic anemia)
AIHD (acquired immune hemolytic
disease)
AILD (angioimmunoblastic
lymphadenopathy with
dysproteinemia)
AIM (L-asparaginase, ifosfamide,
methotrexate)
AIP (acute intermittent porphyria)
air
    bronchogram, a.
    contrast barium enema, a. (ACBE)
    dose, a.
    -equivalent chamber, a.
    exposure, a.
    pollution, a.
    -space disease, a.
    -wall ionization chamber, a.
airborne
airway
AIS (acquired immunodeficiency
syndrome)
AITP (autoimmune thrombocytopenic
purpura)
AJCC (American Joint Committee on
Cancer)
    scale, A.
    staging, A.
AK (above-knee)

amputation, A. (AKA)
akaryocyte
akembe
Akerlund diaphragm
Akiyama procedure
AL-721
ALA (aminolevulinic acid)
ALAD (aminolevulinic acid dehydrase)
Alajouanine syndrome
alanine
    aminotransferase, a. (ALT)
    transaminase, a.
Alanson amputation
alanyl
Albarran gland
Albers-Schönberg disease
albukalin
albumin
    aggregated a.
    blood a.
    bovine a.
    human a.
    iodinated I 125 serum a.
    iodinated I 131 aggregated a.
    iodinated I 131 serum a.
    macroaggregated a. (MAA)
    radioactive a.
    serum a.
albumin autoagglutinating factor
(AAAF)
albumin-bound dye
Albuminar
albuminemia
albuminuria
    Bamberger hematogenic a.
Albumotope I-131
Alcaligenes
    dentrificans, A.
    faecalis, A.
    odorans, A.
Alcian blue
Alcobon
ALD (angioimmunoblastic
lymphadenopathy)
Alder constitutional granulation
anomaly
Alder-Reilly
    anomaly, A.
    body, A.
aldesleukin
aldolase
    deficiency, a.
aldophosphamide

ADDITIONAL TERMS

aldosterone
    -producing antibody, a. (APA)
aldosteronism
    primary a.
aldosteronoma
Aldrich syndrome
alendronate sodium
Aleppo boil
aleukemia
aleukemic
    leukemia, a.
    reticulosis, a.
aleukia
    hemorrhagica, a.
aleukocythemic
aleukocytic
aleukocytosis
Alexan (cytarabine)
Alexander disease
alexia
    cortical a.
alexin
alfacalcidol
alfentanil
Alferon-LDO (interferon alfa-n3)
Alferon-N (interferon alfa-n3)
ALG (antilymphocyte globulin)
alginate
alglucerase (Ceredase)
algorithm
ALHE (angiolymphoid hyperplasia with
  eosinophilia)
alimentary toxic aleukia (ATA)
alimentation
    artificial a.
    parenteral a.
    rectal a.
    total parenteral a. (TPA)
alimentotherapy
aliquot
Alkaban-AQ (vinblastine)
alkalation
alkalimetry
    Engel a.
alkaline phosphatase (ALP)
    leukocyte a. (LAP)
alkaloid
    plant a's
    vinca a's
alkalosis
Alkeran (melphalan)
alkylating

agent, a.
alkylation
alkylator
alkylnitrosamine
ALL (acute lymphoblastic leukemia)
    regimen, A.
ALL (acute lymphocytic leukemia)
    regimen, A.
allele
    multiple a's
    silent a.
allelic
    exclusion, a.
    gene, a.
allelocatalysis
allelocatalytic
allelomorph
allelotaxis
allergen
allergic angiitis
allergization
allesthesia
Allevyn dressing
Allingham procedure
Allium
alloagglutinin
alloantibody
alloantigen
allogeneic
    antigen, a.
    bone marrow transplant, a.
    cell, a.
    effect factor, a. (AEF)
    grafting, a.
    transplantation, a.
allograft
allogroup
alloimmune
alloimmunization
allometric
allometron
allometry
allonomous
allopathic
allopathy
allophenic
alloplasmatic
alloplast
alloplastic
alloplasty
allopurinol
alloreaction

ADDITIONAL TERMS

alloreactive
allosensitization
allosteric
allosterism
allotope
allotoxin
allotransplantation
allotype
    Am a's
    Gm a's
    Inv a's
    Km a's
    Oz a.
allotypy
alloxan
    -Schiff reaction, a.
alloxantin
all-pyrimidine
all-trans-retinoic acid (tretinoin or TRA)
ALM (acral lentiginous melanoma)
Almeida disease
aloe vera plant
Aloe Vesta
aloetic
alogia
aloin
ALOMAD (Adriamycin, Leukeran,
  Oncovin, methotrexate, actinomycin D,
  dacarbazine)
alopecia
    androgenetica, a.
    drug-induced a.
    male pattern a.
    radiation-induced a.
    x-ray a.
alopecic
Alouette amputation
ALP (alkaline phosphatase)
ALP (antilymphocyte plasma)
alpha
    1 antiplasmin, a.
    2 antiplasmin, a.
    1 antitrypsin, a.
    cells, a.
    chain, a.
    chain disease, a.
    chain marker, a.
    chamber, a.
    decay, a.
    difluoromethylornithine, a.
    5-dihydrotestosterone, a.
    emitter, a.

-fetoglobin, a.
-fetoprotein, a. (AFP)
-fetoprotein radioimmunodetection
  with Tc 99m, a.
-globulin, a.
heavy chain disease, a.
helix, a.
interferon, a. (IFN-A)
2 interferon, a. (IFN-alpha 2)
lipoprotein, a.
2 macroglobulin, a.
-methyldopa, a.
-methylparatyrosine, a.
particle spectrum, a.
particles, a.
pulse analyzer, a.
radiation, a.
ray, a.
-TGI, a. (teroxirone)
thal-1-gene, a.
thal-1-trait, a.
thal-2-gene, a.
thal-2-trait, a.
thalassemia 1, a.
thalassemia 2, a.
thalassemia trait, a.
1-thymosin, a.
-tocopherol, a.
Alpha-Beta (alpha tocopherol and beta
  carotene)
Alpha Nine clotting agent (human factor
  IX)
alphavirus
alprazolam
ALS (antilymphocyte serum)
Alsever solution
ALT (alanine aminotransferase)
alteplase
ALT-RCC (autolymphocyte-based
  treatment for renal cell carcinoma)
altretamine (Hexalen or
  hexamethylmelamine or HMM)
Altrigen
ALU-1 family
Aluminostomy
aluminum
    ion contamination, a.
ALV (avian leukosis virus)
    -induced B-cell lymphoma, A.
alveolar
    -cell carcinoma, a.
    infiltrate, a.

ADDITIONAL TERMS

alveolar—*Continued*
 lymphoma, a.
 mucosa, a.
 soft part sarcoma, a. (ASPS)
alveolectomy
alymphia
alymphocytic
alymphocytosis
alymphoplasia
 thymic a.
alymphopotent
alymphopotentiation
ALZ-50
Am (americium)
Am (alpha chain marker) allotype
AMA (antimyosin monoclonal antibody)
 -Fab, A. (antimyosin monoclonal
 antibody with Fab fragment)
amacrine
amanita toxin
amantadine
Amapari virus
amastia
amaurosis
 cat's eye a.
amaurotic
amazia
AmB (amphotericin B or Fungizone)
ambenonium chloride
amber
 codon, a.
 mutation, a.
Ambisome
amboceptor
ambomycin
ambruticin
Ambystoma
 tigrinum, A.
ameba
amebiasis
amebic
amebocyte
ameboma
amegakaryocyte
amegakaryocytic
 thrombocytopenia, a.
amelanosis
amelanotic
ameloblast
ameloblastic
 fibroma, a.
 fibro-odontoma, a.
 fibrosarcoma, a.

 sarcoma, a.
ameloblastoma
 melanotic a.
 pigmented a.
 pituitary a.
American Blood Commission (ABC)
American Cancer Society (ACS)
American Joint Committee on Cancer
 (AJCC)
 scale, A.
 staging, A.
American mandrake
American Rolland
American trypanosomiasis
American Urologic System cancer
 staging classification
americium (Am)
Amersham intracavitary radium
 applicator
Ames
 assay, A.
 test, A.
ametantrone acetate
amethopterin (methotrexate)
AMF (autocrine motility factor)
 -stimulated motility, A.
AmFAR (American Foundation for AIDS
 Research)
amianthosis
Amicar
amidine-lyase
amidinotransferase
amidohydrolase
amido-ligase
amifostine (ethiofos)
amikacin sulfate
Amikin
Amin Aid
aminacrine hydrochloride
amine precursor uptake and
 decarboxylation (APUD)
 cell tumor, a. (APUDoma)
amino acid
 adenylate, a.
 analysis, a.
 analyzer, a.
 sequence analyzer, a.
aminoacidemia
aminoacidopathy
aminoacyl-tRNA synthetase
o-aminoazotoluene
p-aminobenzoic acid (PABA)
aminocaproic acid

ADDITIONAL TERMS

aminoglutethimide (AGT or Cytadren or Elipten)
aminoglycoside
aminogram
p-aminohippurate sodium, p.
p-aminohippuric acid (PAHA)
aminohydrolase
aminohydroxybenzoic acid
aminohydroxypropylidene diphosphonate
aminoimidazolecarboxamine
aminolevulinate dehydratase, a.
5-aminolevulinate synthase, a.
aminolevulinic acid
aminopeptidase
aminopolypeptidase
aminopterin sodium
aminopteroylglutamic acid
aminopurine
aminosalicylate
　　calcium, a.
　　potassium, a.
　　sodium, a.
p-aminosalicylic acid salts
aminosidine sulfate
aminosis
Aminosol
Aminosyn
aminothiadiazole (ATDA)
aminotransferase
amiodarone
amiphenazole HCl
amitosis
AML (acute monocytic leukemia)
AML (acute myeloblastic leukemia)
AML (acute myelocytic leukemia)
AML (acute myelogenous leukemia)
AMLR (autologous mixed lymphocyte reaction)
AMLS (antimouse lymphocyte serum)
AMM (agnogenic myeloid metaplasia)
AMML (acute monomyelocytic leukemia)
AMML (acute myelomonoblastic leukemia)
Amnestrogen
amniocentesis
amniocyte
Amnioplastin
Amniotin

A-mode (amplitude modulation) scan
AMOL (acute monoblastic or monocytic leukemia)
amonafide
amorolfine
amorph
amosite
AMP (adenosine monophosphate) cyclic A.
AMP dialysis
amphibole
amphicarcinogenic
amphileukemic
amphinucleus
amphophil
amphophilic
　　basophil, a.
　　oxyphil, a.
amphotericin B (AmB or Fungizone) lipid complex, a. (ABLC)
amplification gene a.
amplifier T-lymphocyte
Ampligen
amputation
amputee
Amreich vaginal extirpation
AMSA (amsacrine or methaesulfon-m-anisidide)
　　-AZA, A. (amsacrine, 5-azacytidine)
amsacrine (AMSA or m-AMSA)
Amsidyl (acridinyl anisidide or amsacrine)
AMT (autologous marrow transplantation)
amu (atomic mass unit)
AMV (avian myeloblastosis virus)
amyelonic
amygdalin
amygdaloid
amyl nitrite (poppers)
amylase
amyloid
　　degeneration, a.
　　deposition, a.
　　L-chain, a.
　　liver, a.
　　tumor, a.
　　unknown origin, a. of (AUO)
amyloidogenic
amyloidoma
amyloidosis
　　AA a.

ADDITIONAL TERMS

amyloidosis—*Continued*
    AL a.
    cutaneous a.
    idiopathic a.
    immunocyte-derived a.
    immunocytic a.
    immunoglobulin-related a.
    interstitial a.
    lichen a.
    light-chain related a.
    macular a.
    nodular a.
    primary a.
    reactive systemic a.
    secondary a.
ANA (antinuclear antibodies)
anabasis
anabatic
anabolic
    phosphorylation, a.
    steroids, a.
anabolism
Anadrol-50 (oxymetholone)
anaerobe
    facultative a.
    obligate a.
    spore-forming a.
anaerobic
anagen
    effluvium, a.
anagocytic
anagotoxic
anagrelide hydrochloride
anakmesis
anal
    canal, a.
    copulation, a.
    crypt, a.
    erotism, a.
    fisting, a.
    intercourse, a.
    orifice, a.
    penetration, a.
    rimming, a.
    sex, a.
    tear, a.
analbuminemia
analgesia
analgesic
analog
analogue
    folic acid a.
    homologous a.

    metabolic a.
    purine a.
    pyrimidine a.
    somatostatin a.
    substrate a.
analysis
analyzable
analyzer
anamnesis
anamnestic
    response, a.
ANAN (anandron)
Ananase
anandron (ANAN)
anaphase
    flabby a.
anaphylactic
    shock, a.
anaphylactin
anaphylactogen
anaphylactogenesis
anaphylactogenic
anaphylactoid
anaphylatoxin
anaphylaxis
    aggregate a.
anaplasia
    monophasic a.
    polyphasic a.
anaplastic
    astrocytoma, a.
    carcinoma, a.
    seminoma, a.
anaplerosis
anasarca
anasarcous
anascitic
anastomosed
anastomoses (pl. of anastomosis)
anastomosis (pl. anastomoses)
anastomotic
    site, a.
anatherapeusis
anatherapeutic
anazolene sodium
ANC (absolute neutrophil count)
Ancobon (5-FC or 5-flucytosine)
Ancotil
Ancrod
Anderson procedure
andreioma
andreoblastoma
androblastoma

ADDITIONAL TERMS

Andro-Cyp (testosterone)
androgen
    blockade, a.
    synthesis inhibition, a.
androgenic
androgenicity
android
Android-F (fluoxymesterone)
androma
andromimetic
andromorphous
Andronaq (testosterone)
Andronate (testosterone)
Andropository (testosterone)
androstenedione
Andryl (testosterone)
Andy Gump deformity
anechoic
anemia
    achlorhydric a.
    achrestic a.
    achylic a.
    achylica, a.
    acquired hemolytic a.
    acquired iodiopathic sideroblastic
      a.
    acquired sideroachrestic a.
    acute hemolytic a.
    acute myelogenous a.
    Addison a.
    Addison-Biermer a.
    addisonian a.
    African a.
    angiopathic hemolytic a.
    anhematopoietic a.
    anhemopoietic a.
    aplastic a.
    arctic a.
    aregenerative a.
    asiderotic a.
    autoallergic hemolytic a.
    autoimmune hemolytic a. (AIHA)
    Bagdad Spring a.
    Bartonella a.
    Biermer a.
    Biermer-Ehrlich a.
    Blackfan-Diamond a.
    blind loop a.
    brickmaker's a.
    cameloid a.
    cancer-associated a.
    chlorotic a.
    chronic aregenerative a.

chronic disease, a. of
chronic sideroblastic a.
Chvostek a.
cold-antibody autoimmune
    hemolytic a.
congenital a. of newborn
congenital dyserythropoietic a.
congenital Heinz body hemolytic a.
congenital hemolytic a.
congenital hypoplastic a.
congenital nonspherocytic
    hemolytic a.
constitutional aplastic a.
Cooley a.
cow's milk a.
crescent cell a.
cytogenic a.
deficiency a.
dilution a.
dimorphic a.
diphyllobothrium a.
drepanocytic a.
Dresbach a.
drug-induced immune hemolytic a.
dyserythropoietic a.
dyshematopoietic a.
Edelmann a.
Ehrlich a.
elliptocytary a.
elliptocytic a.
elliptocytotic a.
erythroblastic a. of childhood
erythronormoblastic a.
essential a.
Estren-Damashek a.
Faber a.
familial erythroblastic a.
familial megaloblastic a.
Fanconi a.
febrile pleiochromic a.
fetal a.
fish tapeworm a.
folic acid deficiency a.
genetic a.
globe cell a.
glucose-6-phosphate
    dehydrogenase (G6PD) deficiency
    a.
goat's milk a.
ground itch a.
Hayem-Widal a.
Heinz body hemolytic a's
hemolytic a.

ADDITIONAL TERMS

anemia—*Continued*
  hemolytic a. of newborn
  hemorrhagic a.
  hemotoxic a.
  hereditary nonspherocytic
    hemolytic a.
  hereditary sideroachrestic a.
  Herrick a.
  hookworm a.
  hyperchromatic a.
  hyperchromic a.
  hypersplenic a.
  hypochromic a.
  hypochromic microcytic a.
  hypochromica siderochrestica
    hereditaria, a.
  hypoferric a.
  hypoplastic a.
  icterohemolytic a.
  idiopathic hypochromic a.
  idiopathic myelophthisic a.
  immune hemolytic a.
  infantum pseudoleukemica, a.
  infectious a.
  infectious hemolytic a.
  intertropical a.
  iron-deficiency a.
  irradiation a.
  isochromic a.
  Jaksch a.
  lead a.
  Lederer a.
  leukoerythroblastic a.
  lymphatica, a.
  macrocytic a.
  macrocytic achylic a.
  macrocytic a. of pregnancy
  malignant a.
  Marchiafava-Micheli a.
  Mediterranean a.
  megaloblastic a.
  megalocytic a.
  metaplastic a.
  microangiopathic hemolytic a.
  microcytic a.
  milk a.
  miner's a.
  mountain a.
  myelopathic a.
  myelophthisic a.
  neonatal a.
  neonatorum, a.
  nonspherocytic hemolytic a.

  normochromic a.
  normocytic a.
  nosocomial a.
  nutritional a.
  osteosclerotic a.
  ovalocytic a.
  pernicious a.
  phenylhydrazine a.
  physiologic a.
  polar a.
  posthemorrhagic a.
  primaquine-sensitive a.
  primary a.
  primary erythroblastic a.
  primary refractory a.
  primary refractory megaloblastic a.
  pseudoleukemica infantum, a.
  pure red cell a.
  pyridoxine-responsive a.
  radiation a.
  refractoria sideroblastica, a.
  refractory a.
  refractory sideroblastic a.
  Runeberg a.
  schistocytic hemolytic a.
  scorbutic a.
  secondary a.
  secondary refractory a.
  septic a.
  sickle cell a.
  sideroachrestic a.
  sideroblastic a.
  sideropenic a.
  simple achlorhydric a.
  slaty a.
  spastic a.
  spherocytic a.
  splenetica, a.
  splenic a.
  spur-cell a.
  T-cell acute lymphoblastic a.
  target cell a.
  toxic hemolytic a.
  traumatic cardiac hemolytic a.
  trophoneurotic a.
  tropical a.
  tunnel a.
  Von Jaksch a.
  warm-antibody autoimmune
    hemolytic a.
anemic
  anoxia, a.
  hypoxia, a.

ADDITIONAL TERMS

necrosis, a.
anemotrophy
anergic
anergy
anerythroplasia
anerythroplastic
anerythropoiesis
anerythropoietic
anerythroregenerative
anetoderma
aneuploid
aneuploidy
aneurysm
aneurysmal
 bone cyst, a.
ANF (antinuclear factor)
angiitis
 allergic granulomatous a.
 necrotizing a.
angioaccess
angioblast
angioblastic
 meningioma, a.
angioblastoma
angiocavernous
angiochondroma
angiocyst
angiodermatitis
angioendothelioma
angiofibroma
 juvenile a.
 nasopharyngeal a.
angiogenesis
 tumor a.
angiogenesis factor
angiogenic
angioglioma
angiogliomatosis
angiogliomatous
angiogranuloma
angiohemophilia
angioid streak
angioimmunoblastic
 lymphadenopathy with
  dysproteinemia, a. (AILD)
angiokeratoma
angioleiomyoma
angioleucitis
angiolipoleiomyoma
angiolipoma
angiolupoid
angiolymphangioma
angiolymphitis

angiolymphoid
 hyperplasia with eosinophilia, a.
 (ALHE)
angioma
 arteriale racemosum, a.
 arteriovenous a. of brain
 capillary a's
 cavernosum, a.
 cavernous a.
 cherry a's
 cutis, a.
 fissural a.
 hypertrophic a.
 lymphaticum, a.
 plexiform a.
 senile a's
 serpiginosum, a.
 simple a.
 spider a.
 telangiectatic a.
 venosum racemosum, a.
 venous a. of brain
angiomatoid
angiomatosis
 bacillary epithelioid a. (BEA)
 cerebroretinal a.
 encephalofacial a.
 encephalotrigeminal a.
 hepatic a.
 retina, a. of
 retinocerebral a.
angiomatous
angiomyolipoma
angiomyoma
angiomyoneuroma
angiomyosarcoma
angiomyxoma
angionecrosis
angioneoplasm
angioneuromyoma
angionoma
angioreninoma
angioreticuloendothelioma
angioreticuloma
angiosarcoma
 hepatic a.
 myxomatodes, a.
angiotensin
 amide, a.
 -converting enzyme, a. (ACE)
 -I, a.
Angstrom unit
anguidine

ADDITIONAL TERMS

anhematopoietic anemia
anicteric
aniline
    cancer, a.
anilinguist
anilingus
anilinism
anion gap
anionic surfactant
aniridia
    -Wilms tumor syndrome, a.
anisakiasia
Anisakis
    marina, A.
anisocytosis
anisohypercytosis
anisohypocytosis
anisokaryosis
anisoleukocytosis
anisonormocytosis
anisopoikilocytosis
anisoylated plasminogen streptokinase
  activator complex (APSAC)
anlage
ANLL (acute nonlymphocytic leukemia)
ANLL (acute nonlymphoid leukemia)
Ann Arbor staging classification
annihilate
annihilation
    coincidence detection, a. (ACD)
    peak, a.
    photons, a.
    radiation, a.
    reaction, a.
annular phased array
anochromasia
anode
    hooded a.
    rotating a.
anodic
anodyne
anodynia
anol
anomalous
anomaly
    Alder constitutional granulation a.
    Alder-Reilly a.
    May-Hegglin a.
    Pelger nuclear a.
    Pelger-Huet nuclear a.
    Undritz a.
anorectal
anorectic

anorectitis
anorectocolonic
anorectum
anorexia
    -cachexia syndrome, a.
    nervosa, a.
    paraneoplastic a.
anorexiant
anorexic
anorexigenic
anoscope
anoscopic
anoscopy
anosigmoidoscope
anosigmoidoscopy
anosmatic
anosmia
anoxemia
anoxemic
anoxia
    altitude a.
    anemic a.
    anoxic a.
    fulminating a.
    histotoxic a.
    neonatorum, a.
    stagnant a.
anoxiate
anoxic
    anoxia, a.
ansamycin (LM427)
Ansbacher unit
antagonism
antagonist
    folic acid a.
    metabolic a.
    sulfonamide a.
antecedent
    plasma thromboplastin a. (PTA)
antecolic
antemetic
antephase
antherpetic
anthophyllite
6,10-anthracenedicarboxyaldehyde
anthracenediones
anthraconecrosis
anthracosilicosis
anthracosis
anthracotic
anthracycline
anthramycin
anthranecrosis

ADDITIONAL TERMS

anthraquinone
anthrasilicosis
anthrax
    toxin system, a.
anthropometry assessment
antiagglutinin
antiaggressin
antianaphylaxis
antiandrogen (RU-23908)
antianemia factor
antianemic
antiantibody
antianti-factor VIII
antiantitoxin
antiautolysin
antibacterial
antibaryon
antibasement membrane
    antibody, a. (ABMA)
Antibason
anti-B4-blocked ricin
antiblastic
antibody (Ab)
    A33 a.
    acetylcholine receptor a's
    agglutinating a.
    anaphylactic a.
    anti-acetylcholine receptor
     (anti-AChR) a's
    antibasement membrane a.
    antibombesin a.
    anti-CALLA hybridoma a.
    anti-CD5 monoclonal a.
    anticentromere a.
    anticytoplasmic a.
    anti-D a.
    anti-DNA a.
    anti-EA a.
    antifibrin a.
    antiganglioside a.
    antiglomerular basement
     membrane (anti-GEM) a's
    anti-HCV a.
    anti-idiotype a.
    anti-J2 26 monoclonal a.
    anti-La a.
    anti-Leu 2a a.
    anti-Leu 3a a.
    antileukemia a.
    antimelanoma XMMME-001-RTA
     a.
    antimicrosomal a's
    antimitochondrial a.

    anti-MY9 monoclonal a.
    antineutral glycolipid a.
    antinuclear a's (ANA)
    antipeptide a.
    antiphosphotyrosine a.
    antireceptor a's
    anti-Ro a.
    antisheep erythrocyte a.
    anti-Sm a.
    antisulfatide a.
    anti-T cell a.
    antithyroglobulin a's
    antithyroid a's
    atypical a.
    auto-anti-idiotypic a's
    autoimmune a.
    autologous a.
    B1 a.
    B2 a.
    bimodal a's
    bispecific a.
    bivalent a.
    blocking a.
    CD11/l8 a.
    CEAker monoclonal a.
    cell-bound a.
    cell-fixed a.
    cell-mediated a.
    clonal a's
    CMV triclonal a's
    cold a.
    cold-reactive a.
    combining-site a.
    complement-fixing a.
    complete a.
    cross-reacting a.
    cryptosporidiosis a.
    cytophilic a.
    cytotoxic a.
    cytotropic a.
    defective a.
    designer a's
    desmoplakian a.
    Donath-Landsteiner a.
    duck virus hepatitis yolk a.
    Duffy blood a.
    enhancing a.
    F19 a.
    F31 a.
    ferritin-conjugated a.
    fluorescent a.
    Forssman a.
    HAb23 a.

ADDITIONAL TERMS

antibody—*Continued*
heteroclitic a.
heterocytotropic a.
heterogenetic
heterophil a.
heterophile a.
homocytotropic a.
human antimurine a.
humanized a's
humoral a's
HYB-24 a.
hybrid a.
hybridoma a.
idiotype a.
IgA a's
IgG 2A monoclonal a.
IgM a's
IgM-RF a.
immobilizing a.
immune a.
incomplete a.
inhibiting a.
islet cell a's
isophil a.
Kell a.
Kidd a.
leukoagglutinating a.
Lewis a.
lym-1 monoclonal a.
lymphocytotoxic a.
maternal a.
mitochondrial a's
monoclonal a's
natural a's
neutralizing a.
nonprecipitation a.
nuclear a's
OncoScint CR103 monoclonal a.
OncoScint OV103 monoclonal a.
opsonizing a's
Orthoclone OKT3 monoclonal a.
Ortho-mune a.
P-K (Prausnitz-Küstner) a's
polyclonal a.
Prausnitz-Küstner (P-K) a's
precipitating a.
protective a.
rat a's
reaginic a.
Rh a's
rodent-human chimeric a's
saline a's
sensitizing a's

skin-sensitizing a's
splenic a's
SQM1 a.
thyroid-stimulating hormone–
    displacing a's
TI-23 monoclonal a.
triclonal a's
TSH-displacing a's (TDA)
univalent a.
VESP.2 a.
VESP8.2 a.
warm a.
warm-reactive a.
XMMME-001-RTA a.
antibody catabolism
antibody deficiency syndrome
antibody-dependent cell-mediated
    cytotoxicity (ADCC)
antibody half-life
antibody molecules
antibody titer
antibombesin
anti-CALLA hybridoma antibody
anticancer
anticarcinogen
anticarcinogenic
anticholinergic
a1-antichymotrypsin
anticipatory
    grief, a.
    immune suppression, a.
    nausea, a.
    nausea and vomiting, a. (ANV)
anticoagulant
    circulating a.
    lupus-type a.
anticoagulation
anticoagulative
anticoagulin
anticodon
anticomplement
anticomplementary
anticytolysin
anticytotoxin
anti-D antibody
anti-DC5 monoclonal antibody
antidiuretic hormone (ADH)
anti-DNA (antideoxyribonuclease)
anti-DNAse B assay
anti-EA (early antigen) antibody
antielectron
antiemesis
antiemetic

ADDITIONAL TERMS

antienzyme
antiestrogen
antifactor disorder
antifibrin
    antibody imaging, a.
antifibrinolytic
antifol
    Baker a.
antifolate
antifolic acid
antifungal
antiganglioside
    antibody, a.
antigen
    A a.
    A1 a.
    A2 a.
    ABH a.
    ABO a.
    acetone-insoluble a.
    acquired a.
    allogeneic a.
    alum-precipitated a.
    Am a's
    Au (Australia) a.
    Australia (Au) a.
    autologous a.
    B1 a.
    B2 a.
    B3 a.
    BA a.
    BA-1 a.
    bacterial a.
    B-cell differentiation a.
    blood-group a's
    Boivin a.
    Bw4 a.
    Bw4/Bw6 a.
    Bw6 a.
    C a.
    C100-3 a.
    CALLA (common acute
        lymphoblastic leukemia) a.
    capsular a.
    carcinoembryonic a. (CEA)
    cat-scratch a.
    CD a.
    CD4 a.
    cell-surface a.
    Chido-Rodgers a.
    chimeric a.
    class I, II, III a's
    common a.

common acute lymphoblastic
    leukemia a. (CALLA)
common leukocyte a's
complete a.
compound a.
conjugated a.
Cost a.
cross-reacting a.
cryptococcal a.
D a.
delta a.
differentiation a.
Duffy a.
E a.
endogenous a.
exogenous a.
extractable nuclear a's (ENA)
F19 a.
F31 a.
febrile a's
fetal carcinoembryonic a.
fetal sulfoglycoprotein a.
FL160 a.
flagellar a.
Forssman a.
Frei a.
Fy a.
G250 a.
Gm a's
H a.
H-2 a's
Hangar-Rose skin test a.
HBA71 a.
hepatitis a.
hepatitis-associated a. (HAA)
hepatitis B core a. (HBcAg)
hepatitis B e a. (HBeAg)
hepatitis B surface a. (HBsAg)
heterogeneic a.
heterogenetic a.
heterologous a.
heterophil a.
heterophile a.
histocompatibility a's, major and
    minor
HIV a.
HLA a's (human leukocyte
    antigens)
HLA-B a's
Hollinghead a.
homologous a.
HTLV (human T-cell
    lymphotrophic virus) membrane a.

ADDITIONAL TERMS

antigen—*Continued*
  human leukocyte a.
  human lymphocyte a. (HLA)
  human milk fat globule a.-2
  human thymus lymphocyte a.
  Hy a.
  H-Y a.
  I a.
  I adult a.
  Ia a.
  idiotypic a.
  inhalant a.
  Inv group a.
  isogeneic a.
  isophile a.
  Ja a.
  Js a.
  K a.
  Kaproski a.
  Kell a.
  Kidd a.
  Km a's
  Knops a.
  Kveim a.
  Landsteiner-Wiener a.
  LD (lymphocyte-defined) a's
  LEa a.
  LEb a.
  leukocyte common a.
  low-incidence a.
  Luke a.
  Lutheran a.
  Ly a's
  Lyb a's
  lymphocyte-defined (LD) a's
  lymphogranuloma venereum a.
  Lyt a's
  M a.
  M344 a.
  major histocompatibility a's
  McCoy a.
  middle T a.
  Miltenberger a.
  minor histocompatibility a's
  Mitsuda a.
  mucin-type a's
  N a.
  NB150 a.
  nominal a.
  nuclear a's
  O a.
  oncoembryonic a's
  oncofetal a's

onconeural a's
organ-specific a.
Ox a.
Oz a.
P a.
pan-B-cell a.
pancreatic oncofetal a. (POA)
panhematolymphoid a.
partial a.
phytohemagglutinin a. (PHA)
plasma cell a.
plate-specific a.
pollen a.
Pr a.
private a's
proliferating cell nuclear a.
prostate-specific a's
public a's
Qa a.
recall a.
Rh a.
Rho a.
Ri-80 a.
Rodgers a.
SA-85-1 a.
SD (serodefined) a's
SD (serologically defined) a's
self-a.
sequestered a's
serodefined (SD) a's
serologically defined (SD) a's
serum hepatitis (SH) a.
SH (serum hepatitis) a.
shock a.
skin-specific histocompatibility a.
Sm a.
soluble a.
somatic a.
species-specific a.
SS (Sjögren syndrome) a.
SS-A a.
SS-B a.
surface a.
Swann a.
synthetic a.
T a.
T-cell differentiation a.
T-dependent a.
T-independent a.
Tac a.
TAG 72 a.
TATA a. (tumor-associated
  transplantation antigen)

ADDITIONAL TERMS

Tg a.
theta a.
Thomsen-Friedenreich a.
Thy 1 a.
thymus-dependent a.
thymus-independent a.
thymus-leukemia (TL) a.
tissue polypeptide a. (TPA)
tissue-specific a.
Tj a.
TL (thymus leukemia) a.
Tm a.
transplantation a's
tumor-associated a. (TAA)
tumor-associated transplantation a.
    (TATA)
tumor-specific a. (TSA)
tumor-specific transplantation a.
    (TSTA)
tumor-specific transplantation
    resistance a.
V a.
VDRL a.
Vi a.
viral capsid a.
Vr a.
Vs a.
xenogeneic a.
Xga a.
Yk (York) a.
Yo a.
York (Yk) a.
Yt a.
Z a.
antigen-antibody
    complex, a.
    crossed electrophoresis, a.
    reaction, a.
antigen-binding capacity (ABC)
antigen-combining site
antigen excess
antigen gain
antigen predictor
antigen presentation
antigen-presenting
    cell, a. (APC)
    site, a.
antigen unit
antigenemia
antigenemic
ANTI-GENES
antigenic
    antibody lattice formation, a.

-binding receptor, a.
deletion, a.
determinant, a.
determination, a.
drift, a.
expression, a.
modulation, a.
reversible, a.
antigenicity
antigenotherapy
antiglobulin
    consumption test, a.
    reagent, a.
    test, a. (AGT)
antigoitrogenic
antigrowth factor
anti-HCV (hepatitis C virus) antibody
antihemagglutinin
antihemolysin
antihemolytic
antihemophilic
    factor, a. (AHF)
    globulin, a. (AHG)
antihemorrhagic
antiheterolysin
antihistamine
anti-HIV
antihormonal
antihuman
    globulin, a.
    lymphocyte serum, a.
antihyperglycemic
anti-Ia serum
anti-icteric
anti-idiotype
anti-idiotypic
    antibody, a.
anti-immune
anti-isotype
anti-J2 25 monoclonal antibody
anti-La antibody
antileprosy
antileprotic
antilepton
anti-Leu
    -2A antibody, a.
    -3A antibody, a.
antileukemia
    antibody, a.
antileukemic
antileukocidin
antileukocytic
antileukoprotease

ADDITIONAL TERMS

antileukotoxin
antilymphocyte
    globulin, a. (ALG)
    serum, a. (ALS)
antilymphocytic
antimelanoma antibody XMMME-001-RTA
antimeristem
antimeson
antimessenger
antimetabolite
antimethemoglobinemic
antimicrobial
antimitochondrial antibody
antimoniotungstate (HPA-23)
antimonium tungstate (HPA-23)
antimouse lymphocyte serum (AMLS)
antimutagen
anti-MY9
    -blocked ricin, a.
    BMT (bone marrow transplant)
      protocol, a.
    monoclonal antibody, a.
antimycobacterial
antimyosin monoclonal antibody (AMA)
    Fab fragment, a. with (AMA-Fab)
antinausea
antinauseant
antineol
antineoplastic
antineoplaston
antineutral
    glycolipid antibody, a.
antineutrino
antineutron
antineutrophilic cytoplasmic antibody
antinuclear
    antibodies, a. (ANA)
    factor, a. (ANF)
antioncogene
antioncogenic
antioncotic
antioxidant
antiparticle
antipernicious anemia factor (APAF)
antiphagocytic
antiphosphotyrosine
    antibody, a.
antiplasmin
antiplastic
antiplatelet
antipneumococcal
antipodal

antipolycythemic
antiporcine Factor VIII
antiport
antiproliferative
antiprothrombin
antiproton
antiprotozoal
antipyogenic
antipyrine
antiradiation
antiretroviral
anti-Rh agglutinin
anti-RHO-D titer
anti-Ro antibody
antisense
    antibody, a.
    DNA sequence, a.
    oligodeoxynucleotide, a.
    RNA, a.
    strand, a.
antisera (pl. of antiserum)
antiserum (pl. antisera)
    anaphylaxis, a.
antisheep
    erythrocyte antibody, a.
    red blood cells, a.
antisickling
anti-Sm (anti-Smith) antibody
anti-Smith (anti-Sm) antibody
antistreptococcal
antistreptolysin O (ASO)
    titer, a.
antisulfatide
    antibody, a.
anti-T12 allogeneic BMT (bone marrow transplant) protocol
anti-TAP-72 immunotoxin
antitemplate
antithesis
antithetic
antithrombin (AT)
    III, a.
antithromboplastin
antithymocyte
    globulin, a. (ATG)
    serum, a. (ATS)
antithyroglobulin (ATG)
antitoxin
antitryptic reaction
antituberculin
antituberculotic
antituberculous
antitumor

ADDITIONAL TERMS

antitumorigenic
antivenom
antivimenten
antiviral
antivirotic
Antoni type A and B cells
antrectomy
antroduodenectomy
antrotomy
Antrypol
anuclear
anucleated
ANUG (acute necrotizing ulcerative
  gingivitis)
anuresis
anuria
anuric
anus
ANV (anticipatory nausea and vomiting)
anxiety
anxiolytic
anxious
AOPA (ara-C, Oncovin, prednisone,
  asparaginase)
AOPE (Adriamycin, Oncovin,
  prednisone, etoposide)
AP (acid phosphatase)
AP (Adriamycin, Platinol)
AP-1 protein complex
APA (aldosterone-producing adenoma)
APACHE (acute physiology and chronic
  health evaluation) score
APAF (antipernicious anemia factor)
APC (AMSA, chlorambucil, prednisone)
APC (antigen-presenting cell)
APCC (activated prothrombin complex
  concentrates)
APD (disodium pamidronate)
APE (Adriamycin, Platinol, etoposide)
apepsia
aphagia
    algera, a.
aphagopraxia
aphasia
    expressive a.
    subcortical a.
    transcortical a.
aphasic
apheresis
aphtha (pl. aphthae)
aphthae (pl. of aphtha)
    Bednar a.
    cachectic a.

aphthoid
aphthous
    stomatitis, a.
    ulcer, a.
aphthovirus
apinoid cancer
APL (acute promyelocytic leukemia)
aplasia
    Estren-Damshek familial a.
    pure red cell a.
    thymic a.
    thymic-parathyroid a.
aplasmic
aplastic
    anemia, a.
    crisis, a.
Aplisol
Aplitest
aplysia toxin
apnea
apneic
APO (Adriamycin, prednisone, Oncovin)
apocrine
    gland, p.
    metaplasia, a.
    neoplasia, a.
apoenzyme
apoferritin
apolipoprotein
apoplasmatic
apoprotein
apoptosis
aposome
apotransferrin
apple-core lesion
applicator
APR (abdominoperineal resection)
apraxia
apraxic
apron
    lead a.
aprotinin
APRT (adenine
    phosphoribosyltransferase)
APSAC (anisoylated plasminogen
    streptokinase activator complex)
Apt test
APTT (activated partial thromboplastin
    time)
APUD (amine precursor uptake and
    decarboxylation)
    cells, A.
APUDoma (also written apudoma)

ADDITIONAL TERMS

APUDoma—*Continued*
    esophageal A.
apurinic acid
apytalia
apytalism
Aquaplast IC mode
ara-A (adenosine arabinoside)
ara-AC (fazarabine)
ara-adenine
ara-C (cytarabine or cytosine
  arabinoside)
ara-C+ADR (cytarabine, Adriamycin)
ara-C+DNR+PRED+HP (cytarabine,
  daunorubicin, prednisolone,
  mercaptopurine)
ara-C+6TG (cytarabine, thioguanine)
ara-CDP
ara-CMP
ara-CTP
ara-U (arabinosyluracil)
ara-UMP
ara-UTP
arabinosyl-5-azacytidine
arabinosylcytosine
arachidonate
    5-lipoxygenase, a.
    12-lipoxygenase, a.
arachidonic acid
arachnoid cyst
arachnoiditis
arborization
arbovirus
arc
    paired a's
    rotational a.
ARC (AIDS-related complex)
ARCA (acquired red cell aplasia)
archiblastoma
arctic anemia
ARD (AIDS-related disease)
ARDS (adult respiratory distress
  syndrome)
Aredia (pamidronate disodium)
aregenerative
    anemia, a.
Arenaviridae
arenavirus
areola (pl. areolae)
areolae (pl. of areola)
areolar
    cancer, a.
areolitis
ARF (acute renal failure)

argatroban
argema
argentaffin
    carcinoma, a.
argentaffinoma
    bronchus, a. of
    syndrome, a.
arginase
arginine
    carboxypeptidase, a.
    hydrochloride, a.
    synthetase, a.
    tolerance test, a.
    vasopressin, a.
    vasopressin-secreting tumor, a.
argininemia
argininosuccinate
    lyase, a.
    synthetase, a.
argininosuccinic acid (ASA)
argininosuccinicacidemia
argininosuccinicaciduria
arg-leu codon
argon (Ar)
    laser, a.
argyremia
argyrophil
ariboflavinosis
arildone
armed
    leukocytes, a.
    macrophages, a.
Armstrong disease
Arneth grouping of polymorphonuclear
  neutrophils
Arnold
    bodies, A.
    nerve, A.
Aroclor
aromatase
    inhibitor, a.
aromatization
arprinocid
array
    annular phased a.
    linear phased a.
    linear sequenced a.
arrhenoblastoma
arrhenoma
Arrow-Howes multi-lumen catheter
ARS (acute radiation syndrome)
ARS (AIDS-related syndrome)
arsenic trioxide

ADDITIONAL TERMS

arsenism
arsine
ars/trs gene
ART (automated reagin test)
arterial
    blood flow, a.
    blood gases, a. (ABGs)
    blood pressure, a. (ABP)
    line, a.
arteriogram
arteriography
arteritis
    giant cell a.
    temporal a.
arthralgia
arthritides (pl. of arthritis)
arthritis (pl. arthridites)
    acute gouty a.
    acute rheumatic a
    acute secondary a.
    acute suppurative a.
    AIDS a.
    atrophic a.
    bacterial a.
    Bekhterev a.
    blenorrhagic a.
    chronic inflammatory a.
    chronic villous a.
    climactic a.
    cricoarytenoid a.
    crystal-induced a.
    deformans, a.
    degenerative a.
    enteropathic a.
    erosive a.
    exudative a.
    fungal a.
    fungosa, a.
    gonococcal a.
    gonorrheal a.
    gouty a.
    hemophilic a.
    hypertrophic a.
    infectious a.
    Jaccoud a.
    juvenile rheumatoid a. (JRA)
    Lyme a.
    mutilans, a.
    mycotic a.
    neuropathic a.
    nodosa, a.
    pauperum, a.
    proliferative a.

    psoriatic a.
    pyogenic a.
    Reiter a.
    rheumatoid a. (RA)
    sarcoid a.
    septic a.
    sicca, a.
    suppurative a.
    syphilitic a.
    tuberculous a.
    uratic a.
    venereal a.
    vertebral a.
    viral a.
arthrocele
arthrocentesis
arthrodesis
arthroempyesis
arthrogram
arthrography
arthroncus
Arthus
    phenomenon, A.
    reaction, A.
    -type reaction, A.
artifact
artifactitious
artifactual
artificial
    alimentation, a.
    anus, a.
    blood, a.
    immunity, a.
    kidney, a.
    larynx, a.
    lung, a.
    radioactive isotope, a.
    radioactivity, a.
    saliva, a.
    sphincter, a.
    stoma, a.
    voice box, a.
ARV (AIDS-related virus)
Arvin
arylamine
arylaminopeptidase
arylesterase
arylformamidase
arylsulfatase
AS-101
ASA (argininosuccinic acid)
5-ASA (mesalamine)
Asacol

ADDITIONAL TERMS

asbestiform
asbestos
    bodies, a.
    carcinogen, a.
    exposure, a.
asbestosis
Ascher syndrome
ascites
    adiposus, a.
    bloody a.
    chylous a.
    exudative a.
    hemorrhagic a.
    hydremic a.
    malignant a.
    milky a.
    transudative a.
ascitic
    fluid, a.
ascitogenous
Ascoli reaction
ascorbate
    cyanide test, a.
    reductase, a.
ascorbemia
ascorbic acid
asemia
    graphica, a.
    mimica, a.
    verbalis, a.
asepsis
aseptic
    necrosis, a.
A-SHAP (Adriamycin, Solu-Medrol,
    high-dose ara-C, Platinol)
Ashkenazi Jewish patient
asialia
asialo GM1 glycoprotein
asiderosis
asiderotic
Askin tumor
ASN (L-asparaginase)
Asnase
ASO (antistreptolysin-O) titer
ASP (L-asparaginase)
L-asparaginase (ASN or ASP or Elspar)
aspartate
    aminotransferase, a. (AST)
    carbamoyl transferase, a.
    transaminase, a.
aspartic acid
aspartocin
aspartylglucosaminuria

Aspegic
aspergilloma
aspergillomycosis
aspergillosis
aspergillotoxicosis
Aspergillus
    bouffardi, a.
    cookei, A.
    flaux, A.
    fumigatus, A.
    glaucus, A.
    gliocladium, A.
    mucoroides, A.
    niger, A.
    restrictus, A.
    terreus, A.
aspergillustoxicosis
Asperkinase
asperlin
aspermia
Aspilia
aspirating needle
aspiration
    biopsy, a.
    biopsy cytology, a. (ABC)
    cytology, a.
    needle, a.
asplenia
asplenism
assay
    biological a.
    blastogenesis a.
    Boyden chamber a.
    CA15-3 RIA a.
    cell-mediated lympholysis (CML) a.
    CH50 a.
    competitive binding a.
    complement a.
    complement binding a.
    double antibody sandwich a.
    E (erythrocyte) rosette a.
    EAC (erythrocyte, antibody, and
        complement-coated) rosette a.
    ELISA a. (enzyme-linked
        immunosorbent assay)
    enzyme-linked immunosorbent a.
        (ELISA)
    erythropoietin a.
    Factor III multimer a.
    four-point a.
    glycosylated hemoglobin a.
    hemagglutination inhibition a.
        (HIA)

ADDITIONAL TERMS

hemolytic complement a.
hemolytic plaque a.
human tumor cloning a.
human tumor clonogenic a.
human tumor colony-forming a.
human tumor stem cell a.
immune a.
immune adherence
    hemagglutination a. (AHA)
immunochemical a.
immunofluorescent a.
immunoradiometric a.
indirect a.
Jerne plaque a.
LAL (limulus amebocyte lysate) a.
limulus amebocyte lysate (LAL) a.
lymphocyte proliferation a.
microbiological a.
microcytotoxicity a.
microencapsulation a.
microhemagglutination a.–
    Treponema pallidum (MHA-TP)
mixed lymphocyte culture (MLC) a.
plaque-forming cell a.
polyethylene glycol precipitation a.
radioligand a.
radioreceptor a.
Raji cell a.
RAST inhibition a.
staphylococcal protein A-binding a.
stem cell a.
thyroid radioisotope a. (TyRIA)
total complement a.
Treponema pallidum
    hemagglutination a. (TPHA)
whole complement a.
AST (antistreptolysin titer)
AST (aspartate aminotransferase)
astasia
astatine
asteroid
    body, a.
asthenia
asthenic
Astler-Coller
    modification of Dukes C
    classification, grades B2, B3, C,
    A.
    rectal system, A.
    tumor staging, A.
ASTRA profile
Astrafer
astral ray

astroblast
astroblastoma
astrocyte
    fibrous a's
    gemistocytic a.
    plasmatofibrous a's
    protoplasmic a's
astrocytin
astrocytoma, grades 1 through 4
    anaplastic a.
    fibrillare, a.
    gemistocytic a.
    glioblastoma multiforme, a.
    hypothalamic a.
    pilocytic a.
    protoplasmaticum, a.
astrocytosis
astroglia
astrokinetic
astroma
astrosphere
asymmetrical
asymmetry
asymptomatic
    seropositive, a.
    shedding, a.
AT (adjunctive therapy)
AT (antithrombin)
ATA (alimentary toxic aleukia)
Atabrine
atactic
ataxia
    -pancytopenia syndrome, a.
ataxoadynamia
ATD (autoimmune thyroid disease)
ATDA (aminothiadiazole)
atelectasia
atelectasis
atelectatic
ATG (antithymocyte globulin)
ATG (antithyroglobulin)
Atgam
AtheroCath
atherogenesis
atheroma
athrepsia
athreptic
    immunity, a.
Athrombin-K
athymia
athymism
athyrea
athyroidemia

ADDITIONAL TERMS

athyrosis
athyrotic
ATL (acute tumor lysis)
ATL (adult T-cell leukemia)
ATL (adult T-cell lymphoma)
ATLL (adult T-cell leukemia/
 lymphoma)
ATN (acute tubular necrosis)
aTNM (autopsy staging of tumor, nodes,
 and metastasis)
atom
 activated a.
 asymmetric carbon a.
 Bohn a.
 excited a.
 helium a.
 hydrogen a.
 ionized a.
 Na a.
 nuclear a.
 recoil a.
 Rutherford a.
 stripped a.
 tagged a.
atom-activated abscess
atom-chipping
atom counter
atom-tracing spectrometer
atomic
 absorption spectrometry, a.
 absorption spectroscopy, a. (AAS)
 accelerator, a.
 bomb, a.
 cluster, a.
 cocktail, a.
 energy, a.
 dust, a.
 fallout, a.
 mass, a.
 mass unit, a.
 nucleus, a.
 number, a.
 pile, a.
 radiation, a.
 shell, a.
 spectrum, a.
 theory, a.
 volume, a.
 weight, a.
atomism
atomization
atonia
atonic

neurogenic bladder, a.
atony
atopic
atopy
atovaquone
ATP (adenosine triphosphate)
ATPase (adenosine triphosphatase)
atransferrinemia
atresia
atretic
atrophied
atrophy
ATS (antithymocyte serum)
attenuated
attenuation
atticoantrotomy
Atvogen
atypia
atypical
 lipoma, a.
 lymphocytes, a.
Au (Australia)
 antigen, A.
 antigenemia, A.
Au (gold)
 ^{195}Au
 ^{198}Au
 ^{198}Au grains
 ^{198}Au irradiation
 ^{198}Au ophthalmic applicator
 ^{199}Au
Auberger
 blood group system, A.
 factor, A.
Auchincloss-Madden mastectomy
Auer
 bodies, A.
 rods, A.
AUG codon
Auger electron
AUL (acute undifferentiated leukemia)
AUO (amyloid of unknown origin)
aurantiasis cutis
Aureoloid-198
Aureotope
auroparticle
aurora particle
 counter, a.
aurotherapy
aurothioglucose
Ausab
 EIA, A.
 radioimmunoassay, A.

ADDITIONAL TERMS

Auscell test
Ausria H-125 test
Austin and Van Slyke method
Australia antigen
Aust-tect test system
Auszyme monoclonal
AUTO 4-HC protocol
  (cyclophosphamide, busulfan,
  4-hydroperoxycyclophosphamide)
autoagglutination
autoagglutinin
autoantibody
    antiplatelet a.
autoanticomplement
autoantigen
auto-anti-idiotypic antibodies
autoantitoxin
autoarcesis
autobacteriophage
autobiotic
autobody
autocatalysis
autocatalytic
autochthonous
autoclasia
autoclasis
autoclastic
autocrine
    excretion, a.
    motility factor, a. (AMF)
    secretion, a.
    stimulation, a.
autocytolysin
autocytolysis
autocytolytic
autocytometer
autocytotoxin
autoerythrocyte sensitization syndrome
autoerythrophagocytosis
autogenesis
autogenetic
autogenous
autograft
autohemagglutination
autohemagglutinin
autohemic
autohemolysin
autohemolysis
autohemolytic
autohemotherapy
autohemotransfusion
autoimmune
    disease, a.

hemolytic anemia, a. (AHA or
  AIHA)
leukopenia, a.
pancytopenia, a.
polyendocrine-candidiasis
  syndrome, a.
thrombocytopenia, a.
thrombocytopenic purpura, a.
  (AITP)
thyroid disease, a. (ATD)
thyroiditis, a.
thyroidosis, a.
autoimmunity
autoimmunization
autoinfection
autoinfusion
autoinoculation
autointerference
autoisolysin
autoleukoagglutinin
AutoLogic gamma counting system
autologous
    antibody, a.
    blood, a.
    bone graft, a.
    bone marrow transplantation, a.
    (ABMT)
    clot, a.
    fat graft, a.
    hematopoietic reconstitution, a.
    marrow transplantation, a. (AMT)
    platelets, a.
    transfusion, a.
    transplant, a.
    typing, a.
autolymphocyte
    -based treatment for renal cell
    carcinoma, a. (ALT-RCC)
    serum, a. (ALS)
autolysate
autolysin
autolysis
autolysosome
autolytic
autolyze
automated
    immunoprecipitation, a.
    reagin test, a.
autonephrectomy
autonomic
    ataxia, a.
    nerve block, a.
    neuropathy, a.

ADDITIONAL TERMS

autophagosome
autophagy
autopharmacologic
autopharmacology
Autoplex
autoprothrombin
    I, a.
    II, a.
    C, a.
autopsied
autopsy
autoradiography
autoreactive
autoregulation
autoreinfusion
autosensitization
autosensitized
autosepticemia
autoserum
autosome
autosplenectomy
autotherapy
autothromboagglutinin
autotoxemia
autotoxicosis
autotoxin
autotransfusion
autotransplantation
autovaccination
autovaccine
autovaccinotherapy
auxesis
auxospore
AV (Adriamycin, vincristine)
AV (arginine vasopressin)
AV (avian virus)
avarol
avarone
avian
    adenovirus, a.
    erythroblastosis virus, a.
    leukemia virus, a.
    leukosis virus, a. (ALV)
    leukosis virus-induced B-cell
      lymphoma, a.
    myeloblastosis virus, a. (AMV)
    virus, a. (AV)
Avicenna gland
avidin-biotin system
avidity
Avinar
Avitene
    sandwich, A.

Avlosulfon (dapsone)
AVM (Adriamycin, vinblastine,
    methotrexate)
AVM (Adriamycin, vincristine,
    mitomycin-C)
Avogadro number
AVP (actinomycin D, vincristine,
    Platinol)
AVP (Adriamycin, vincristine,
    procarbazine)
avridine
axes (pl. of axis)
axilla (pl. axillae)
axillae (pl. of axilla)
axillary
    adenopathy, a.
    contents, a.
    fat pad, a.
    involvement, a.
    lymph node, a.
    lymphadenopathy, a.
    nodal dissection, a.
    sweep, a.
    tail of Spence, a.
axis (pl. axes)
axon
Axsain
ayahuasca
Ayerza
    disease, A.
    syndrome, A.
Ayve spatula
ayw1, ayw2, ayw4, aywr (hepatitis B
    surface antigen subdeterminants)
5-AZ
AZA (azathioprine)
5-AZA (5-azacytidine)
Azactam
5-azacytidine (5-AZA)
8-azaguanine (8-azg)
azalides
azanidazole
azarabine
azarole
azaserine
azathioprine (AZTP)
5-azauracil (5-AzU)
6-azauracil (6-AzU)
5-azauridine (5-AzUR)
6-azauridine (6-AzUR)
5-AZC (azacitidine)
AzdU (azidouridine)
azetepa

ADDITIONAL TERMS

8-azg (8-azaguanine)
3′-azido-3′-deoxythymidine
azidodideoxyuridine
azidothymidine (AZT)
azidouridine (AzdU)
Azimexon
aziridinylbenzoquinone (AZQ)
azithromycin
Azlin (azlocillin)
azlocillin (Azlin)
azoic diazo dye
azole
azoospermia
azotemia
azotomycin
Azovan Blue
azoxymethane
AZQ (aziridinylbenzoquinone or
  diaziquone)
AZT (azidothymidine)
AZTP (azathioprine)
aztreonam
5-AzU (5-azauracil)
6-AzU (6-azauracil)
5-AzUR (5-azauridine)
6-AzUR (6-azauridine)
azure B dye
azurophile
  granules, a.
azurophilia
azygoesophageal
azygogram
azygography
azygos
  nodes, a.
  vein, a.

B

B1, 2, 3 antigen
B16
  cell line, B.
  melanoma syngeneic, B.
B16 melanoma
B-carotene
B-cell
  acute lymphoblastic leukemia, B.
  (B-ALL)
  antigen receptors, B.
  associated antigen, B.
  bursal-derived cell, B.
  chronic lymphocytic leukemia, B.
  differentiation factor, B. (BCDF)
  growth factor, B. (BCGF)

immunoglobulin, B.
insulinoma, B.
leukemia, B.
lymphocytosis, B.
lymphoma, B.
mitogen, B.
neoplasm, B.
restricted antigen, B.
B-chain gene complex
B-endorphin
B-lymphocyte
  stimulatory factor, B. (BSF)
B-lymphoma
B-mode (brightness mode)
  echography, B.
B-pleated sheet fibril
Ba (barium)
BA-1 antigen
Babesia
  microti, B.
babesiasis
babesiosis
Babinski-Nageotte syndrome
baboon
bacillary
  epithelioid angiomatosis, b. (BEA)
bacille Calmette-Guérin (BCG)
bacillemia
bacilli (pl. of bacillus)
bacilliform
bacillus (pl. bacilli)
  Battey b.
  Boas-Oppler b.
  Calmette-Guérin b.
  Chauveau b.
  coliform b.
  colon b.
  Döderlein b.
  Ducrey b.
  dysentery b.
  Escherich b.
  Friedländer b.
  Gartner b.
  Ghon-Sachs b.
  Hansen b.
  Hoffman b.
  Klebs-Loeffler b.
  Koch-Weeks b.
  lepra b.
  Morgan b.
  Newcastle-Manchester b.
  paracolon b.
  Pfeiffer b.

ADDITIONAL TERMS

bacillus—*Continued*
  Preisz-Nocard b.
  Schmitz b.
  Schmorl b.
  Shiga b.
  tetanus b.
  tubercle b.
  Weeks b.
  Welch b.
  Whitmore b.
backcross
backflow
background radiation
backscatter
baclofen
BACO (bleomycin, Adriamycin, CCNU, Oncovin)
BACOD (bleomycin, Adriamycin, cyclophosphamide, Oncovin, dexamethasone)
BACON (bleomycin, Adriamycin, CCNU, Oncovin, nitrogen mustard)
BACOP (bleomycin, Adriamycin, cyclophosphamide, Oncovin, prednisone)
BACT (BCNU, ara-C, cyclophosphamide, 6-thioguanine)
BACT (bleomycin, Adriamycin, cyclophosphamide, tamoxifen)
Bactec
bacteremia
bacteria (pl. of bacterium)
  acid-fast b. (AFB)
  coliform b.
  hemophilic b.
bacterial
  recombination, b.
bactericidal
bactericide
bactericidin
bacterioagglutinin
bacteriocarcinogenic
bacteriohemagglutinin
bacterioid
bacteriolysin
bacteriolysis
bacterio-opsonin
bacteriopexy
bacteriophage
bacteriophytoma
bacterioplasmin
bacterioprecipitin
bacteriopsonin

bacteriorhodopsin
bacteriotoxemia
bacterium (pl. bacteria)
Bacteroides
  asaccharolyticus, B.
  bivius, B.
  fragilis, B.
  funduliformis, B.
  melaninogenicus, B.
  pneumosintes, B.
  praeacutus, B.
  putredinis, B.
  splanchnicus, B.
  thetaiotaomicron, B.
  ureolyticus, B.
  vulgatus, B.
Bactigen S. pneumoniae test
bactin-3
BactoAgar
Bactocill
Bactrim
baculovirus
Bafverstedt syndrome
BAGF (brachioaxillary bridge graft fistula)
Bagdad Spring anemia
Bagshawe regimen
Bakamjian flap
Baker antifol
bakkola (a fungus used in cancer treatment)
BAL (British antilewisite)
BAL (bronchoalveolar lavage)
balanced electrolyte solution (BES)
Balb/C
  mice, B.
  sarcoma virus, B.
balding
  male pattern, b. in
baldness
  male pattern b.
BALF (bronchoalveolar lavage fluid)
Balint syndrome
Balkan
  nephritis, B.
  nephropathy, B.
B-ALL (B-cell acute lymphoblastic leukemia)
ball
  myoma, b.
  -valve carcinoid tumor, b.
balloon cells
Balser fatty necrosis

ADDITIONAL TERMS

Balzer type
BAM/BLITZ (B4 blocked ricin)
 protocol
Bam HI
 restriction enzymes, B.
 recognition site, B.
Bamberger hematogenic albuminuria
bamboo bodies
Bamfolin
bamnidazole
BAMON (bleomycin, Adriamycin,
 methotrexate, Oncovin, nitrogen
 mustard)
banding
 G (Giemsa) b.
 Q (quinacrine) b.
 R (reverse) b.
Banti
 disease, B.
 syndrome, B.
BAP (bleomycin, Adriamycin,
 prednisone)
barb
barbed
 hook, b.
 wire, b.
Barcroft apparatus
bare lymphocyte syndrome
Bargen streptococcus
barium (Ba)
 cyanoplatinate, b.
 enema, b.
 meal, b.
 sulfate, b.
 swallow, b.
Barrett
 esophagus, B.
 metaplasia, B.
barrier
Barron pump
Bart hemoglobin
Bartonella
 anemia, B.
 bacilliformis, B.
bartonellosis
Bartter syndrome
baryon
basal cell
 cancer, b.
 carcinoma, b.
 dysplasia, b.
 epithelioma, b.
 hyperplasia, b.

 nevus syndrome, b.
basaloid
 carcinoma, b.
basaloma
base pairs (bp)
Basedow disease
basement membrane
 zone, b.
Basex syndrome
Basham mixture
basic fuchsin dye
Basidiomycetes
basiloma
basisphenoid
baso (basophil)
basocyte
basocytopenia
basocytosis
basoerythrocyte
basoerythrocytosis
basopenia
basophil
 beta b.
 Crooke-Russell b's
 delta b.
basophil chemotactic factor (BCF)
basophilia
basophilic
 adenoma, b.
 erythroblast, b.
 erythrocyte, b.
 leukemia, b.
 leukocyte, b.
 stippling, b.
basophilism
basophilopenia
basosquamous cell carcinoma
Bassen-Kornzweig syndrome
Basset operation
BAT (brain-adjacent tumor)
bat wing appearance
Batson
 hypothesis, B.
 plexus, B.
battery
 hepatitis b.
 tests, b. of
Battey
 -avium complex, B.
 bacillus, B.
 factor, B.
batteyin
BAU (benzylacyclouridine)

ADDITIONAL TERMS

bauxite pneumoconiosis
BAVIP (bleomycin, Adriamycin, vinblastine, imidazole carboxamide, prednisone)
Bay region concept
Bayes theorem
Bayle granulation
Baylor rapid autologous transfusion (BRAT) system
Bazex
    disease, B.
    syndrome, B.
BBB (blood-brain barrier)
B4 blocked ricin
BBVP-M (BCNU, bleomycin, VePesid, prednisone, methotrexate)
BCAVe (bleomycin, CCNU, Adriamycin, Velban)
BCD (bleomycin, cyclophosphamide, dactinomycin)
BCDF (B-cell differentiation factors)
BCF (basophil chemotactic factor)
BCG (bacille Calmette-Guérin vaccine or TheraCys or Tice)
BCGF (B-cell growth factor)
BCL2 gene
BCNU (bis-chloronitrosourea or carmustine)
BCOP (BCNU, cyclophosphamide, Oncovin, prednisone)
BCP (BCNU, cyclophosphamide, prednisone)
BCVP (BCNU, cyclophosphamide, vincristine, prednisone)
BCVPP (BCNU, cyclophosphamide, vinblastine, procarbazine, prednisone)
506BD
Bdellovibrio
B-DNA right-handed helix
B-DOPA (bleomycin, dacarbazine, Oncovin, prednisone, Adriamycin)
Be (beryllium)
BEA (bacillary epithelioid angiomatosis)
BEAC (BCNU, etoposide, ara-C, cyclophosphamide)
BEAM (brain electrical activity map)
beam
    electron b.
    neutron b.
    photon b.
    proton b.
    radiation b.
    useful b.

    x-ray b.
beam alignment
beam barrier
beam collimation
beam energies
beam modification
beam-shaping blocks
beam shield
beam splitter
beam therapy
beamtherapy
Beard treatment
Bearn-Kunkel syndrome
Bearn-Kunkel-Slater syndrome
Beau line
BEB (blind esophageal brushing)
Beck gastrostomy
Becker
    factor, B.
    nevus, B.
Beckwith syndrome
Beckwith-Weidemann syndrome
Beclard amputation
becquerel (Bq)
Becquerel rays
Bednar aphthae
bedfast
bedridden
bedsore
beechwood cellulose
beefy-red tongue
Béguez César disease
behavioral
    approach, b.
    modification, b.
    research, b.
    technique, b.
Behçet disease
Behla bodies
Behnken unit
Behring law
beige mice
BEIR (biological effects of ionizing radiations)
Belganyl (suramin)
Bell treatment
belladonna
belly bath intraperitoneal chemotherapy
below-knee amputation (BKA)
Belt prostatectomy
BEMP (bleomycin, Eldisine, mitomycin, Platinol)
Bence Jones

ADDITIONAL TERMS

bodies, B.
protein, B.
proteinemia, B.
proteinuria, B.
Benedikt syndrome
benign
adenoma, b.
adenomatous polyp, b.
chondroblastoma, b.
cystic teratoma, b.
disease, b.
lesion, b.
mesenchymoma, b.
monoclonal gammopathy, b. (BMG)
prostatic hypertrophy, b. (BPH)
tumor, b.
benignant
benignity
Bennet small corpuscles
Bennett
classification, B.
disease, B.
benoxaprofen
bentonite flocculation test
benzanthracene
benzene
ring, b.
benzimidazole
benzodepa
benzo(a)pyrene
benzol
benzoylpas calcium
benzomorphan
benzotherapy
3, 4-benzpyrene
benzquinamide
benzyl
analogue of serotonin, b.
antiserotonin, b.
benzylacyclouridine (BAU)
BEP (bleomycin, etoposide, Platinol)
bereaved
bereavement
Berger disease
Bergh staging system
Bergman sign
Bergonie-Tribondeau law
Berkson bias
Berkson-Gage calculation
Bernard-Soulier
disease, B.
syndrome, B. (BSS)
Berrens factor

berry cell
Berry-Dedrick phenomenon
Berubigen
berylliosis
beryllium (Be)
BES (balanced electrolyte solution)
Bessey-Lowry unit
Bessey-Lowry-Brock unit
Besnier-Boeck disease
beta
activity, b.
-alpha biosynthetic globin ratio, b.
basophil, b.
carotene, b.
cells, b.
chain, b.
decay, b.
emission, b.
emitter, b.
endorphin, b.
-globin synthesis, b.
globulin, b.
-glucuronidase, b.
-glycerophosphatase, b.
-hCG (human chorionic
gonadotropin) hormone, b.
hemolysis, b.
interferon, b.
irradiation applicator, b.
-lactam antibiotics, b.
-lapachone, b.
-lipoprotein, b.
-lysin, b.
2-microglobulin, b.
-oxybutyric acid, b. (BOBA)
particles, b.
-pleated sheet, b.
radiation, b.
ray, b.
ray applicator, b.
ray spectrograph, b.
ray spectrometer, b.
receptor, b.
subunit radioimmunoassay, b.
thalassemia, b.
betaglycan
betahistine HCl (Serc)
Betaseron (human recombinant beta
interferon)
betatron
irradiation, b.
betel
cancer, b.

ADDITIONAL TERMS

betel—*Continued*
    quid, b.
bethanechol chloride
Bethesda
    system, B.
    unit, B.
BeV (billion electron volts)
bevatron
B factor
BF (blastogenic factor)
BFN (biologic false-negative)
BFP (biologic false-positive)
BFU (burst-forming unit)
BFU-E (burst-forming unit—erythroid)
Bg blood group system
BGLF4 gene
B-hCG (beta-human chorionic
    gonadotropin)
BHD (BCNU, hydroxyurea, dacarbazine)
BHDV (BCNU, hydroxyurea,
    dacarbazine, vincristine)
Bianchi syndrome
Biaxin (clarithromycin)
BIB (biliointestinal bypass)
Bicarbolyte
bicellular
Bicibon
BiCNU (carmustine)
bidermoma
Biermer
    anemia, B.
    disease, B.
Biermer-Ehrlich anemia
Bifidobacterium
    adolescentis, B.
    bidifum, B.
    eriksonii, B.
B-IFN (beta-interferon)
bifunctional
bile
Bilharzia
bilharzial
bilharziasis
bilharzic
bilharzioma
bili (bilirubin)
Bili light
biliary
    cirrhosis, b.
    duct, b.
    obstruction, b.
    tract, b.
bilineage

leukemia, b.
biliointestinal bypass (BIB)
biliopancreatic bypass (BPB)
bilirubin
    direct b.
    indirect b.
bilirubinemia
biliverdin
    reductase, b.
biliverdinic acid
billion electron volts (BeV)
Billroth I, II, or III procedure
bimodal antibodies
binary fission
binder
binding energy
Binet staging system
bioactive
bioassay
bioavailability
bioblast
biochemical
    biopsy, b.
    epidemiology, b.
    heterogene, b.
    marker, b.
    metastasis, b.
    racial index, b.
    response modifiers, b. (BRMs)
biochemistry
biochemorphology
Biodel Implant/BCNU
biofeedback
Bio Foam Eggcrate
biohazard
biologic
    effects of ionizing radiation, b.
        (BEIR)
    false-negative, b. (BFN)
    false-positive, b. (BFP)
    half-life, b.
    implant, b.
    marker, b.
    response markers, b.
    response modifier, b. (BRM)
biological
    therapy, b.
    warfare, b.
biology
    cellular b.
    molecular b.
    radiation b.
bioluminescence

ADDITIONAL TERMS

bioluminescent
biomarker
biomedical
biomedicine
biomembrane
biomicroscope
biomicroscopy
biomodulation
biomodulin
biomolecule
bionucleonics
biophysical
biophysics
bioplasm
bioplast
biopsied
biopsy
    aspiration b.
    aspiration cytology b.
    biochemical b.
    bite b.
    blind b.
    bone b.
    bone marrow b.
    bronchial brush b.
    brush b.
    chorionic villus b.
    closed pleural b.
    cold knife conization b.
    cone b.
    contralateral b.
    core b.
    cup b.
    cytological b.
    endomyocardial b.
    endoscopic b.
    excisional b.
    exploratory b.
    fine needle b.
    incisional b.
    intranasal b.
    Jamshidi needle b.
    liver b.
    lymph node b.
    mediastinal node b.
    Menghini needle b.
    nasal cavity b.
    needle b.
    needle core b.
    open b.
    open lung b.
    paranasal sinus b.
    percutaneous b.

    percutaneous needle b.
    pleural b.
    pre-excisional b.
    prostate needle b.
    punch b.
    scalene node b.
    skinny needle b.
    sponge b.
    sternal b.
    surface b.
    testicular b.
    transbronchial lung b.
    trephine b.
    Tru-Cut needle b. (TNB)
    wedge b.
    wide b.
biopsychosocial
bioptome
Biopty
    cut needle, B.
    gun, B.
biopyoculture
biosafety
Biosearch 8600 automated DNA
  synthesizer
biospectrometry
biospectroscopy
biostatistics
biostimulation
biosynthesis
biosynthetic
biosynthetize
BioTac biopsy cannula
biotaxis
biotin
    -avidin-peroxidase
      immunoperoxidase, b.
BIP (bleomycin, ifosfamide, Platinol)
biphasic
biphenotypic
    leukemia, b.
bipotentiality
biotinylated
biotransformation
biotrepy
Biotropin
biphosphonate APD
biplane
    sector probe, b.
    view, b.
Birbeck granule
Bird sign
birds' nest lesion

ADDITIONAL TERMS

BIRG-587 (nevirapine)
bisantrene hydrochloride
bischlorethylnitrosourea (BCNU)
bisexual
bisexuality
bispecific antibody
bis-perfluorobutyl ethylene (F44E)
bisphosphoglycerate
    mutase, b.
    phosphatase, b.
    synthetase, b.
bisulfan
bite biopsy
Bittner
    agent, B.
    milk factor, B.
bivalency
bivalent
Bivona voice prosthesis
bizarre leiomyoma
Bizzozero
    cells, B.
    corpuscles, B.
    platelets, B.
BKA (below-knee amputation)
BK-mole syndrome
black
    -bile diffusion theory, b.
    cancer, b.
    hairy tongue, b.
    light, b.
    lung, b.
    phthisis, b.
    tongue, b.
Blackfan-Diamond
    anemia, B.
    syndrome, B.
bladder
    biopsy, b.
    carcinoma, b.
    carcinoma classification, b.
    incontinence, b.
Blakemore-Sengstaken tube
blast
    cell, b.
    cell leukemia, b.
    crisis, b.
    transformation, b.
    wave, b.
blastema
blastic
    crisis, b.
    leukemia, b.

    metastasis, b.
blastin
blastocyte
blastocytoma
blastoderm
blastogenesis
    assay, b.
blastogenic
    factor, b. (BF)
blastoma
    pluricentric b.
    unicentric b.
blastomatoid
blastomatosis
blastomatous
blastomere
blastomogenic
blastomogenous
Blastomyces
    brasiliensis, B.
    coccidioides, B.
    dermatitidis, B.
blastomycosis
    cutaneous b.
    North American b.
    South American b.
    systemic b.
bleach kit
bleeder (hemophiliac)
bleeder's disease
bleeding
    diathesis, b.
    time, b.
Blenoxane (bleomycin)
BLEO (bleomycin)
BLEO-MOPP (bleomycin, nitrogen
    mustard, Oncovin, procarbazine,
    prednisone)
bleomycin sulfate (Blenoxane or BLM)
    sterile b. sulfate
blepharectomy
blepharoadenoma
blepharoatheroma
blepharoncus
Blessig cysts
blind esophageal brushing (BEB)
blind loop
    anemia, b.
    syndrome, b.
BLITZ protocol (monoclonal antibodies)
BLM (bleomycin sulfate)
blocked ricin
blocking

ADDITIONAL TERMS

antibody, b.
factor, b.
blocks
    Cerrobend b.
    customized b.
    lead b.
Bloedorn applicator
Blom-Singer
    valve, B.
    voice prosthesis, B.
Blondlot rays
blood
    -brain barrier, b. (BBB)
    buffy coat culture, b.
    cell, b.
    chemistry, b.
    coagulation factors I through XIII,
      b.
    component therapy, b.
    count, b.
    crossmatching, b.
    culture, b.
    doping, b.
    dust, b.
    dust of Miller, b.
    dyscrasia, b.
    exchange, b.
    expander, b.
    gas, b.
    gas analysis, b.
    group, b.
    group antigen, b.
    island, b.
    islets, b.
    lakes, b.
    -letting, b.
    level, b.
    loss, b.
    patch, b.
    picture, b.
    plasma, b.
    platelets, b.
    poisoning, b.
    pool scan, b.
    products, b.
    pressure, b.
    serum, b.
    shunting, b.
    smear, b.
    sugar, b.
    -thymus barrier, b.
    transfusion, b.
    tumor, b.

    type, b.
    typing, b.
    urea nitrogen, b. (BUN)
    volume, b.
    warmer, b.
blood group
    ABO b.
    Auberger b.
    Bg b.
    Cartwright b.
    Colton b.
    Cost-Sterling b.
    Diego b.
    Dombrock b.
    Duffy b.
    Gerbich b.
    H b.
    HI b.
    high-frequency b.
    I b.
    Ii b.
    Kell b.
    Kidd b.
    Landsteiner b.
    Lewis b.
    low-frequency b.
    Lutheran b.
    McLeod b.
    MN b.
    P b.
    Rh b.
    Sciana b.
    Sid b.
    Stoltzfus b.
    Vel b.
    Wright b.
    Xg b.
    Xga b.
Bloodgood disease
Bloom syndrome
blot test
    Southern b.
    Western b.
blotting
blubbery lip syndrome
blue
    dome cyst, b.
    nevus, b.
    rubber bleb nevus, b.
blueberry
    lips, b.
    nodules, b.
Blumberg sign

ADDITIONAL TERMS

Blumenthal disease
Blumer rectal shelf
blunt duct adenosis
blush
    tumor b.
BLV (bovine leukemia virus)
Blym transforming gene
BMD (bone marrow depression)
B-MOPP (bleomycin, mechlorethamine,
    Oncovin, procarbazine, prednisone)
BMP (BCNU, methotrexate,
    procarbazine)
BMT (bone marrow transplantation)
BMY-27857
BMY-28090 (elsamitrucin)
BMY-40900
BNCT
BNL (breast needle localization)
BOAP (bleomycin, Oncovin, Adriamycin,
    prednisone)
Boas-Oppler bacillus
BOBA (beta-oxybutyric acid)
Bocca neck dissection
Bodansky unit
Bodin-Gibb staging system
body
    Alder-Reilly b.
    Amato b's
    amygdaloid b.
    Arnold b's
    asbestos b's
    asbestosis b's
    Aschoff b's
    asteroid b.
    Auer b's
    bamboo b's
    Behla b's
    Bence Jones b's
    Bracht-Wachter b's
    Cabot ring b's
    Call-Exner b's
    cancer b's
    Councilman b's
    Cowdry-type A intranuclear
      inclusion b's
    crescent b's
    Deetjen b's
    Dohle b's
    Dohle inclusion b's
    Donne b's
    Dutcher b.
    Ehrlich hemoglobinemic
      b's

    elementary b.
    ferruginous b's
    fibrin b's
    fuchsin b's
    gamma-Favre b's
    Gordon elementary b.
    Harting b's
    Heinz b.
    Heinz-Ehrlich b's
    Howell b's
    Howell-Jolly b's
    immune b.
    inclusion b's
    inner b's
    Jolly b's
    Leishman-Donovan b.
    Lipschutz b's
    malpighian b's
    Masson b's
    Mott b's
    Muller dust b's
    Neill-Mooser b's
    Nissl b's
    Pappenheimer b's
    Phi b's
    Pick b's
    Plimmer b's
    psammoma b.
    Reilly b's
    Russell b's
    Schaumann b's
    Verocay b's
    Weibel-Palade b's
    X b.
    zebra b.
body defense
body fluid
body mass
    index, b.
body pharmacy
body section radiography
body surface area (BSA)
Boeck
    disease, B.
    sarcoid, B.
    sarcoidosis, B.
boggy
BOH butyroid
Bohn nodule
Bohr
    atom, B.
    effect, B.
    equation, B.

ADDITIONAL TERMS

theory, B.
Boiven antigen
BOLD (bleomycin, Oncovin, lomustine,
  dacarbazine)
Boltzmann
    constant, B.
    equation, B.
bolus
bolused
bomb
    atomic b.
    cobalt b.
    hydrogen b.
    nuclear b.
    plutonium b.
    thermonuclear b.
bombard
bombardment
Bombay phenotype
bombesin
    GRP immunoreactivity, b.
Bomgart stomal bag
bone
    block, b.
    cancer, b.
    cell, b.
    cyst, b.
    density, b.
    destruction, b.
    erosion, b.
    graft, b.
    metastases, b.
    pain, b.
    radiation absorption, b.
    resorption, b.
    sarcoma, b.
    scan, b.
    tumor, b.
bone marrow
    aspirate, b.
    aspiration, b.
    autografting, b.
    biopsy, b.
    cell pool, b.
    depression, b. (BMD)
    embolism, b.
    failure, b.
    harvest, b.
    infiltration, b.
    infusion, b.
    mast cells, b.
    match, b.
    needle, b.

pressure, b.
progenitor cell, b.
purging, b.
relapse, b.
scan, b.
stem cell, b.
suppression, b.
tap, b.
toxicity, b.
transplantation, b. (BMT)
Bonefos
Bonifacio anticancer goat serum
Bonine
Bonnevie-Ullrich syndrome
Bonnier syndrome
BONP (bleomycin, Oncovin, Natulan,
  prednisolone)
bony
    metastases, b.
    pain, b.
    tenderness, b.
boomerang DNA amplification
Boorman gastric cancer typing system,
  types I through IV
boost
    dose, b.
    field, b.
    radiation, b.
    shrinking field technique, b.
boosted
booster
    dose, b.
    immunization, b.
BOP (BCNU, Oncovin, prednisone)
BOP (bleomycin, Oncovin, Platinol)
BOPAM (bleomycin, Oncovin,
  prednisone, Adriamycin,
  mechlorethamine, methotrexate)
BOPP (BCNU, Oncovin, procarbazine,
  prednisone)
Bordet-Gengou
    agar, B.
    phenomenon, B.
    reaction, B.
boring
    cancer, b.
    pain, b.
bornelone
borocaptate sodium B10
boron
    counter, b.
    neutron capture, b.
boronated antibody

ADDITIONAL TERMS

Borrelia
  burgdorferi, B.
  lymphocytoma, B.
Borrmann classification
boss
bosselated
bosselation
bossing
Boston Children's Hospital staging
  system
botryoid sarcoma
botryomycosis
Böttcher crystals
Bouin solution
bound
  antigen, b.
  electron, b.
Bourneville disease
Bovin fixation
bovine
  adenovirus, b.
  albumin, b.
  aortic endothelial cells, b.
  bone, b.
  colloid, b.
  colostrum, b.
  dialyzable leukocyte extract, b.
  gamma globulin, b.
  lentivirus, b.
  leukemia virus, b. (BLV)
  papilloma virus, b.
  pituitary extract, b.
  red blood cells, b.
  serum albumin, b. (BSA)
  thyrotropin, b.
bowel
  incontinence, b.
  perforation, b.
  preparation, b.
  wall, b.
  wall penetration, b.
Bowen
  disease, B.
  precancerous dermatosis, B.
  tumor, B.
bowenoid
  carcinoma of vulva, b.
boxcar effect
boy-in-a-bubble disease
Boyden chamber
bp (base pairs)
BPA (burst-promoting activity)
BPB (biliopancreatic bypass)

BPD (bronchopulmonary dysplasia)
BPH (benign prostatic hypertrophy)
Bq (becquerel)
brachioaxillary bridge graft fistula
  (BAGF)
brachioproctic
  erotism, b. (anal fisting)
Bracht-Wachter lesion
brachytherapy
bracken fern
Bradshaw test
bradycinesia
bradycinetic
  analysis, b.
bradykinin
bradylalia
Bragg peak
brain
  abscess, b.
  -adjacent tumor, b. (BAT)
  biopsy, b.
  cancer, b.
  -dead, b.
  death, b.
  edema, b.
  metastases, b.
  scan, b.
  stem, b.
  stem glioma, b.
  tumor, b.
brain stem
braking radiation
branched chain
branchial cleft cyst
branchiogenic
branchiogenous
branchioma
Branhamella
  catarrhalis, B.
BRAT (Baylor rapid autologous
  transfusion)
  system, B.
Braun pouch
Braun-Jaboulay
  gastrectomy, B.
  gastroenterostomy, B.
brawny edema
breakpoint
  cluster region, b.
breakthrough
  bleeding, b.
  pain, b.
breast

ADDITIONAL TERMS

biopsy, b.
carcinoma, b.
fibrocystic disease, f.
implant, b.
lump, b.
mammography, b.
mammoplasty, b.
needle localization, b. (BNL)
reconstruction, b.
removal, b.
self-examination, b. (BSE)
tumor, b.
breast cancer
adenoid cystic b.
carcinoid b.
ductal b.
glycogen-rich clear cell b.
inflammatory b.
in situ, b.
intracystic b.
lobular b.
male b.
mammographically occult b.
microinvasive b.
mucinous b.
multicentric b.
multifocal b.
oat cell b.
occult b.
papillary b.
preclinical b.
secretory b.
signet ring b.
squamous cell b.
sudoriferous b.
tubular b.
breastfed
breastfeeding
Brecher and Cronkite technique
breeder reactor
Brenner
nodule, B.
tumor, B.
brequinar sodium
Breslow microstaging system
Bricker procedure
Bricker-Modlin technique
Brieger cachexia reaction
Brigham brain tumor
Brill-Symmers disease
brilliant cresyl blue
brim sign
brinolase

Brinton disease
Brissaud-Sicard syndrome
Bristowe syndrome
British antilewisite (BAL)
BRM (biologic response modifier)
Broca
amnesia, B.
motor speech area, B.
Broders
grading system, B.
index, grades 1 to 4, B.
Brodmann areas
broken-straw sign
bromatherapy
bromatotherapy
bromelain
bromocriptine
5-bromodeoxyuridine (broxuridine or
BUdR)
5-bromo-2'-deoxyuridine
5-bromouracil
Brompton
cocktail, B.
mixture, B.
solution, B.
bronch (bronchoscopy)
bronched (received or performed
bronchoscopy)
bronchi (pl. of bronchus)
bronchial
adenoma, b.
brush biopsy, b.
brushings, b.
carcinoma, b.
lavage, b.
tree, b.
washings, b.
bronchiectasis
bronchiolar
bronchiole
bronchoalveolar
brushings, b.
carcinoma, b.
lavage, b. (BAL)
lavage fluid, b. (BALF)
washings, b.
bronchoalveolitis
bronchoblastomycosis
bronchodilator
bronchoesophageal
bronchoesophagoscopy
bronchofiberoscope
bronchofibroscopy

ADDITIONAL TERMS

bronchogenic
  adenocarcinoma, b.
  carcinoma, b.
  cyst, b.
  oat cell carcinoma, b.
bronchogram
bronchography
  Cope b.
bronchomediastinal
  lymphatic trunks, b.
bronchomycosis
bronchopathy
bronchopneumonia
bronchopulmonary
  aspergillosis, b.
  cyst, b.
  dysplasia, b. (BPD)
  node, b.
bronchoradiography
bronchoscope
  fiberoptic b.
  rigid b.
bronchoscopy
  aspiration b.
  flexible fiberoptic b.
bronchospasm
bronchospastic
  component, b.
bronchospirography
bronchospirometry
bronchus (pl. bronchi)
bronze baby syndrome
bronzed
  disease, b.
  skin, b.
Brooke
  disease, B.
  tumor, B.
bropirimine (ABPP)
Broviac catheter
brown
  sputum, b.
  tumor, b.
Brown dermatome
Brown-Pearce tumor
Brown-Roberts-Wells (BRW) CT
  stereotaxic guide
Brown-Séquard syndrome
broxuridine
bruceantin
Brucella
  canis, B.

melitensis, B.
brucellosis
Bruel & Kjaer ultrasound scanner
Brugia
  malayi, B.
  pahangi, B.
bruise
bruising
  easy b.
bruit
brunnescence
brunnescent
Bruns syndrome
Brunschwig operation
brush
  biopsy, b.
  cells, b.
  cytology, b.
brushings
  washings, b. and
Bruton
  agammaglobulinemia, B.
  disease, B.
  -type infantile X-linked
    agammaglobulinemia, B.
BRW (Brown-Roberts-Wells) CT
  stereotaxic guide
Bryce sign
BSA (body surface area)
BSA (bovine serum albumin)
BSE (breast self-examination)
BSF (B-lymphocyte stimulatory factor)
BSGF (brachiosubclavian bridge graft
  fistula)
BSO (buthionine sulfoximine)
BSRL (buserelin)
BSS (Bernard-Soulier syndrome)
BT (BCNU, triazinate)
BU (busulfan)
Bu factor
bubbicle
bubble
  agent, b.
  -boy disease, b.
bubo
buccal
  cavity, b.
  mucosa, b.
Buchler afterloading system
Buckley syndrome
Bucky-Potter diaphragm
Budd-Chiari syndrome

ADDITIONAL TERMS

BUdR (bromodeoxyuridine or
   broxuridine)
   radiosensitizer, B.
buffalo hump
Buffalo orphan prototype
buffer
buffering
buffy
   coat, b.
   coat smear, b.
   crust, b.
Bufrolin
Buhl desquamative pneumonia
bulky
   lesion, b.
   tumor, b.
bulla (pl. bullae)
bullae (pl. of bulla)
bullous
   lesion, b.
   pemphigoid, b.
   pemphigoid antigen, b.
   pyoderma, b.
Buminate
BUN (blood urea nitrogen)
Bunge amputation
bur
   drill, b.
   hole, b.
Burkitt
   -like lymphoma, B.
   lymphoma, B.
   staging, B. (grades A, B, C, D)
   tumor, B.
   -type acute lymphoblastic
      leukemia, B.
   -type acute lymphocytic leukemia,
      B.
Burnet
   acquired immunity, B.
   theory, B.
Burnett applicator
Burns space
Burow
   solution, B.
   triangle, B.
burr cell
burred
burring
bursa (pl. bursae)
   -equivalent tissue, b.
bursae (pl. of bursa)

burst
   -forming unit, b. (BFU)
   -forming unit—erythroid, b. (BFU-
      E)
   -promoting activity, b. (BPA)
Buruli ulcer
Busacca nodules
Buschke-Lowenstein tumor
buserelin (BSRL)
busulfan (BU or MeliBu or Myleran)
Butchart staging system
buthionine sulfoximine (BSO)
L-buthionine sulfoximine (BSO)
butorphanol
Butter cancer
butter yellow
butterfly
   appearance, b.
   astrocytoma, b.
   needle, b.
   rash, b.
   shadow, b.
   -type glioma, b.
butyl
   -DNJ, b. (deoxynojirimycin)
   nitrate, b.
butylated
   hydroxytoluene, b.
butyroid
buyer's club
buyo cheek cancer
BVAP (BCNU, vincristine, Adriamycin,
   prednisone)
BV-ara-U
BVCPP (BCNU, vinblastine,
   cyclophosphamide, procarbazine,
   prednisone)
BVD (BCNU, vincristine, dacarbazine)
BVDS (bleomycin, Velban, doxorubicin,
   streptozocin)
BVPP (BCNU, vincristine, procarbazine,
   prednisone)
BW 12C
BW 30lU (piritrexim)
BW 566C80
BW A770U (crisnatol mesylate)
BW B759U (DHPG)
bypass
   duodenal b.
   fundoesophageal b.
   gastric b.
   intestinal b.

ADDITIONAL TERMS

bypass—*Continued*
   jejunoesophageal b.
   jejunoileal b.
bypassed
bystander
   innocent b.

C
   C antigen
   C100-3 antigen
   C-band
   C-banding
C-cell hyperplasia
C8166 cell line
C3 complement receptor
C factor
C Harlem hemoglobin
C3 nephritic factor
C particle
C peptide
C3 proactivator (C3PA)
   convertase, C. (C3PAase)
C protein
C-reactive protein (CRP)
C3 receptor
C region
C substance
C-terminal
   assay, C.
   constant region, C.
C-type
   retrovirus, C
   RNA virus, C.
CA 15-2 antigen serum tumor marker
CA 15-2 RIA (radioimmunoassay)
CA 15-3 antigen serum tumor marker
CA 19-9 antigen serum tumor marker
CA 72-4 antigen serum tumor marker
CA-125
   assay, C.
   cancer antigen, C.
CAA (constitutional aplastic anemia)
CABOP (cyclophosphamide,
   Adriamycin, bleomycin, Oncovin,
   prednisone)
Cabot ring bodies
CABS (CCNU, Adriamycin, bleomycin,
   streptozotocin)
CAC (cisplatin, ara-C, caffeine)
cachectic
   diarrhea, c.
cachectin
cachexia

cancerous c.
hypophyseal c.
hypophysioprivia, c.
lymphatic c.
malarial c.
paraneoplastic c.
pituitary c.
saturnine c.
strumiprivia, c.
uremic c.
cachexia reaction
cacoethic
cacogeusia
cacotrophy
cactinomycin
CACP (cisplatin)
CAD (cyclophosphamide, Adriamycin,
   dacarbazine)
CAD (cytosine arabinoside,
   daunorubicin)
cadaver
   blood transfusion, c.
   bone transplant, c.
CADD-PLUS infusion pump
CADIC (cyclophosphamide, Adriamycin,
   DTIC)
cadmium (Cd)
CAE (cyclophosphamide, Adriamycin,
   etoposide)
CAF (cyclophosphamide, Adriamycin,
   5-fluorouracil)
cafe-au-lait spot
caffeine
   analogue, c.
CAFFI (cyclophosphamide, Adriamycin,
   5-fluorouracil by continuous infusion)
CAFP (cyclophosphamide, Adriamycin,
   5-fluorouracil, prednisone)
CAFTH (cyclophosphamide,
   Adriamycin, 5-fluorouracil, tamoxifen,
   Halotestin)
CAFVP (cyclophosphamide, Adriamycin,
   5-fluorouracil, vincristine, prednisone)
Cajal
   cell, C.
   method, C.
calcific
   change, c.
   density, c.
   shadow, c.
calcification
   metastatic c.
   non-neoplastic c.

ADDITIONAL TERMS

calcified
  density, c.
  epithelioma, c.
  granuloma, c.
  leiomyoma, c.
  lesion, c.
  lymph node, c.
  mass, c.
  uterine fibroid, c.
calcifying
  fibroma, c.
  giant cell tumor, c.
  hematoma, c.
Calcimar
calcitonin
calcium
  channel blocker, c.
  trisodium pentetate, c.
Calcium Chel 330
calculation of survival rates
  actuarial method, c. by (life-table
    method)
  direct method, c. by
  life-table method, c. by (actuarial
    method)
calculi (pl. of calculus)
calculus (pl. calculi)
Caldwell view
Caldwell-Luc procedure
CALF (cyclophosphamide, Adriamycin,
  leucovorin calcium, 5-fluorouracil)
calf thymus extract
CALF-E (cyclophosphamide,
  Adriamycin, leucovorin calcium,
  5-fluorouracil, ethinyl estradiol)
CALG (Cancer and Acute Leukemia
  Group)
calibrate
calibration
calicheamicin
calicheamicinone
californium (Cf)
  neutron brachytherapy, c.
  252 radioisotope, c.
calipers
Call-Exner bodies
CALLA (common acute lymphoblastic
  leukemia antigen)
  -positive leukemia, C.
  + T-Ig phenotype, C.
Callender classification
Callison fluid
Calmette test

Calmette-Guérin bacillus
calmodulin
caloradiance
calorescence
calusterone
calutron
calvacin
calvities
Calymmatobacterium
  granulomatis, C.
CAM (cell adhesion molecule)
CAM (chorioallantoic membrane)
  assay, C.
CAM (cyclophosphamide, Adriamycin,
  methotrexate)
CAMB (cyclophosphamide, Adriamycin,
  methotrexate, bleomycin)
CAMELEON (cytosine arabinoside,
  high-dose methotrexate, leucovorin,
  Oncovin)
Campbell de Morgan spots
cameloid anemia
CAMEO (cyclophosphamide,
  Adriamycin, methotrexate, etoposide,
  Oncovin)
Cameray gamma camera
Ca_2 metal ion
Camey ileocystoplasty
CAMF (cyclophosphamide, Adriamycin,
  methotrexate, 5-fluorouracil)
CAMF (cyclophosphamide, Adriamycin,
  methotrexate, folic acid)
CAMLO (cytosine arabinoside,
  methotrexate, leucovorin, Oncovin)
cAMP (adenosine 3′,5′-cyclic phosphate)
cAMP (cyclic AMP)
CAMP (cyclophosphamide, Adriamycin,
  methotrexate, procarbazine)
camptothecin
Campylobacter
  cinaedi, C.
  coli, C.
  fennelliae, C.
  fetus, C.
  jejuni, C.
  pyloris, C.
campylobacteriosis
canal
  Cloquet c.
  Hyrtl c.
canal ray
cancellous
  bone, c.

ADDITIONAL TERMS

cancer
   acinar c.
   acinous c.
   adenoid c.
   à deux, c.
   adrenal cortex c.
   alveolar c.
   ampullary c.
   aniline c.
   apinoid c.
   aplastic thyroid c.
   areolar c.
   atrophicans, c.
   betel c.
   bile duct c.
   biliary duct c.
   black c.
   bladder c.
   bone c.
   boring c.
   brain c.
   branchiogenous c.
   breast c,
   Butter c.
   buyo cheek c.
   cecal c.
   cellular c.
   cerebriform c.
   cervical lymph node c.
   cervical stump c.
   chimney-sweep's c.
   chondroid c.
   claypipe c.
   cloacogenic c.
   colloid c.
   colon c.
   colorectal c.
   conjugal c.
   contact c.
   corset c.
   cribriform c.
   cystic c.
   de nova c.
   dendritic c.
   dermoid c.
   dhoti c.
   duct c.
   dye workers' c.
   en cuirasse, c.
   encephaloid c.
   endocrine pancreatic c.
   endometrial c.
   endothelial c.

   epidermal c.
   epidermoid c.
   epiesophageal c.
   epithelial c.
   esophageal c.
   exocrine pancreatic c.
   extragonadal germ cell c.
   extrapulmonary small cell c.
   familial c.
   follicular thyroid c.
   fungous c.
   glandular c.
   green c.
   hard c.
   hematoid c.
   in situ, c.
   invasive c.
   jacket c.
   kang c.
   kangri c.
   latent c.
   lip c.
   lymph node c.
   male breast c.
   medullary c.
   medullary thyroid c.
   melanotic c.
   metastatic c.
   microinvasive c.
   mule-spinners' c.
   nasopharyngeal c.
   neuroendocrine c.
   non–small cell lung c.
   occult c.
   ovarian c.
   pancreatic c.
   paraffin c.
   periampullary c.
   pipe-smoker's c.
   pitchworkers' c.
   prostate c.
   renal c.
   retrograde c.
   roentgenologist's c.
   scirrhous c.
   small cell lung c.
   snuff c.
   soft c.
   solanoid c.
   soot c.
   spider c.
   spindle cell c.
   T-helper c.

ADDITIONAL TERMS

tar c.
telangiectatic c.
testicular c.
thyroid c.
tubular c.
uroepithelial c.
urothelial c.
uterine c.
vaginal c.
villous duct c.
vulvar c.
Cancer and Acute Leukemia Group
  (CALG)
cancer and steroid hormone (CASH)
cancer-associated anemia
cancer bodies
cancer cachexia
cancer cell
cancer cell collector
cancer chemotherapy
cancer classification
cancer cluster
cancer control window (CCW)
cancer family
cancer-free (CF)
    white mouse, c. (CFWM)
cancer gene
cancer genetics
cancer grading
Cancer Information Center (CIS)
cancer juice
cancer milk
cancer nests
cancer phobia
cancer reaction
cancer risk
cancer serum
cancer serum index (CSI)
cancer spread
cancer staging
canceremia
cancericidal
cancerigenic
cancerin
cancerism
cancerocidal
cancerogenic
cancerophobia
cancerous
    cachexia, c.
    growth, c.
    lesion, c.
    mass, c.

tissue, c.
cancerphobia
cancer-ulcer
cancriform
cancroid
cancrology
cancrum
    nasi, c.
    oris, c.
    pudendi, c.
Candida
    albicans, C.
    stomatitis, C.
candidal
    arthritis, c.
    esophagitis, c.
    proctitis, c.
    stomatitis, c.
    vaginitis, c.
candidiasis
candle
    cesium c. implant
    vaginal c.
Caner-Decker syndrome
canine
    adenovirus, c.
    -transmissible tumor, c.
canker sore
Cannabic
cannabidiol
cannabinoid
cannabinol
cannabis
Cannon ring
cannula (pl. cannulae)
cannulae (pl. of cannula)
cannulation
Cantell alpha interferon
Cantor tube
CAO (cyclophosphamide, Adriamycin,
    Oncovin)
CAP (cyclophosphamide, Adriamycin,
    Platinol)
CAP (cyclophosphamide, Adriamycin,
    prednisone)
CAP-I (cyclophosphamide, Adriamycin,
    Platinol)
CAP-II (cyclophosphamide, Adriamycin,
    high-dose Platinol)
Capastat Sulfate
CAP-BOP (cyclophosphamide,
    Adriamycin, procarbazine, bleomycin,
    Oncovin, prednisone)

ADDITIONAL TERMS

CAPD (continuous ambulatory
   peritoneal dialysis)
capillary
   electrophoresis, c.
   fragility, c.
   leak syndrome, c.
   permeability, c.
   refill, c.
Caplan syndrome
capping enzyme
CAPPr (cyclophosphamide, Adriamycin,
   Platinol, prednisone)
CAPR (combined abdominoperineal
   resection)
capreomycin sulfate
capsaicin
capsulectomy
capsuloma
caracemide
Carazzi hematoxylin
carbamate
   -linked, c.
carbaminohemoglobin
carbamoylation
Carbarsone
carbetimer
carbidopa
carbimazole
carbogen
carbohemoglobin
carbon
   14, c.
   black, c.
carbonate
   ferrous c.
   dehydratase, c.
carboplatin (Paraplatin)
Carbovir
carboxyhemoglobin
carboxyhemoglobinemia
carboxylation
carboxypeptidase
   G, c.
carbuncle
   malignant c.
Carcalon
carcinelcosis
carcinemia
carcinoembryonic antigen (CEA)
carcinogen
   chemical c.
   proximate c.
   ultimate c.

carcinogenesis
   chemical c.
   foreign-body c.
   multistage c.
carcinogenic
carcinogenicity
carcinoid
   adenoma of bronchus, c.
   flush, c.
   heart disease, c.
   syndrome, c.
   tumor, c.
carcinology
carcinolysin
carcinolysis
carcinolytic
carcinoma (pl. carcinomata)
   acinar c.
   acinar cell c.
   acinic cell c.
   acinose c.
   acinous c.
   adenocystic c.
   adenoid cystic c.
   adenoid squamous cell c.
   adenomatosum, c.
   adenosquamous c.
   adrenal cortex, c. of
   alveolar c.
   alveolar cell c.
   alveolar mucoid c.
   ameloblastic c.
   anaplastic c.
   apocrine c.
   argentaffin c.
   argyrophil cell c.
   Bartholin gland c.
   basal cell c.
   basocellulare, c.
   basaloid c.
   basosquamous cell c.
   bile duct c.
   Bowen c.
   bowenoid c.
   branchiogenic c.
   breast c.
   bronchioalveolar c.
   bronchiolar c.
   bronchioloalveolar c.
   bronchogenic c.
   cavitary c.
   cecal c.
   cerebriform c.

ADDITIONAL TERMS

ceruminous c.
cervical c.
cholangiocellular c.
chorionic c.
ciliated cell c.
clear cell c.
cloacogenic c.
colloid c.
colon c.
colorectal c.
comedo c.
contralateral synchronous c.
corpus c.
cribriform c.
cutaneum, c.
cylindrical c.
cylindrical cell c.
cylindromatous c.
cystic c.
duct c.
ductal c.
durum, c.
Ehrlich ascites c. (EAC)
embryonal cell c.
encephaloid c.
en cuirasse, c.
endometrial c.
endometrioid c.
epibulbar c.
epidermoid c.
epimyothelial c.
epitheliale adenoides, c.
Epstein-Barr nasopharyngeal c.
erectile c.
erysipelatoides, c.
esophageal c.
ex ulcere, c.
exophytic c.
extrahepatic biliary c.
fibrinolamellar c.
fibrolamellar liver cell c.
fibrosum, c.
focal lobular c.
follicular c.
gallbladder c.
gastric c.
gelatiniform c.
gelatinous c.
giant cell c.
gigantocellulare, c.
glandular c.
glassy cell c.
glycogen-rich clear cell c.

granulosa cell c.
hair-matrix c.
hematoid c.
hepatobiliary c.
hepatocellular c.
Hurthle cell c.
hyaline c.
hypernephroid c.
infantile embryonal c.
infiltrating ductal cell c.
inflammatory c.
in situ, c. (CIS)
insulin-secreting c.
intercalated duct c.
intermediate c.
intracystic breast c.
intraductal c.
intraepidermal c.
intraepithelial c.
intrahepatic bile duct c.
invasive c.
islet cell c.
jejunal c.
juvenile c.
kangri burn c.
Krompecher c.
Kulchitsky-cell c.
large-cell c.
laryngeal c.
latent c.
lateral aberrant thyroid c.
lenticular c.
lenticulare, c.
leptomeningeal c.
Lewis lung c.
lipid-rich c.
lipomatous c.
liver cell c.
lobular c.
lobular c. in situ
lung c.
lymphoepithelial c.
medullare, c.
medullary c.
medullary thyroid c.
melanotic c.
meningeal c.
Merkel cell c.
mesometanephric c.
mesonephric c.
metaplastic c.
metastatic c.
metatypical c.

ADDITIONAL TERMS

carcinoma—*Continued*

microinvasive c.
mixed hepatocellular c.
molle, c.
mucinous c.
muciparum, c.
mucocellulare, c.
mucoepidermoid c.
mucosum, c.
mucous c.
multicentric c.
myxomatodes, c.
nasopharyngeal c.
neuroendocrine c.
nevoid basal cell c.
nigrum, c.
non-Bowen squamous cell c.
noninfiltrating intraductal c.
noninfiltrating lobular c.
nonkeratinizing c.
non–small cell bronchogenic c.
oat cell c.
occult c.
odontogenic c.
oncocytic cell c.
oncoplastic c.
ossificans, c.
osteoid c.
ovarian c.
pancreatic c.
papillary c.
parathyroid c.
periportal c.
pipe-smoker's c.
pleomorphic large-cell c.
polypoid c.
poorly differentiated c.
preclinical c.
preinvasive c.
prickle cell c.
primary c.
prostatic c.
pultaceous c.
recurrent c.
renal cell c.
reserve cell c.
residual c.
salivary duct c.
sarcomatodes, c.
sarcomatoid c.
scar c.
schneiderian c.
scirrhous c.

scroti, c.
sebaceous c.
secondary c.
secretory c.
signet-ring cell c.
simplex, c.
small-cell c.
small-cell bronchogenic c.
solanoid c.
solid c.
spheroidal cell c.
spindle cell c.
Spiroptera c.
spongiosum, c.
squamous c.
squamous cell c. (SCC)
string c.
stump c.
subglottic c.
subungual epidermoid c.
sudoriferous c.
superficial multicentric basal cell c.
supraglottic c.
sweat gland c.
telangiectaticum, c.
telangiectodes, c.
thymic c.
thyroid c.
trabecular c.
transglottic c.
transitional cell c.
tuberosum, c.
tuberous c.
tubular c.
undifferentiated c.
undifferentiated epidermoid c.
undifferentiated squamous cell c.
ureteral c.
urethral c.
urothelial transitional cell c.
uterine c.
V-2 c.
vaginal c.
varicoid c.
verrucous c.
verrucous squamous cell c.
villosum, c.
villous c.
vulvar squamous cell c.
Walker c.
well-differentiated c.
wolffian duct c.
yolk-sac c.

ADDITIONAL TERMS

carcinomata (pl. of carcinoma)
carcinomatoid
carcinomatophobia
carcinomatosis
carcinomatous
    leptomeningitis, c.
    pericarditis, c.
    tumor, c.
carcinomelcosis
carcinophilia
carcinophilic
carcinophobia
carcinophobic
carcinosarcoma
    embryonal c.
carcinosis
    miliary c.
    pleurae, c.
    pulmonary c.
carcinostatic
carcinous
cardiac
    tamponade, c.
    toxicity, c.
cardiomyopathy
Caremark infusion system
CARET (Carotene and Retinol Efficacy
    Trial)
CA15-2 RIA
carina (pl. carinae)
carinae (pl. of carina)
carinal
Carl Smith disease
carmustine (BCNU or BiCNU)
Carney triad
carnidazole
Carnitor
Caroli disease
carotenase
carotene
    beta c.
Carotene and Retinol Efficacy Trial
    (CARET)
carotenemia
carotenoid
carotenosis
carotid body tumor
carotin
Carprofen
carrier
    -free, c.
    -free radioisotope, c.
Carrion disease

Carrisyn (acemannan)
carrot juice
Cartwright
    blood group system, C.
    factor, C.
carubicin
caruncle
Cas-Br-E virus
cascade
    electron c.
    metastatic c.
cascade hypothesis
cascade transformer
case control study
caseating
caseation
Casec
casein
    kinase II, c.
caseous
    lesion, c.
    necrosis, c.
CASH (cancer and steroid hormone)
Casodex
C-asparaginase (Crasnitin)
Caspersson type B cells
cassette mutagenesis
cast
CAST (color allergy screening test)
Castananzi solution
castanospermine
Castle intrinsic factor
Castleman disease
castrate
castration
casual sex
CAT (chloramphenicol
    acetyltransferase)
    expression gene, C.
CAT (computerized axial tomography)
    scan, C.
CAT (cytosine arabinoside, Adriamycin,
    6-thioguanine)
CAT (cytosine arabinoside, thioguanine)
catabasis
catabatic
catabolic
    half-life, c.
catabolism
    antibody c.
catagen
CAT-A-KIT (catecholamine assay kit)
catalase

ADDITIONAL TERMS

catalysis
catalyst
Catapres (clonidine)
catecholamine
catenation
cathartic
cathemoglobin
cathepsin
    C/P185, c.
    D, c.
    E, c.
Cath-Secure tape
cation
cationic
cationogen
cathode
    luminescence, c.
    ray, c.
    stream, c.
cathodic
cat's eye reflex
cat-scratch
    antigen, c.
    disease, c. (CSD)
    fever, c.
cautery
cauterization
CAV (cyclophosphamide, Adriamycin,
    Velban)
CAV (cyclophosphamide, Adriamycin,
    vincristine)
Cavaliere factor
cavalryman osteoma
CAVe (CCNU, Adriamycin, Velban)
cavernous
    hemangioma, c.
    lymphangioma, c.
CAVH (continuous arteriovenous
    hemofiltration)
cavitation
cavitating
Cavitron ultrasonic aspirator (CUSA)
cavography
CAVP (cyclophosphamide, Adriamycin,
    VM-26, prednisone)
CAVP-I (cyclophosphamide,
    Adriamycin, vincristine, prednisone)
CAVP-16 (cyclophosphamide,
    Adriamycin, VP-16)
CAVPM (cyclophosphamide,
    Adriamycin, VP-16, prednisone,
    methotrexate)

CAVU (continuous arteriovenous
    ultrafiltration)
CB 1348
CB10-277
CBC (complete blood count)
CBF (cerebral blood flow)
CBG (corticosteroid-binding globulin)
c-bic gene
C3b INA (C3b inactivator)
C3b inactivator (C3b INA)
    accelerator, C.
CBL (chronic basophilic leukemia)
CBPPA (cyclophosphamide, bleomycin,
    procarbazine, prednisone, Adriamycin)
CBV (cyclophosphamide, BCNU,
    VePesid)
CBV (cyclophosphamide, BCNU, VP-16-
    213)
CBVD (CCNU, bleomycin, vinblastine,
    dexamethasone)
CCAT (conglutinating complement
    absorption test)
CCAVV (CCNU, cyclophosphamide,
    Adriamycin, vincristine, VP-16)
CCF (crystal-induced chemotactic
    factor)
CCFE (cyclophosphamide, cisplatin,
    5-fluorouracil, estramustine)
CCM (cyclophosphamide, CCNU,
    methotrexate)
CCMA (CCNU, cyclophosphamide,
    methotrexate, Adriamycin)
CCNU (lomustine)
    methyl C. (semustine)
CCNU-OP (CCNU, Oncovin, prednisone)
CCOB (CCNU, cyclophosphamide,
    Oncovin, bleomycin)
CCT (cranial computed tomography)
CCV (CCNU, cyclophosphamide,
    vincristine)
CCV-AV (CCNU, cyclophosphamide,
    vincristine--Adriamycin, vincristine)
CCVB (CCNU, cyclophosphamide,
    vincristine, bleomycin)
CCVPP (CCNU, cyclophosphamide,
    Velban, procarbazine, prednisone)
CCVV (cyclophosphamide, CCNU,
    VP-16, vincristine)
CCVVP (cyclophosphamide, CCNU,
    VP-16, vincristine, Platinol)
CCW (cancer control window)
Cd (cadmium)

ADDITIONAL TERMS

CD (cluster of differentiation)
CD (cytarabine, daunorubicin)
CD4
   antigen, C.
   cells, C.
   helper cells, C.
   IgG, C.
   lymphocyte, C.
   positive lymphocyte, C.
   Pseudomonas exotoxin, C.
   receptor, C.
   recombinant soluble, C. (Receptin
     or rsCD4)
   T-cell, C.
CD4+ cells
CD5+ monoclonal antibody
CD5-T lymphocyte
   immunotoxin, C. (XomaZyme-H65)
CD8 cells
CD8+ cells
CD11/18 monoclonal antibody
CD18 antigen
cdA (chlorodeoxyadenosine)
2-cdA (2-chlorodeoxyadenosine)
CDA (congenital dyserythropoietic
   anemia)
C-DAK
   artificial kidney, C.
   dialyzer, C.
CDC (carboplatin, doxorubicin,
   cyclophosphamide)
CDC (Centers for Disease Control)
cdc-2 kinase
CDDP (cis-diamminedichloroplatinum)
CDDP (cisplatin)
CDE (cyclophosphamide, doxorubicin,
   etoposide)
cDNA (complementary DNA)
   cloning, c.
cDNA (copy DNA)
   cloning, c.
CDP (cytidine diphosphate)
CDR (complementarity-determining
   region)
Ce (cerium)
CEA (carcinoembryonic antigen)
   -125, C.
   level, C.
   -Roche assay, C.
   -Tc 99m, C.
CEAker monoclonal antibody
CEB (carboplatin, etoposide, bleomycin)

CECA (cisplatin, etoposide,
   cyclophosphamide, Adriamycin)
cecal
cecectomy
cecitis
cecocolostomy
cecoileostomy
cecopexy
cecoplication
cecosigmoidostomy
cecostomy
cecotomy
cecum
cedar cone extract
Cedecea
   davisae, C.
CeeNu (CCNU or lomustine)
Ceetolan Concentrate
CEF (cyclophosphamide, epirubicin,
   5-fluorouracil)
cefamandole
cefazolin
cefepime
cefmetazole (Zefazone)
ceforanide
cefprozil (Cefzil)
ceftazidime
ceftriaxone
cefuroxime
Cefzil
CEL (chronic eosinophilic leukemia)
Celbenin
Celestin tube
celiac
celibacy
celibate
celiectomy
celioacography
celiocentesis
celioma
celiomyomectomy
celiomyomotomy
celioscope
celioscopy
celiothelioma
cell
   A c.
   Abbe-Zeiss counting c.
   absorptive c.
   accessory c's
   acid c.
   acidophilic c.

ADDITIONAL TERMS

cell—*Continued*
  acinar c's
  acinous c's
  acoustic hair c.
  active protein c's
  adelomorphous c's
  adherent c.
  adipose c.
  adventitial c's
  agger nasi c's
  air c's
  algoid c's
  alpha c's
  alveolar c's
  amacrine c's
  ameboid c's
  amine precursor uptake and
    decarboxylation (APUD) c's
  amphophilic c.
  antibody-dependent cytotoxic c's
  antigen-presenting c's
  antigen-reactive c's
  antigen-sensitive c's
  Antoni type A and B c's
  apocrine c's
  APUD (amine precursor uptake and
    decarboxylation (APUD) c's
  argentaffin c's
  argyrophilic c's
  Arias-Stella c's
  arkyochrome c.
  Armanni-Ebstein c's
  Aschoff c's
  B c's (B-lymphocytes)
  balloon c's
  band c.
  basal c.
  basal granular c's
  basophilic c.
  beaker c.
  berry c.
  beta c's
  Betz c's
  Bevan-Lewis c's
  blast c.
  blood c's
  bone marrow c's
  bristle c's
  bronchic c.
  brood c.
  burr c.
  C c's
  Cajal c.

  calciform c.
  cameloid c.
  capsule c.
  Caspersson type B c's
  castration c's
  caudate c's
  caveolated c's
  CD 4 c.
  CD 4 helper c.
  CD 4+ c.
  CD 8 c.
  CD 8+ c.
  central c's
  centroacinar c's
  chalice c.
  chief c's
  CHO c's
  chromaffin c's
  chromophobe c's
  chromophobic c's
  Clara c.
  Clarke c's
  Claudius c's
  clear c's
  cleavage c's
  cleaved c's
  clump c's
  CMS-5 c's
  coated c's
  columnar c.
  commissural c's
  committed c.
  connective tissue c's
  contrasuppressor c's
  corneal c.
  Corti c's
  COS c's
  counting c.
  crenated c's
  crescent c's
  Crooke c's
  cuboidal c's
  Custer c's
  cylindrical c's
  cytotoxic T c's
  D c's
  daughter c.
  Davidoff c's
  delta c's
  demilune c's
  dendritic c's
  dendritic epidermal c's
  differentiated c's

ADDITIONAL TERMS

Dorothy Reed c's
Downey c's
dust c's
Edelmann c.
effector c.
elementary c.
emigrated c.
encasing c's
endocrine c's
endothelioid c's
enterochromaffin c.
ependymal c's
epithelial c's
epithelioid c's
erythroid c's
eukaryotic c's
F c's
fat c's
Ferrata c.
foam c's
follicular center c's
follicular dendritic c's
follicular epithelial c's
foreign body giant c's
Foulis c's
Fuller c.
fusiform c.
G c's
gametoid c's
gamma c's
Gaucher c.
Gegenbaur c.
germinal c.
ghost c.
Giannuzzi c's
giant c.
gitter c's
Gley c's
glia c's
glitter c's
glomerular c.
glomus c.
goblet c.
gonadotroph c.
gonadotropic c.
Goormaghtigh c's
granular c.
granulosa c's
granulosa-lutein c's
grape c.
hairy c.
Hammar myoid c's
hand-mirror c.

heckle c.
Heidenhain c's
HeLa c's
helmet c.
helper c's
hematopoietic c's
hepatic c's
heteromeral c's
hilus c's
Hodgkin c's
Hoechst 33342 c's
Hofbauer c's
homozygous typing c's (HTC)
Hurthle c's
hybrid c's
hybridoma c's
hyperchromatic c.
I-c.
immunologically competent c.
immunoreactive c's
inclusion c's
inducer c.
inflammatory c.
intercapillary c.
interdigitating c's
interfollicular c's
interstitial c's
intracytoplasmic inclusion c's
irreversibly sickled c's
islet c's
juvenile c.
juxtaglomerular c's
K (killer) c's
Karpas T c's
karyochrome c's
killer (K) c's
killer T c's
Kulchitsky c's
Kupffer c's
L c's
lacunar c.
Langerhans c's
Langhans c's
Langhans giant c's
large-granule c's
LE c.
Leishmann chrome c's
lepra c.
Leydig c's
littoral c's
Loevit c.
longiradiate c's
lutein c's

ADDITIONAL TERMS

cell—*Continued*
  Lyl B c.
  lymph c.
  lymphadenoma c's
  lymphoid c.
  lymphoreticular c's
  M c's
  Marchand c.
  marrow c.
  Martinotti c's
  mast c.
  mastoid c's
  matrix c's
  maturation B c's
  mediator c.
  memory c's
  Merkel c's
  Merkel-Ranvier c's
  mesenchymal c's
  mesothelial c's
  Meynert c's
  migratory c's
  Mikulicz c's
  mitral c.
  mixed c's
  mononuclear c.
  Mooser c.
  morular c.
  mossy c.
  mother c.
  Mott c.
  mouth c's
  mucous c's
  mucosal c's
  mulberry c.
  Müller c's
  mycosis c.
  myeloid c.
  myeloma c.
  myoepithelial c's
  myoepithelioid c's
  Nageotte c's
  natural killer (NK) c's
  Neumann c's
  neuroendocrine c's
  neuroepithelial c's
  neuroglial c's
  neuronal c's
  neutrophilic c.
  nevus c.
  Niemann-Pick c's
  NK (natural killer) c's
  noble c's

nonadherent c's
nonnucleated c's
nucleated c's
nucleated red blood c's
null c's
oat c's
oat-shaped c's
osseous c's
osteoprogenitor c's
owl's eye c's
oxyntic c's
oxyphil c's
oxyphilic c's
packed human blood c's
packed red blood c's
Paget c.
pagetoid c.
pancreatic polypeptide (PP) c.
Paneth c's
parafollicular c's
paraluteal c's
paralutein c's
parenchymal hepatic c's
parenchymal liver c's
parent c.
parietal c's
paroxysmal nocturnal hemoglobin
  (PNH) c's
pathologic c's
pavement c's
peripheral stem c's
perithelial c.
pessary c.
phagocytic c's
pheochrome c's
photoreceptor c's
physaliferous c's
Pick c's
pigment c.
pineal c's
plaque-forming c's
plasma c's
pluripotent myeloid stem c's
PNH (paroxysmal nocturnal
  hemoglobin) c's
polychromatic c's
polychromatophil c's
polyhedral c's
polyplastic c.
PP (pancreatic polypeptide) c.
pre-B c's
precursor c.
pre-T c's

ADDITIONAL TERMS

prickle c.
primitive granulosa c's
primitive wandering c's
principal c's
progenitor c's
prolactin c.
pulmonary epithelial c's
pulpar c.
Purkinje c's
pus c.
pyramidal c.
pyrrhol c's
RA (ragocyte) c.
ragocyte (RA) c.
Raji c's
reactive c's
red c.
red blood c.
Reed c's
Reed-Sternberg giant c's
resting c.
resting wandering c.
reticular c's
reticuloendothelial c.
reticulum c.
reversible sickled c.
rhagiocrine c.
Rh-negative c's
Rieder c.
Rindfleisch c's
rod c's
rosette c's
Rouget c's
round c.
S c's
sarcogenic c's
satellite c's
scavenger c's
Schultze c's
Schwann c.
segmented c.
seminoma c.
senescent c's
sensitized c.
sentinel c's
Sézary c.
shadow c.
sickle c.
signet-ring c.
silver c's
skeletogenous c.
small-granule c's
smudge c's

somatic c's
somatotropic c's
sperm c.
spiculated c's
spider c.
spindle c.
spur c.
squamous c.
stab c.
staff c.
star c's
stave c's
stellate c's
stem c.
Sternberg giant c's
Sternberg-Reed c's
stipple c.
supporting c's
suppressor c's
sustentacular c's
sympathicotrophic c's
syncytial c's
synovial c's
T c's
T4 c's
T8 c's
T-cytotoxic c's
T-suppressor c's
tadpole c's
target c.
tart c.
tautomeral c's
Tdth c's
tegmental c's
theca c's
theca-lutein c's
Thoma-Zeiss counting c.
thymic epithelial c.
thymus nurse c.
thyroidectomy c's
thyrotroph c.
thyrotropic c.
Touton giant c.
trophochrome c's
Türk c.
Ty c's
Tzanck c.
U937 histiocytic lymphoma c's
ultimobranchial c's
unipotential stem c's
vacuolated c.
vasofactive c's
vasoformative c's

ADDITIONAL TERMS

cell—*Continued*
veil c's
veiled c's
ventricular c.
veto c's
virgin c's
von Kupffer c's
wandering c's
Warthin-Finkeldey c's
wasserhelle c's
water-clear c.
white c.
white blood c.
xanthoma c.
xenoplated tumor c's
zymogenic c's
cell adhesion molecule (CAM)
cell assay test
cell bank
cell binding
cell-bound antibody
cell counter
cell-counting chamber
cell culture
cell cycle
cell-cycle nonspecific
cell death
cell differentiation
cell envelope
cell-fixed antibody
cell fractions
cell growth cycle
cell homing
cell interaction (CI) genes
cell kill
cell kinetics
cell lines
cell marker
cell maturation
cell-mediated
immunity, c. (CMI)
lympholysis, c. (CML)
cell migration
cell mimicry
cell morphology
cell nests
cell population
cell receptor
cell recruitment
cell replication
cell sorter
cell sorting
cell strain

cell surface marker
cell washing
Cellano phenotype
Cellolite patty
Cell-Saver Haemolite
celltrifuge
cellular
adaptation, c.
biochemistry, c.
blue nevus, c.
cancer, c.
differentiation, c.
-embolic theory, c.
genes, c. (c-onc)
genetics, c.
immune deficiency, c.
immunity, c.
immunodeficiency syndrome, c.
(CIDS)
rejection, c.
retinoic acid–binding protein-I, c.
(CRABP-I)
suppression, c.
theory, c.
cellularity
cellule
claire, c.
cellulicidal
cellulifugal
cellulipetal
cellulitis
cellulofibrous
cellulotoxic
cellulous
CEM (cytosine arabinoside, etoposide,
methotrexate)
cementification
cementifying fibroma
cementoblastoma
cementofibroma
cementoma
CEM/HIV-1 cell line
Centers for Disease Control (CDC)
centigray (cGy)
centimorgan (cM)
centistoke
Centovir
Centoxin
central
amaurosis, c.
amputation, c.
ataxia, c.
axis, c.

ADDITIONAL TERMS

axis depth dose, c.
axis midplane dose, c.
lesion, c.
venous catheter, c. (CVC)
centrifugal
centrifugation
centrifuge
centriole
centrocyte
centrocytic
centromere
centrosome
Centry
CEP (CCNU, etoposide, prednimustine)
CEP (cyclophosphamide, etoposide,
   Platinol)
cephalin cholesterol flocculation
cephalosporin
cephalosporinase
ceramide glucosidase
cercaria
cercariasis
cercarienhullenreaktion
cereal fiber
cerebellar
   ataxia, c.
   degeneration, c.
cerebellopontine angle tumor
cerebellum
cerebral
   amaurosis, c.
   atrophy, c.
   convexity, c.
   hemorrhage, c.
   syndrome, c.
   tumor, c.
cerebriform
   cancer, c.
   carcinoma, c.
   cells, c.
cerebroma
cerebrospinal fluid (CSF)
Ceredase (alglucerase)
Cerenkov
   counter, C.
   radiation, C.
cerium (Ce)
ceroma
Cerrobend
   blocks, C.
   castings, C.
   cutouts, C.
   mantle blocks, C.

mask, C.
Cerubidine (daunorubicin)
ceruloplasmin
ceruminoma
Cervex-Brush
cervical
   biopsy, c.
   cancer, c.
   carcinoma, c.
   cone, c.
   conization, c.
   cyst, c.
   dysplasia, c.
   intraepithelial neoplasia grades I,
      II, III, c. (CIN)
   lymph nodes, c.
   lymphadenopathy, c.
   metaplasia, c.
   stump, c.
cervicectomy
cervices (pl. of cervix)
cervicitis
cervix (pl. cervices)
   uteri, c.
Cesamet
cesium (Cs)
   137, c.
   applicator, c.
   cylinder, c.
   implant, c.
   insertion, c.
   intracavitary c. implantation
   needle, c.
Cestan syndrome
Cestan-Chenais syndrome
CET (coefficient of equivalent thickness)
cetiedil citrate
Cetus trial
Cf (californium)
   252 radioisotope, C.
CF (cancer-free)
CF (Christmas factor)
CF (cisplatin, 5-fluorouracil)
CF (citrovorum factor)
CF (complement factor)
CF (leucovorin)
CFA (complement-fixing antibody)
CFIDS (chronic fatigue and immune
   dysfunction syndrome)
CFL (cisplatin, 5-fluorouracil,
   leucovorin calcium)
CFM (cyclophosphamide, 5-fluorouracil,
   mitoxantrone)

ADDITIONAL TERMS

c-fms oncogene
C-fos
CFP (cyclophosphamide, 5-fluorouracil, prednisone)
CFPT (cyclophosphamide, 5-fluorouracil, prednisone, tamoxifen)
CFT (complement-fixation test)
CFU (colony-forming unit)
CFU-C (colony-forming unit—culture)
CFU-E (colony-forming unit—erythroid)
CFU-Eos (colony-forming unit—eosinophils)
CFU-G (colony-forming unit—granulocytes)
CFU-GMEMM (colony-forming unit—granulocyte-macrophage, erythroid, megakaryocyte, multipotential)
CFU-GM (colony-forming unit—granulocyte-macrophage)
CFU-L (colony-forming unit—lymphoid)
CFU-M (colony-forming unit—macrophage)
CFU-S (colony-forming unit—spleen)
CFWM (cancer-free white mouse)
CGD (chronic granulomatous disease)
CGL (chronic granulocytic leukemia)
cGMP (cyclic guanosine monophosphate)
CGP (circulating granulocyte pool)
CGR Medical Corporation
    AGC Curieton afterloader, C.
    Saturn III accelerator, C.
CGS 16949A
cGy (centigray)
C3H
    mammary tumor, C.
    melanoma, C.
C'H50 (total hemolytic complement)
CHA (congenital hypoplastic anemia)
CHAD (cyclophosphamide, hexamethylmelamine, Adriamycin, DDP)
Chagas disease
chain
    branched c.
    closed c.
    H (heavy) c.
    heavy (H) c.
    J (joining) c.
    joining (J) c.
    kappa c.
    L (light) c.
    lambda c.

    lateral c.
    light (L) c.
    side c.
chain-initiation codons
chain-reacting pile
chain reactor
chain scission
chain-termination codons
chain terminator
chaining
chalicosis
chalone
chancre
chancriform
chancroid
Chaoul
    therapy, C.
    tube, C.
CHAP (cyclophosphamide, Hexalen, Adriamycin, Platinol)
Charcot joint
Charcot-Leyden crystals
Charcot-Robin crystals
charge-exchange accelerator
C Harlem hemoglobin
CHART (continuous hyperfractionated accelerated radiotherapy)
Chase diet
CH50 assay
c-Harvey-ras oncogene
chaulmoogra oil
chaulmoogric acid
Chaussier areola
CHBA (congenital Heinz body hemolytic anemia)
CHD (cyclophosphamide, hexamethylmelamine, DDP)
CHD-R (cyclophosphamide, hexamethylmelamine, DDP, radiotherapy)
Check-Flo introducer
checker colony
Chediak-Higashi
    anomaly, C.
    syndrome, C.
Chee medium
cheilectomy
cheilocarcinoma
cheiloplasty
cheilostomatoplasty
chelate
chelating agent
chelation

ADDITIONAL TERMS

chelator
chemical
   carcinogen, c.
   carcinogenesis, c.
   exposure, c.
   pneumonitis, c.
   spill, c.
   warfare, c.
chemicophysics
chemiluminescence
chemo (chemotherapy)
chemoattractant
chemobiotic
ChemoCap
chemocoagulation
chemodectoma
chemoembolization
chemoendocrine
chemohormonal
chemoimmunology
chemokinesis
chemokinetic
chemopallidectomy
chemopallidothalamectomy
Chemo-Port catheter
chemoprevention
chemopreventive
chemoprophylaxis
chemoprotector   .
chemoradiation
chemoradiotherapy
chemoreceptor
   trigger zone, c. (CTZ)
chemoresistance
chemoresistant
chemosensitive
chemosensitivity
chemosensitizer
chemoserotherapy
chemosis
chemosmosis
chemosurgery
chemotactic
chemotaxis
chemothalamectomy
chemotherapeutic
   agents, c.
   drugs, c.
   index, c. (CI)
chemotherapeutics
chemotherapy
   combination c.
   cytotoxic c.

   intraperitoneal c.
   intrathecal c.
   single-agent c.
chemotherapy code for evaluation of
  progress
   −2 definitely worse
   −1 probably worse
   0 no change since last scan
   +1 probably better
   +2 definitely better
chemotherapy drugs
chemotherapy-induced
chemotherapy protocol
chemotrophic
chemotropic
chemotropism
Chernobyl accident
cherry
   angioma, c.
   -picking procedure, c.
Cherry-Crandall procedure
Chesapeake hemoglobin
chest wall cancer
chew (snuff or tobacco)
chewing tobacco
CHEX-UP (cyclophosphamide,
  hexamethylmelamine, 5-fluorouracil,
  Platinol)
CHF (cyclophosphamide,
  hexamethylmelamine, 5-fluorouracil)
Chi site
Chiari syndrome
chiasma
chiasmatic
Chiba needle
Chicago
   classification, C.
   disease, C.
chick-cell agglutination
chief
   agglutinin, c.
   cell, c.
   cell adenoma, c.
Chiffelle and Putt method
Child classification
Child-Turcotte classification
childhood cancer
chimera
   radiation c.
chimeric
   antibody, c.
chimerism
chimney-sweep's cancer

ADDITIONAL TERMS

Chinese
    Compound Q, C.
    cucumber, C.
    hamster, C.
    trichosanthin, C.
CHIP (cis-dichlorotranshydroxy-bis-
    isopropylamine platinum IV)
CHIP (iproplatin)
Chiron strip
chitin synthetase
Chlamydia
    psittaci, C.
    trachomatis, C.
chlamydial
chloracetate esterase
chloral hydrate
chlorambucil (CLB or Leukeran)
chloramphenicol acetyltransferase
    (CAT)
chlordiazepoxide
Chlorella
chlorhexidine gluconate mouthrinse
chloride
chlormadinone
chlormethine
2-chlorocordycepin
2-chlorodeoxyadenosine (2-CdA)
chloroerythroblastoma
chloroleukemia
chlorolymphosarcoma
chloroma
chloromethyl ether
chloromyeloma
chloronitrosurea
chloroquine
    hydrochloride, c.
    phosphate, c.
chlorotrianisene (Tace)
chlorozotocin (DCNU)
CHL+PRED (chlorambucil,
    prednisone)
Chl-VPP (chlorambucil, vinblastine,
    procarbazine, prednisone)
CHO (cyclophosphamide,
    hydroxydaunomycin, Oncovin)
CHO cells
choana (pl. choanae)
choanae (pl. of choana)
CHOB (cyclophosphamide,
    hydroxydaunomycin, Oncovin,
    bleomycin)
chocolate
    agar, c.

cyst, c.
CHOD (cyclophosphamide,
    hydroxydaunomycin, Oncovin,
    dexamethasone)
cholangioadenoma
cholangiocarcinoma
cholangiocellular
    carcinoma, c.
cholangiocholecystocholedochectomy
cholangioenteric
cholangioenterostomy
cholangiogastrostomy
cholangiogram
cholangiography
cholangiohepatoma
cholangiojejunostomy
cholangioma
cholangiopancreatography
    endoscopic retrograde c.
cholangitis
cholanthrene
cholecystectomy
cholecystocolostomy
cholecystocolotomy
cholecystoduodenostomy
cholecystogastric
cholecystogastrostomy
cholecystogram
cholecystography
cholecystoileostomy
cholecystojejunostomy
cholecystokinin
cholecystopyelostomy
cholecystosonography
cholecystostomy
    percutaneous c.
choledochal
choledochous
choledochoduodenostomy
choledochogram
choledochography
choledochojejunostomy
choledocholithiasis
choledochoscope
choledochoscopy
choledochography
cholegram
cholegraphy
cholelithiasis
cholepathia
cholescintigram
cholescintigraphy
cholestasis

ADDITIONAL TERMS

cholestatic
  jaundice, c.
cholesteatoma
cholesterol
cholesterosis
choline
  treatment, c.
cholinergic
cholinesterase
chondroadenoma
chondroangioma
chondroblastoma
chondrocarcinoma
chondroectodermal
chondroendothelioma
chondrofibroma
chondroid cancer
chondroitinase
chondrolipoma
chondroma
  -enchondroma, c.
  joint c.
  juxtacortical c.
  periosteal c.
  pulmonary c.
  sarcomatosum, c.
  synovial c.
  true c.
chondromatosis
  synovial c.
chondromyoma
chondromyxoma
chondromyxoid
  fibroma, c.
chondromyxosarcoma
chondronecrosis
chondrosarcoma
  central c.
  clear cell c.
  mesenchymal c.
chondrosarcomatosis
chondrosarcomatous
chondrosteoma
chop amputation
CHOP (cyclophosphamide, Halotestin,
  Oncovin, prednisone)
CHOP (cyclophosphamide,
  hydroxydaunomycin, Oncovin,
  prednisone)
CHOP-BLEO (cyclophosphamide,
  hydroxydaunomycin, Oncovin,
  prednisone, bleomycin)
Chopart amputation

CHOPE (cyclophosphamide, Halotestin,
  Oncovin, prednisone, etoposide)
CHOR (cyclophosphamide,
  hydroxydaunomycin, Oncovin,
  radiotherapy)
chordoblastoma
chordocarcinoma
chordoepithelioma
chordoma
chordosarcoma
chorellin
chorioadenoma
  destruens, c.
chorioallantoic membrane (CAM)
  assay, c.
chorioangiofibroma
chorioangioma
chorioblastoma
choriocarcinoma
chorioepithelioma
  malignum, c.
chorioma
choriomeningitis
  lymphocytic c.
chorionepithelioma
chorionic
  carcinoma, c.
  gonadotropin, c.
  villus biopsy, c.
chorioretinitis
choristoblastoma
choristoma
choroid plexus
choroidal
  melanoma, c.
choroidectomy
Chou and Fasman method
Chou and Talalay method
c-H-ras oncogene
Christmas
  disease, C.
  factor, C. (CF)
chromaffin
  cells, c.
chromaffinoblastoma
chromaffinoma
  medullary c.
chromaffinopathy
chromargentaffin
chromatid
chromatin
chromatogram
chromatography

ADDITIONAL TERMS

chromatography—*Continued*
  adsorption c.
  affinity c.
  column c.
  exclusion c.
  gas c.
  gas-liquid c.
  gas-solid c.
  gel-filtration c.
  gel-permeation c.
  high-performance liquid c.
  ion-exchange c.
  molecular sieve c.
  paper c.
  partition c.
  thin-layer c.
chromatokinesis
chromatophil
chromatophore
chromatophoroma
chromatophoromatosis
chromatophorotropic
chromatotaxis
chromic phosphate (P32)
Chromitope
  chloride, C.
  phosphate, C.
  sodium, C.
chromium (Cr)
  -51 labeled serum albumin, c.
  -51 tagged red cells, c.
  red cell mass, c.
Chromobacterium
  violaceum, C.
chromoblast
chromoblastomycosis
chromoclastogenic
chromocyte
chromogranin
chromoma
chromomere
chromomycosis
chromonucleic acid
chromophil
chromophilic
chromophobe
  adenoma, c.
chromophobic
  adenoma, c.
chromoprotein
chromosomal
  abnormality, c.
  damage, c.

  manipulation, c.
  mutation, c.
  rearrangement, c.
  translocation, c.
chromosome
  accessory c's
  acentric c.
  acrocentric c.
  autosomal c.
  daughter c's
  dicentric c.
  double-minute c.
  gametic c.
  homologous c's
  m c.
  metacentric c.
  mitochondrial c.
  nucleolar c's
  Ph (Philadelphia) c.
  Philadelphia (Ph) c.
  ring c.
  sex c's
  small c.
  somatic c.
  submetacentric c.
  supernumerary c.
  X c.
  Y c.
chromosome aberration
chromosome banding
chromosome breakage
chromosome deletion
chromosome inversion
chromosome manipulation
chromosome map
chromosome rearrangement
chromosome translocation
chromosome walking
chromotherapy
chromotope sodium
chromotoxic
chronic
  anemia, c.
  fatigue and immune dysfunction
    syndrome, c. (CFIDS)
  granulocytic leukemia, c. (CGL)
  granulomatous disease, c. (CGD)
  lymphadenopathy syndrome, c.
  lymphocytic leukemia, c. (CLL)
  malaise, c.
  myelocytic granulocytic leukemia,
    c.
  myelocytic leukemia, c. (CML)

ADDITIONAL TERMS

myelogenous leukemia, c. (CML)
myeloid leukemia, c.
chrysarobin
chrysiasis
chrysophanic acid
chrysophoresis
chrysotherapy
chrysotile
Churg-Strauss syndrome
Chvostek anemia
CHVP (cyclophosphamide,
   hydroxydaunomycin, VM-26,
   prednisone)
chylangioma
chyle
chylothorax
chylous
      anemia, c.
chymase
chymotrypsin
Ci (curie)
CI (cell interaction)
      gene, C.
CI (chemotherapeutic index)
CI-898 (trimetrexate)
CIA (CCNU, isophosphamide,
   Adriamycin)
Cibacalcin
CIC (circulating immune complexes)
cicatrices (pl. of cicatrix)
cicatricial
      fibromatosis, c.
      fibrosarcoma, c.
      pemphigoid, c.
cicatricotomy
cicatrix (pl. cicatrices)
      hypertrophic c.
      vicious c.
cicatrization
ciclamycin O
CID (combined immunodeficiency
   disease)
CID (cytomegalic inclusion disease)
cidal
CIDS (cellular immunodeficiency
   syndrone)
CIE (counterimmunoelectrophoresis)
CIF (clonal inhibitory factor)
CIg (cytoplasmic immunoglobulin)
cigarette
      addiction, c.
      filter, c.
      smoking, c.

Ci-hr (curie-hour)
cilastatin sodium
ciliary body melanoma
ciliated metaplasia
Cilofungin
cimetidine
CIN (cervical intraepithelial neoplasia)
      grades I, II, III, C.
cinchona bark
cinebronchogram
cinecholedochogram
cinecystogram
cinedensigram
cinedensigraphy
cine-esophagram
cinefluorogram
cinefluorography
cinematoradiogram
cinematoradiography
cinemicrography
cinephlebogram
cineradiogram
cineroentgenofluorogram
cineroentgenofluorography
cineroentgenogram
cineroentgenography
cingula (pl. of cingulum)
cingulectomy
cingulotomy
cingulum (pl. cingula)
cinoxate
Cipro (ciprofloxacin)
ciprofloxacin
circulating
      anticoagulants, c.
      antigen, c.
      atypical lymphocytes, c.
      gene pool, c.
      granulocyte pool, c. (CGP)
      immune complexes, c. (CIC)
      red cells, c.
circumanal
circumoral
circumscribed
      lesion, c.
      precancerous melanosis of
         Dubreuilh, c.
cirrhosis
      biliary c.
      macronodular c.
cirrhotic
cis
      -acting, c.

ADDITIONAL TERMS

cis—*Continued*
  activity, c.
  asymmetry, c.
  -DDP, c.
    (diamminedichloroplatinum)
  -diamminedichloroplatinum, c.
    (CDDP)
  -element, c.
  -platinum, c. (cisplatin)
  -position, c.
  -retinoic acid, c.
  -rotamer, c.
  -trans test, c.
CIS (Cancer Information Service)
CIS (carcinoma in situ)
CISCA (cisplatin, cyclophosphamide,
  Adriamycin)
CISCAii/VBiv (cisplatin,
  cyclophosphamide, Adriamycin,
  vinblastine, bleomycin)
cisplatin (CDDP or cis-platinum or DDP
  or Platamine or Platinol)
cis-platinum (CDDP or cisplatin or DDP
  or Platamine or Platinol)
cistern
cisternogram
cisternography
  radionuclide c.
  RISA (radioiodinated serum
    albumin) c.
cistron
citrate
  cupric c.
  phosphate dextrose, c.
  phosphate dextrose adenine, c.
  synthetase, c.
citrated plasma
citric acid
Citrobacter
  amalonaticus, C.
  freundii, C.
  intermedius, C.
citrovorum
  factor, c. (CF or leucovorin)
  rescue, c.
cJun gene
c-Kirsten-ras oncogene
CL 286558
clamoxyquin hydrochloride
Clara
  cells, C.
  hematoxylin, C.
Claricid

clarithromycin
Clark
  classification, C. (levels I through
    V)
  level of invasion, C.
Clark-Collip method
Clarke cell
clasmatocyte
clasmatocytoma
clasmatocytosis
clasmatodendrosis
clasmatosis
clasmocytic
  lymphoma, c.
clasmocytoma
Class I, II, III antigens
classification
  autopsy c.
  clinical c.
  pathologic c.
  retreatment c.
classification of leukemia (FAB —
  French/American/British)
    FAB-M1 myeloblastic, with no
      differentiation
    FAB-M2 myeloblastic, with
      differentiation
    FAB-M3 promyelocytic
    FAB-M5 monocytic
    FAB-M6 erythroleukemia
clastogenic
clathrin
Clausin method
claypipe cancer
CLB (chlorambucil)
clear cell
  adenocarcinoma, c.
  carcinoma, c.
  chondrosarcoma, c.
clearance
cleavage
cleave
cleaved cell
Cleocin
Cleveland procedure
Clinacox
clindamycin
clinical
  remission, c.
  staging, c.
  trials, c.
Clinitron air bed
Clinoril

ADDITIONAL TERMS

Clitocybe
   illudens, C.
clitoridectomy
clitoris
clivus
CLL (chronic lymphocytic leukemia)
cloaca (pl. cloacae)
cloacae (pl. of cloaca)
cloacogenic
   anal cancer, c.
   carcinoma, c.
clofazimine
clofibrate
clonal
   deletion theory, c.
   development, c.
   expansion, c.
   inhibitory factor, c. (CIF)
   selection theory of Burnet, c.
clonality
clone
   neoplastic c.
cloned
   gene, c.
clonidine hydrochloride
cloning
   DNA c.
   molecular c.
cloning vector
clonogenic
   assay, c.
   technique, c.
clonorchiasis
clonotype
Cloquet
   canal, C.
   node, C.
Clorox bleach
   assay, C.
   prophylaxis, C.
   technique, C.
clonotypic
closed
   amputation, c.
   chain, c.
   needle biopsy, c.
clostridial
Clostridium
   bifermantans, C.
   botulinum, C.
   butyricum, C.
   cadaveris, C.
   clostridiiforme, C.

difficile, C.
novyi, C.
perfringens, C.
ramosum, C.
septicum, C.
sphenoides, C.
sporogenes, C.
tertium, C.
tetani, C.
welchii, C.
clot
   lysis, c.
   retraction, c.
clotrimazole
clotting
   agent, c.
   factors, c.
   parameters, c.
   time, c.
cloud chamber
Cloudman melanoma
Clough and Richter syndrome
clozapine
clumped
   cells, c.
   platelets, c.
clumping
cluster
   cancer c.
   differentiation, c. of (CD)
clustering
C&M (cocaine and morphine)
Cm (curium)
   242, C.
   244, C.
cM (centimorgan)
CMC (cyclophosphamide, methotrexate, CCNU)
CMC-VAP (cyclophosphamide, methotrexate, CCNU, vincristine, Adriamycin, procarbazine)
CMF (cyclophosphamide, methotrexate, 5-fluorouracil)
CMF-AV (cyclophosphamide, methotrexate, 5-fluorouracil, Adriamycin, vincristine)
CMFAVP (cyclophosphamide, methotrexate, 5-fluorouracil, Adriamycin, vincristine, prednisone)
CMF-BLEO (cyclophosphamide, methotrexate, 5-fluorouracil, bleomycin)
CMF-FLU (cyclophosphamide,

ADDITIONAL TERMS

CMF-FLU—*Continued*
methotrexate, 5-fluorouracil,
fluoxymesterone)
CMFH (cyclophosphamide,
methotrexate, 5-fluorouracil,
hydroxyurea)
CMFP (cyclophosphamide,
methotrexate, 5-fluorouracil,
prednisone)
CMFpT (cyclophosphamide,
methotrexate, 5-fluorouracil, low-dose
prednisone, tamoxifen)
CMFPTH (cyclophosphamide,
methotrexate, 5-fluorouracil,
prednisone, tamoxifen, Halotestin)
CMFP-VA (cyclophosphamide,
methotrexate, 5-fluorouracil,
prednisone, vincristine, Adriamycin)
CMFT (cyclophosphamide,
methotrexate, 5-fluorouracil,
tamoxifen)
CMF-TAM (cyclophosphamide,
methotrexate, 5-fluorouracil,
tamoxifen)
CM-5-FU (cyclophosphamide,
methotrexate, 5-fluorouracil)
CMFV (cyclophosphamide,
methotrexate, 5-fluorouracil,
vincristine)
CMFVAT (cyclophosphamide,
methotrexate, 5-fluorouracil,
vincristine, Adriamycin, testosterone)
CMFVP, also known as Cooper CMFVP,
Cooper regimen, and SWOG CMFVP
(cyclophosphamide, methotrexate,
5-fluorouracil, vincristine, prednisone)
CMH (cyclophosphamide, m-AMSA,
hydroxyurea)
CMI (cell-mediated immunity)
CML (cell-mediated lympholysis)
CML (chronic myelocytic leukemia)
CML (chronic myelogenous leukemia)
C-MOPP (cyclophosphamide,
mechlorethamine, Oncovin,
procarbazine, prednisone)
c-mos oncogene
CMP (CCNU, methotrexate,
procarbazine)
CMP (cytidine monophosphate)
CMPF (cyclophosphamide,
methotrexate, prednisone,
5-fluorouracil)
CMS-5 cells

CMV (cisplatin, methotrexate,
vinblastine)
CMV (cytomegalovirus)
colitis, C.
hepatitis, C.
immune globulin, C.
mononucleosis, C.
prophylaxis, C.
retinitis, C.
triclonal antibodies, C.
c-myc
gene, c.
messenger run, c.
CNHD (congenital nonspherocytic
hemolytic disease)
CNF (cyclophosphamide, Novantrone,
5-fluorouracil)
CNOP (cyclophosphamide, Novantrone,
Oncovin, prednisone)
CNS (central nervous system)
fluid, C.
leak, C.
leukemia, C.
lymphoma, C.
prophylaxis, C.
Co (cobalt)
48, C.
56, C.
57, C. (bleomycin)
58, C.
59, C.
60, C.
60 eye plaque, C.
60 moving strip, C.
60 ophthalmic applicator, C.
60 teletherapy, C.
137 teletherapy, C.
Co(III) mustard complex
CoA (coenzyme A)
transferase, C.
coadunation
coagglutination
coagulability
coagulable
coagulant
coagulase
coagulate
coagulation
acute disseminated intravascular c.
blood c.
chronic disseminated intravascular
c.
diffuse intravascular c. (DIC)

ADDITIONAL TERMS

disseminated intravascular c.
(DIC)
coagulation cascade
coagulation factor
coagulation pathway
coagulation time
coagulative
coagulogram
coagulometer
coagulopathy
   consumption c.
   paraneoplastic c.
coal
   soot, c.
   tar, c.
   worker's pneumoconiosis, c.
co-alcohol fractionation
coalesce
coalescence
COAP (cyclophosphamide, Oncovin,
ara-C, prednisone)
COAP-BLEO (cyclophosphamide,
Oncovin, ara-C, prednisone, bleomycin)
coated
   pits, c.
   vesicles, c.
coatomer
CoA-transferase
coaxial sheath cut-biopsy needle
COB (cisplatin, Oncovin, bleomycin)
cobalamin
   adenosyltransferase, c.
cobalt (Co)
   -48, c.
   -57, c. (bleomycin)
   -58, c.
   -59, c.
   -60, c. (eye plaque)
   -60, c. (isotope)
   -60, c. (ophthalmic applicator)
   -60, c. (single x-ray beam)
   -60, c. (teletherapy unit)
   markers, c.
   moving strip, c.
   salipyrine, c.
   -201 c.-60 source
   therapy, c.
cobaltosis
cobaltous
   chloride, c.
Cobatope-57
Cobe double blood pump
COBMAM (cyclophosphamide, Oncovin,

bleomycin, methotrexate, Adriamycin,
MeCCNU)
cocaine
   baby, c.
   metabolites, c.
cocainism
cocainomania
co-capping
cocarcinogen
cocarcinogenesis
Coccidioides
   immitis, C.
coccidioidoma
coccidioidomycosis
Cockcroft-Walton voltage multiplier
cockscomb cervix
coctoantigen
cocto-immunogen
coctolabile
coctoprecipitin
coctostabile
cocultivation
coculture
Codasa
code
   genetic c.
   triplet c.
code sequence
codeine
Codman
   triangle, C.
   tumor, C.
codominance
codominant
   genes, c.
codon
   chain-initiation c.
   chain-termination c.
   nonsense c.
Codroxomin
coefficient
   equivalent thickness, c. of (CET)
   sedimentation c.
   volume c.
coelomic metaplasia
coenzyme
   I, c.
   II, c.
   A, c. (CoA)
   Q, c. (CoQ)
   R, c. (CoR)
cofactor
   platelet c.

ADDITIONAL TERMS

COF/COM (cyclophosphamide,
Oncovin, 5-fluorouracil plus
cyclophosphamide, Oncovin,
methotrexate)
coffee enema
coffee-grounds
    emesis, c.
    material, c.
    vomitus, c.
Coffey-Humber treatment
cognate
coherence
coherent
cohesion
cohesive
Cohnheim theory
cohort
    label, c.
    life table, c.
    study, c.
co-immunoprecipitation
coin lesion
coincidence counter
coinheritance
coital
coitus
CO_2 laser
Colaspase
colchicine
cold
    agglutination, c.
    agglutinin, c.
    antibody, c.
    cone, c.
    conization, c.
    cup forceps, c.
    fission, c.
    hemagglutinin, c.
    hemolysin test, c.
    -insoluble proteins, c.
    knife, c.
    light, c.
    nodule, c.
    -reacting antibody, c.
coldsore
Cole
    energy loss formula, C.
    hematoxylin, C.
colectomy
Coley toxin
colicolitis
colinearity
Colistin

colitis
collagen
    vascular disease, c.
collagenase
collapse therapy (for tuberculosis)
Collet syndrome
Collet-Sicard syndrome
collimation
collimator
    rotational axis, c.
Collins
    classification, C.
    law, C.
    solution, C.
colliquation
    ballooning c.
    reticulating c.
colliquative
collision tumor
Collison fluid
colloid
    cancer, c.
    carcinoma, c.
    cyst, c.
    degeneration, c.
    technetium isotope, c.
colloidal
    chromic phosphate, c.
    gold, c.
    P-32, c.
    silica, c.
ColloKit
colloma
Collostat
coloanal
colocalization
colocolostomy
colocutaneous
    colofixation, c.
    fistula, c.
coloenteritis
colon
    cancer, c.
    perforation, c.
    resection, c.
colonization
colonopathy
colonoscope
colonoscopy
colony
    counter, c.
    -forming cells, c.
    -forming unit—culture, c. (CFU-C)

ADDITIONAL TERMS

-forming unit—eosinophils, c.
(CFU-Eos)
-forming unit—erythroid, c. (CFU-
E)
-forming unit—granulocyte, c.
(CFU-G)
-forming unit—granulocyte-
macrophage, c. (CFU-GM)
-forming unit—granulocyte-
macrophage, erythroid,
megakaryocyte, multipotential, c.
(CFU-GMEMM)
-forming unit—lymphoid, c. (CFU-
L)
-forming unit—macrophage, c.
(CFU-M)
-forming unit—spleen, c. (CFU-S)
-stimulating activity, c. (CSA)
-stimulating factor, c. (CSF)
colopexotomy
colopexy
coloplication
coloproctectomy
coloproctitis
coloproctostomy
colorectal
adenoma, c.
fistula, c.
polyp, c.
cancer, c.
carcinoma, c.
carcinoma antigen, c. (CA19-9)
hemorrhage, c.
mass, c.
colorectitis
colorectostomy
colorectum
Colorgene DNA Hybridization Test
colosigmoidostomy
colostomy
diverting c.
double-barreled c.
end-to-side c.
functioning c.
gun-barrel c.
Hartmann c.
ileotransverse c.
loop c.
Mikulicz c.
permanent c.
sigmoid c.
sigmoid loop c.
terminal c.

transverse c.
Wangensteen c.
wet c.
colostomy bag
colostomy stoma
colovaginal
colovesical
colpectomy
colpocytology
colpomicroscopy
colpomyomectomy
colposcope
colposcopy
colpostat
Colpostats applicator
Colton blood group classification
Columbia Clinical Classification
columnar
Colyonal
Colyte
COM (cyclophosphamide, Oncovin,
MeCCNU)
COM (cyclophosphamide, Oncovin,
methotrexate)
coma
COMA-A (cyclophosphamide, Oncovin,
methotrexate, Adriamycin, ara-C)
comatose
COMB (cyclophosphamide, Oncovin,
MeCCNU, bleomycin)
COMB (cyclophosphamide, Oncovin,
methotrexate, bleomycin)
COMBAP (cyclophosphamide, Oncovin,
methotrexate, bleomycin, Adriamycin,
prednisone)
combination
chemotherapy, c.
index, c.
combined
abdominoperineal resection, c.
(CAPR)
immunodeficiency, c.
immunodeficiency disease, c.
(CID)
modality therapy, c.
combining site antibody
COMe (cyclophosphamide, Oncovin,
methotrexate)
comedo
comedocarcinoma
COMET-A (cyclophosphamide, Oncovin,
methotrexate, leucovorin, etoposide,
ara-C)

ADDITIONAL TERMS

COMF (cyclophosphamide, Oncovin,
  methotrexate, 5-fluorouracil)
comfort care
comitogenic
COMLA (cyclophosphamide, Oncovin,
  methotrexate, leucovorin, ara-C)
Commando
  glossectomy, C.
  procedure, C.
committed
  cell, c.
  progenitor cell, c.
common
  acute lymphoblastic leukemia
    antigen, c. (CALLA)
  variable agammaglobulinemia, c.
  variable hypogammaglobulinemia,
    c. (CVH)
  variable immunodeficiency, c. (CVI)
communal needle
community immunity
COMP (cyclophosphamide, Oncovin,
  methotrexate, prednisone)
compassionate use
Compazine
compensated ionization chamber
compensatory polycythemia
complement
  activation, c.
  assay, c.
  -binding, c.
  cascade, c.
  deficiency, c.
  -dependent, c.
  deviation, c.
  fixation, c. (CF)
  fixation test, c. (CFT)
  -fixing antibody, c. (CFA)
  fragment, c.
  lysis sensitivity test, c.
  -mediated anaphylaxis, c.
  -mediated cytotoxicity, c.
  receptor, c.
  sequence, c.
  system, c.
  unit, c.
complemental
complementary
  bases, c.
  DNA, c. (cDNA)
  genes, c.
complementation
complementophil

complete
  antibody, c.
  blood count, c. (CBC)
  clinical remission, c.
complex
complotype
compluetic reaction
component
  M (macroglobulinemia) c.
  M (myeloma) c.
  plasma thromboplastin c. (PTC)
  secretory c.
component blood therapy
Compound B
compound cyst
Compound Q (CoQ)
Compound R
Compound S (CoS)
compression
  fracture, c.
  spinal cord c.
Compton
  absorption, C.
  effect, C.
  electron, C.
  photon, C.
  scattering, C.
computed tomography (CT)
computerized transaxial tomography
  (CTAT)
ConA (concavalin A)
Concato disease
concavalin A (ConA)
concentrate
  bovine c.
  lyophilized c.
  porcine c.
concentration
concomitant immunity
condom
condylectomy
condyloma (pl. condylomata)
  acuminatum, c.
  latum, c.
condylomata (pl. of condyloma)
Condylox
cone (conization)
  cold c.
cone biopsy
conformational determinant
conformer
congener
congenital

ADDITIONAL TERMS

agammaglobulinemia, c.
anemia of newborn, c.
dyserythropoietic anemia, c. (CDA)
Heinz body hemolytic anemia, c.
 (CHBA)
hypoplastic anemia, c. (CHA)
immunity, c.
nonspherocytic hemolytic disease,
 c. (CNHD)
conglutinating complement absorption
 test (CCAT)
conglutination
conglutinin
conglutinogen
 activating factor, c. (KAF)
Congo red
 stain, C.
 test, C.
conical
conization
 cervical c.
 cold knife c.
conjugated
 antigen, c.
 bilirubin, c.
 estrogens, c.
conjunctivoma
Conn syndrome
connective tissue
connexin 26 (Cx26)
consanguineous
 donor, c.
conservative treatment
consolidation therapy
consolidative
Constant Spring hemoglobin
constipated
constipation
constitutional
 aplastic anemia, c. (CAA)
 hyperbilirubinemia, c.
 thrombopathy, c.
consumption coagulopathy
contact
 activation product, c.
 cancer, c.
 factor, c.
contaminated
contamination
contig (contiguous segment)
 map, c.
contiguous
 exons, c.

gene syndrome, c.
segment, c.
segment map, c.
continuous
 ambulatory peritoneal dialysis, c.
 (CAPD)
 arteriovenous hemofiltration, c.
 (CAVH)
 arteriovenous ultrafiltration, c.
 (CAVU)
 subcutaneous infusion, c. (CSQI)
contraception
contraceptive
contralateral
 radiation, c.
contrast
 agent, c.
 enema, c.
 enhancement, c.
 medium, c.
 study, c.
contrasuppression
contrasuppressor
Contreras method
control fistula
controlled substance
convergent beam irradiation
convertase
convertin
Cooley
 anemia, C.
 disease, C.
Coolidge tube
Coomassie brilliant blue
Coombs
 direct test, C.
 indirect test, C.
Cooper
 CMFVP, C. (cyclophosphamide,
 methotrexate, 5-fluorouracil,
 vincristine, prednisone)
 ligament, C.
 regimen, C.
Cooper-Rand electronic speech aid
cooperator cell
COP (cyclophosphamide, Oncovin,
 prednisolone)
COP (cyclophosphamide, Oncovin,
 prednisone)
COPA (cyclophosphamide, Oncovin,
 prednisone, Adriamycin)
COPAC (CCNU, Oncovin, prednisone,
 Adriamycin, cyclophosphamide)

ADDITIONAL TERMS

COP-B (cyclophosphamide, Oncovin,
prednisone, bleomycin)
COP-BLAM (cyclophosphamide,
Oncovin, prednisone, bleomycin,
Adriamycin, Matulane)
COP-BLEO (cyclophosphamide,
Oncovin, prednisone, bleomycin)
Cope
　　bronchography, C.
　　needle, C.
COPE (cyclophosphamide, Oncovin,
Platinol, etoposide)
copia retroposon
COPP (CCNU, Oncovin, procarbazine,
prednisone)
COPP (cyclophosphamide, Oncovin,
procarbazine, prednisone)
coproantibody
coproporphyria
　　erythropoietic c.
　　hereditary c.
coproporphyrin
coproporphyrinogen
copy DNA (cDNA)
CoQ (Compound Q)
Corbus disease
cord
　　compression, c.
　　tumor, c.
cordotomy
core
　　antigen, c.
　　biopsy, c.
　　electron microscopy, c.
　　particles, c.
　　protein, c.
corepressor
Cormed ambulatory infusion pump
corpora (pl. of corpus)
corps ronds
corpus (pl. corpora)
　　carcinoma, c.
　　luteum cyst, c.
corpuscle
　　Bennet small c.
　　blood c.
　　chyle c.
　　concentric c's
　　Drysdale c.
　　Eichhorst c's
　　Gierke c's
　　Hassall c's
　　Hayem c.

Leber c's
lymph c's
lymphoid c's
Norris c's
Nunn gorged c's
Rainey c's
red c.
reticulated c.
Rohl marginal c's
salivary c.
thymus c's
Vater c's
white c.
corpuscular
　　radiation, c.
correlational studies
Corrigan pneumonia
corset cancer
cortical bone
corticosteroid
corticosterone
corticotroph
corticotropin
　　-releasing factor, c. (CRF)
　　-releasing hormone, c. (CRH)
cortisol
cortisone
Cortrosyn
Corynebacterium
　　diphtheriae, C.
　　genitalium, C.
　　haemolyticum, C.
　　minutissimum, C.
　　ovis, C.
　　parvulum, C.
　　parvum, C.
　　pseudodiphtheriticum, C.
　　pseudotuberculosis, C.
　　pyogenes, C.
　　tenuis, C.
　　xerosis, C.
Corzyme
CoS (Compound S)
COS cells
Cosmegen (dactinomycin)
cosmesis
cosmetic
　　appearance, c.
　　effect, c.
　　surgery, c.
cosmic
　　radiation, c.
　　ray, c.

ADDITIONAL TERMS

ray counter, r.
cosmid
cosmotron
Cost antigen
Cost-Sterling blood group system
costimulatory
cothromboplastin
cotinine
co-trimoxazole
cotton-wool spots
Coulter counter
Coumadin
coumadinize
Councilman bodies
count
  Addis c.
  Arneth c.
  blood c.
  complete blood c. (CBC)
  differential c.
  direct platelet c.
  filament-nonfilament c.
  indirect platelet c.
  manual differential c.
  neutrophil lobe c.
  reticulocyte c.
  Schilling c.
  staff c.
  white blood cell c.
counter
  aurora particle c.
  boron c.
  Cerenkov c.
  cosmic ray c.
  Coulter c.
  crystal c.
  Duke cell c.
  externally quenched c.
  gamma well c.
  Geiger c.
  Geiger-Klemperer c.
  Geiger-Müller c.
  heavy particle c.
  Linson electronic cell c.
  proportional c.
  radiation c.
  Rutherford-Geiger c.
  scintillation c.
  screen-wall c.
  self-quenched c.
  solar gamma ray c.
  solar x-ray c.
  whole-body c.

countercurrent
  exchanger, c.
  immunoelectrophoresis, c. (CIE)
counterelectrophoresis
counterelectrophoretic
counterflow centrifugal elutriation
counterimmunoelectrophoresis (CIE)
counting
  cell, c.
  chamber, c.
  rate meter, c.
  tube, c.
counts per minute (cpm)
counts per second (cps)
course
  chemotherapy, c. of
  dialysis, c. of
  disease, c. of
  radiation, c. of
Courvoisier sign
Courvoisier-Terrier syndrome
Coutard
  law, C.
  method, C.
covalence
covalency
covalent
  bond, c.
covariate
  -survival relationship, c.
cow's milk
  anemia, c.
  immune globulin, c.
Cowden
  disease, C.
  syndrome, C.
Cowdry type A intranuclear inclusion
  bodies
Cox
  proportional hazard, C.
  regression analysis, C.
CP (Cytoxan, Platinol)
CPA (cyclophosphamide)
C3PA (C3 proactivator)
C3PAase (C3 proactivator convertase)
C. parvum (Corynebacterium parvum)
CPB (cyclophosphamide, Platinol,
  BCNU)
CPC (cyclophosphamide, Platinol,
  carboplatin)
CPD (citrate-phosphate-dextrose)
CPDA-1 (citrate-phosphate-dextrose-
  adenine)

ADDITIONAL TERMS

CPDD (cis-platinum
diamminedichloride)
cpm (counts per minute)
CPM (CCNU, procarbazine,
methotrexate)
CPOB (cyclophosphamide, prednisone,
Oncovin, bleomycin)
C-POX vaccine
cps (counts per second)
CPTR (cyproterone)
C1q assay
Cr (chromium)
-51, C.
-51 RBC, C. (chromium-51 tagged
red blood cells)
13-CRA (isotretinoin)
CRABP-I (cellular retinoic acid–binding
protein-I)
cranial
computed tomography, c. (CCT)
irradiation, c.
nerve rhizotomy, c.
craniectomy
craniobuccal cyst
craniofacial
appliance, c.
craniometric
craniopharyngeal
cyst, c.
duct tumor, c.
craniopharyngioma
cranioplastic powder
cranioplasty
craniospinal
irradiation, c. (CSI)
craniotomy
flap, c.
cranium
c-ras oncogene
Crasnitin (C-asparaginase)
crateriform
craterization
CRE (cumulative radiation effect)
creatine
kinase, c.
phosphokinase, c.
phosphotransferase, c.
creatinine
CREG (cross-reactive group)
crenated
erythrocyte, c.
crenation
crenocyte

crenocytosis
crescent
bodies, c.
cell anemia, c.
CRF (corticotropin-releasing factor)
CRF-187
CRH (corticotropin-releasing hormone)
51Cr-heated RBCs (red blood cells)
cribriform
carcinoma, c.
cricoid
cricopharyngeal
cricopharyngeus
cricothyroid
cricothyrotomy
Crigler-Najjar syndrome
crises (pl. of crisis)
crisis (pl. crises)
crisnatol mesylate (BW A770U)
crit (hematocrit)
criteria (pl. of criterion)
criterion (pl. criteria)
Crithidia
fasciculata, C.
lucilliae, C.
crocidolite
Crofton immunization
Crohn
disease, C.
granulomatous enteritis, C.
cromolyn
Cromoral
Cronassial
Crooke
cell, C.
hyaline degeneration, C.
tube, C.
Crooke-Russell basophils
CROP (cyclophosphamide, rubidazone,
Oncovin, prednisone)
CROPAM (cyclophosphamide,
rubidazone, Oncovin, prednisone,
L-asparaginase, methotrexate)
cross
agglutination, c.
-immunity, c.
link, c.
-linkage, c.
-linking, c.
-match, c.
-matching, c.
-reacting, c.
-reacting agglutinin, c.

ADDITIONAL TERMS

-reacting antibody, c.
-reacting antigen, c.
-reaction, c.
-reactivation, c.
-reactive group, c. (CREG)
-reactivity, c.
-sensitivity, c.
-sensitization, c.
-table lateral fields, c.
crossed (crossmatched)
crossed immunoelectrophoresis
crossmatch
crossmatching
crossover trial
CRP (C-reactive protein)
cruciferous
cruciform
cruiser
cruising
Cruveilher
    nodules, C.
    tumor, C.
crymotherapy
cryoablation
cryobank
cryobiology
cryocautery
cryoconization
cryocrit
cryodestruction
cryofibrinogen
cryofibrinogenemia
cryogammaglobulin
cryogen
cryogenics
cryoglobulin
cryoglobulinemia
cryopathic
    hemolytic syndrome, c.
cryophylactic
cryoprecipitability
cryoprecipitate
cryoprecipitated antihemophilic factor
cryoprecipitation
cryopreservation
cryopreserved
cryoprobe
cryoprostatectomy
cryoprotectant
cryoprotective
cryoprotein
cryostat
cryosurgery

cryothalamectomy
cryothalamotomy
cryotherapy
cryoultramicrotomy
crypt
    anal c's
    tonsillar c's
crypto (cryptococcosis or
    cryptosporidiosis)
cryptococcal
    meningitis, c.
cryptococcoma
cryptococcosis
Cryptococcus
    histolyticus, C.
    hominis, C.
    meningitidis, C.
    neoformans, C.
cryptoempyema
cryptoglioma
cryptoleukemia
cryptoradiometer
cryptoradiometry
cryptorchid
cryptorchidectomy
cryptorchidism
cryptosporidial
cryptosporidiosis
    antibody, c.
Cryptosporidium
    listeria, C.
    parvum, C.
cryptosporidium
    immune whey protein concentrate,
    c.
crystal
    counter, c.
    -induced arthritis, c.
    -induced chemotactic factor, c.
    (CCF)
    -lattice constant, c.
    scintillation detector, c.
    violet, c.
crystallographic
crystallography
crystalloid
Cs (cesium)
    -131, C.
    -132, C.
    -134, C.
    -137, C.
    needle, C.
    teletherapy unit, C.

ADDITIONAL TERMS

CS-85
CS-87
CSA (colony-stimulating activity)
CSD (cat-scratch disease)
CSF (cerebrospinal fluid)
CSF (colony-stimulating factor)
CsI (cesium iodide)
CSI (cancer serum index)
CSI (craniospinal irradiation)
CSQI (continuous subcutaneous
 infusion)
c-src
    gene, c.
    protein, c.
csTNM (clinical surgical tumor, nodes,
 and metastasis staging)
CT (computed tomography)
    body scanner, C.
    -directed biopsy, C.
    gantry, C.
    scan, C.
CTAT (computerized transaxial
 tomography)
CTCb (cyclophosphamide, thiotepa,
 carboplatin)
CTCL (cutaneous T-cell lymphoma)
CTL (cytotoxic T-lymphocyte)
cTNM (clinical tumor, nodes, and
 metastasis staging)
CTP (cytidine triphosphate)
CTX (cyclophosphamide)
CTX-Plat (cyclophosphamide, Platinol)
CTZ (chemoreceptor trigger zone)
Cu (copper)
    -61, C.
    -64, C.
    -67, C.
cubical atom
cuboid cell
cucumber
    Chinese c.
cuffing
CUG (cytidine-uridine-guanosine)
    codon, C.
cul-de-sac
culdoscope
culdoscopy
culture
cultured up
cumulative
    dose, c.
    drug action, c.
    genes, c.

    radiation effect, c. (CRE)
    toxicity index, c.
cunnilinctus
cunnilinguist
cunnilingus
curability
curable
curative
    dose, c.
    radiation, c.
    surgery, c.
    treatment, c.
cure rate
curettage
curettement
curettings
curiage
Curie
    law, C.
    therapy, C.
curie (Ci)
curiegram
curie-hour (Ci-hr)
curietherapy
Curietron afterloading system
curioscopy
curium (Cm)
Curling ulcer
Curvularia
CUSA (Cavitron ultrasonic aspirator)
Cushing
    basophilism, C.
    response, C.
    syndrome, C.
cushingoid
Custer cell
customized blocks
Cutait-Turnbull operation
cutaneous
    anthrax, c.
    horn, c.
    needle lavage, c.
    T-cell lymphoma, c. (CTCL)
cut-biopsy needle
cutdown
    catheter, c.
Cutie Pie meter
CV (cisplatin, VP-16)
CVA (cyclophosphamide, vincristine,
 Adriamycin)
CVA-BMP (cyclophosphamide,
 vincristine, Adriamycin, BCNU,
 methotrexate, procarbazine)

ADDITIONAL TERMS

CVAD (cyclophosphamide, vincristine,
Adriamycin, dexamethasone)
CVB (CCNU, vinblastine, bleomycin)
CVC (central venous catheter)
CVD (cisplatin, vinblastine, dacarbazine)
CVEB (cisplatin, Velban, etoposide,
bleomycin)
CVH (common variable
hypogammaglobulinemia)
CVI (carboplatin, VePesid, ifosfamide)
CVI (common variable
immunodeficiency)
CVM (cyclophosphamide, vincristine,
methotrexate)
CVP (cyclophosphamide, vincristine,
prednisone)
CVP-BLEO (cyclophosphamide,
vincristine, prednisone, bleomycin)
CVPP (CCNU, vinblastine, prednisone,
procarbazine)
CVPP (cyclophosphamide, vinblastine,
procarbazine, prednisone)
CVPP-CCNU (cyclophosphamide,
vinblastine, procarbazine, prednisone,
CCNU)
Cx26 (connexin 26)
CxT (concentration x time)
CY (cyclophosphamide or Cytoxan)
CyADIC (cyclophosphamide,
Adriamycin, DTIC)
cyanemia
cyanhematin
cyanhemoglobin
cyanmethemoglobin
cyanmetmyoglobin
cyanoacrylate
cyanobacteria
cyanocobalamin
Co 57 solution, c.
Co 58 solution, c.
Co 60 solution, c.
cyanosed
cyanosis
cyanotic
CYC (cyclophosphamide)
cycasin
cyclamate
cyclic
AMP (adenosine monophosphate),
c.
AMP (adenosine monophosphate)
synthetase, c.
chemotherapy, c.

GMP (guanosine monophosphate),
c.
nucleotides, c.
cyclin
D, c.
gene, c.
cyclizine hydrochloride
cyclobenzaprine
cyclocryotherapy
cyclocytidine
cycloheximide
cyclohexylnitrosourea (CCNU)
cycloisomerase
cycloleucine
cycloligase
cyclomastopathy
cyclomethycaine
sulfate, c.
cyclo-oxygenase
cyclophorometer
cyclophosphamide (CPA or CPM or
CYC or Cycoblastin or Endoxan-Asta
or Neosar or Procytox)
cystitis, c.
Cyclo-Prostin
Cyclops procedure
cycloserine
cyclosporin A (Sandimmune)
cyclosporine
cyclotron
radiation, c.
Cycoblastin (cyclophosphamide)
CyHOP (cyclophosphamide, Halotestin,
Oncovin, prednisone)
cylindrical
carcinoma, c.
cylindroma
cylindromatous
cylindrosarcoma
cyproheptadine
cyproterone (CPTR)
acetate, c.
Cyronine
cyst
adventitious c.
alveolar c's
angioblastic c.
atheromatous c.
Blessig c's
blue dome c.
Boyer c.
branchial cleft c.
branchiogenetic c.

ADDITIONAL TERMS

cyst—*Continued*
bronchogenic c.
bronchopulmonary c.
calcifying odontogenic c.
cervical c.
chocolate c.
colloid c.
compound c.
corpus luteum c.
craniobuccal c.
craniopharyngeal duct c.
dentigerous c.
dermoid c.
duplication c.
endometrial c.
endothelial c.
enteric c.
enterogenous c.
epidermal c.
epidermoid c.
epithelial c.
extravasation c.
exudation c.
false c.
follicular c.
foregut c.
functional ovarian c.
Gartner c.
gartnerian c.
gas c.
gingival c.
Gorlin c.
hemorrhagic c.
inclusion c.
intraepithelial c's
intrapituitary c's
involution c.
Iwanoff c.
lymphoepithelial c.
mediastinal c.
multiloculated c.
multilocular c.
nasopalatine c.
odontogenic c.
ovarian c.
pancreatic c.
paranephric c.
parapelvic c.
parathyroid c.
parovarian c.
pericardial c.
peripelvic c.
pilar c.

pilonidal c.
porencephalic c.
primordial c.
proligerous c.
pseudomucinous c.
pyelogenic c.
radicular c.
Rathke c's
retention c.
saccular c.
Sampson c.
sarcosporidian c.
sebaceous c.
serous c.
soapsuds c's
solitary c.
springwater c.
stafne bone c.
Tarlov c.
thyroglossal duct c.
trichilemmal c.
cystadenocarcinoma
cystadenoma
adamantinum, c.
bile duct c.
mucinous c.
papillary c.
papillary c. lymphomatosum
partim simplex partim papilliferum, c.
pseudomucinous c.
serous c.
cystathionine
cystectomy
cysteine
cystic
adenoma, c.
astrocytoma, c.
breast, c.
cancer, c.
carcinoma, c.
cervicitis, c.
change, c.
chondromalacia, c.
degeneration, c.
differentiated nephroblastoma, c.
disease, c.
epithelioma, c.
fibroma, c.
fibrosis, c.
hygroma, c.
lesion, c.
lymphangioma, c.

ADDITIONAL TERMS

mass, c.
mastitis, c.
mastopathy, c.
medial necrosis, c.
neoplasm, c.
nephroma, c.
odontoma, c.
ovarian mass, c.
ovary, c.
structure, c.
tumor, c.
cystiform
cystigerous
cystinosis
cystitis
  cyclophosphamide c.
  hemorrhagic c.
  radiation c.
cystoadenoma
cystocarcinoma
cystocolostomy
cystoduodenostomy
cystoepithelioma
cystofibroma
cystogram
cystography
cystojejunostomy
cystolutein
cystoma
  myxoid c.
  serosum simplex, c.
cystomatitis
cystomatous
cystometrogram
cystometrography
cystomyoma
cystomyxoadenoma
cystomyxoma
cystophorous
cystoplasty
cystoproctitis
cystoproctostomy
cystoprostatectomy
cystopyelography
cystorectostomy
cystosarcoma
  phyllodes, c.
  phylloides, c.
cystoscope
cystoscopy
cystose
cystostomy
cystourethritis

cystourethrogram
cystourethrography
cystourethroscope
cystourethroscopy
Cytadren (aminoglutethamide)
cytapheresis
cytarabine (Alexan or ara-C or Cytosar
  or cytosine arabinoside)
  hydrochloride, c. (Cytosar-U)
cytembena
cytidine
  deaminase, c.
  diphosphate, c.
  monophosphate, c.
  triphosphate, c.
  -uridine-guanosine, c. (CUG)
cytoanalyzer
cytoarchitectonic
cytoarchitectural
cytoarchitecture
cytobiology
cytobiotaxis
Cytobrush
cytocentrifugation
cytocentrifuge
cytochalasin
  B, c.
cytochemical
cytochemism
cytochemistry
cytochrome
  b5 reductase, c.
  c oxidase, c.
  P-450 reductase, c.
cytocidal
cytocide
cytoclasis
cytoclastic
cytoclesis
cytocletic
cytocrit
cytoctic
cytoctony
cytodiagnosis
cytodiagnostic
cytodieresis
cytodifferentiated
cytodifferentiation
CytoGam (cytomegalovirus immune
  globulin)
cytogenesis
cytogenetic
cytogenic

ADDITIONAL TERMS

cytogenic—*Continued*
 anemia, c.
 marker, c.
cytogenous
cytogeny
cytoglomerator
cytoglucopenia
cytoglycopenia
cytogony
cytohistogenesis
cytohistologic
cytohistology
cytoid
cytokeratin
cytokine
cytokinesis
cytokinetic
cytologic
 aspiration, c.
 atypia, c.
 biopsy, c.
 diagnosis, c.
 T-lymphocyte, c.
cytological
 biopsy, c.
 brush, c.
cytology
 aspiration biopsy c. (ABC)
 brush c.
 exfoliative c.
cytolysate
cytolysin
cytolysis
 antibody-dependent cell-mediated c.
 immune c.
cytolysosome
cytolytic
cytoma
cytomegalic
 inclusion body, c.
 inclusion disease, c. (CID)
cytomegalovirus (CMV)
 hepatitis, c.
 immune globulin, c. (CytoGam)
 pneumonia, c.
 retinitis, c.
cytometaplasia
cytometer
cytometry
cytomorphology
cytomorphosis
cytonecrosis
cytopathic

cytopathogenesis
cytopathogenetic
cytopathogenic
cytopathogenicity
cytopathologic
cytopathology
cytopenia
cytophagocytosis
cytophagous
cytophagy
cytopheresis
cytophil
cytophilic
 antibody, c.
cytophotometer
cytophotometric analysis
cytophotometry
cytophylaxis
cytophysics
cytoplasm
cytoplasmic
 immunoglobulin, c. (CIg)
 inclusion, c.
cytoreductive surgery
Cytosar
Cytosar-U (cytarabine)
cytoscopy
cytosine
 arabinoside, c. (ara-C)
 5-hydroxymethyl c.
cytoskeletal
cytoskeleton
cytosol
 aminopeptidase, c.
cytosolic
 calcium, c.
cytospin smear
cytostasis
cytostatic
cytostromatic
cytotactic
cytotaxigen
cytotaxin
cytotaxis
Cytotec (misoprostol)
cytotherapy
cytotoxic
 agent, c.
 antibody, c.
 chemotherapy, c.
 suppressor, c.
 T cells, c.
 T-lymphocytes, c. (CTL)

ADDITIONAL TERMS

tumor agent, c.
cytotoxicity
    antibody-dependent cell-mediated c.
    antibody-dependent cellular c.
cytotoxin
cytotrophoblast
cytotropic
    antibody, c.
cytotropin
cytotropism
Cytovene (ganciclovir)
Cytoxan (CTX or cyclophosphamide)
    lyophilized, C.
CyVADACT (cyclophosphamide,
    vincristine, Adriamycin, dactinomycin)
CyVADIC (cyclophosphamide,
    vincristine, Adriamycin, DTIC)
CyVMAD (cyclophosphamide,
    vincristine, methotrexate, Adriamycin,
    DTIC)

 d (suffix added to eye classification indicating diffuse retinal involvement without discrete mass)
2,4-D (2,4-dichlorophenoxyacetic acid)
D antigen
D cell
D-deficiency factor
D-deletion syndrome
D-dimers test
D factor
D-loop
D region
Da (dalton)
dA (deoxyadenosine)
D2A (2′,3′-dideoxyadenosine)
DAB (p-dimethylaminoazobenzene)
DAC (5-AZA-2′-deoxycytidine)
dacarbazine (DTIC or DTIC-Dome or
    imidazole carboxamide)
Dacie type II
dacryoadenoscirrhus
dacryoma
dacryoscintigraphy
DACT (dactinomycin)
dactinomycin (actinomycin D or
    Cosmegen or DACT)
dADP (deoxyadenosine diphosphate)
DAF (decay-activating factor)
DAF (decay antibody-accelerating
    factor)

DAG (diacylglycerol)
DAG (dianhydrogalactitol)
daisy-head colony
Dakin solution
Dalacin C
Dalalone
d-ala-peptide T
Dale reaction
Dale-Laidlaw clotting time
dalton (Da)
daltroban
dam
    dental d.
    rubber d.
daminozide
dAMP (deoxyadenosine
    monophosphate)
damping
Dana Farber
    Cancer Institute, D.
    series, D.
danazol (Danocrine)
Dane particles
Danocrine (danazol)
Dansac
    ileal pouch, D.
    karaya seal pouch, D.
    ostomy pouch, D.
Dansyz phenomenon
Dantrium
dantrolene sodium
Danubian endemic familial nephropathy
DAP I (dianhydrogalactitol, Adriamycin,
    Platinol)
DAP II (dianhydrogalactitol,
    Adriamycin, high-dose Platinol)
dappen dish
dapsone
DAP/TMP (dapsone and trimethoprim)
Daraprim
Darier disease
Darier-Roussy sarcoid
Darier-White disease
darkfield
    fluorescent antibody d.
darkfield examination
darkfield microscopy
dark-ground microscopy
Darling disease
Darmstruck lymphoma
Darrow solution
DAT (daunomycin, ara-C,
    6-thioguanine)

database
DATHF (5-deaza-5,6,7,
8-tetrahydrofolate)
dATP (deoxyadenosine triphosphate)
DATVP (daunomycin, ara-C,
thioguanine, vincristine, prednisone)
daughter
cell, d.
cyst, d.
isotope, d.
nuclide, d.
daunoblastina
daunomycin (DNM)
daunorubicin hydrochloride (Cerubidine
or DNR)
Daunoxome (liposomal daunorubicin)
Daussets method
DAV (dibromodulcitol, Adriamycin,
vincristine)
DAVA (desacetyl vinblastine amide or
DVA or vindesine)
DAVH (dibromodulcitol, Adriamycin,
vincristine, Halotestin)
Davidsohn
differential absorption test, D.
sign, D.
dawn phenomenon
Day factor
DBA (dibenzanthracene)
DBA (Dolichos biflorus agglutinin)
DBA/2 mice
dbcAMP (dibutyryl cyclic adenosine
monophosphate)
DBD (dibromodulcitol or mitolactol)
DBM (demineralized bone matrix)
DBM (dibromomannitol)
DBV (dacarbazine, BCNU, vincristine)
DC (daunorubicin, cytarabine)
D&C (dilatation and curettage)
dC (deoxycytidine)
DCCMP (daunorubicin, cyclocytidine,
6-mercaptopurine, prednisone)
dCDP (deoxycytidine diphosphate)
DCF (2′-deoxycoformycin or
pentostatin)
DCM (dichloromethotrexate)
dCMP (deoxycytidine monophosphate)
DCMP (daunorubicin, cytarabine,
6-mercaptopurine, prednisone)
DCNB (dinitrochlorobenzene)
DCT (daunorubicin, cytarabine,
thioguanine)
DCT (direct Coombs test)

dCTP (deoxycytidine triphosphate)
DCV (dacarbazine, CCNU, vincristine)
ddA (dideoxyadenosine)
DDATHF (5,10-dideaza-tetrahydrofolate)
DDAVP (desamino-D-arginine
vasopressin)
DDAVP (desmopressin acetate)
ddC (dideoxycytidine or HIVID)
ddI (dideoxyinosine or Videx)
DDMP (diaminodichlorophenyl-
methylpyrimidine)
DDP (cis-diaminodichloroplatinum or
cisplatin)
DDS (dapsone)
DE (dose equivalent)
deactivation
deactylvinblastine
deallergization
deamidase
deaminase
Dean and Webb titration
10-deaza-aminopterin
5-deaza-5,6,7,8-tetrahydrofolate
(DATHF)
debilitated
debility
debrancher glycogen disease
debride
debridement
debriding
debris
Debrisan
debrisoquine
debulked
debulking
procedure, d.
tumor, d. of
Decadron
DECAL (dexamethasone, etoposide,
cisplatin, ara-C, L-asparaginase)
Decaris
decatenation
decay
alpha d.
beta d.
exponential d.
gamma d.
isomeric d.
nuclear d.
positron d.
radioactive d.
decay-accelerating factor (DAF)
decay-activating factor (DAF)

ADDITIONAL TERMS

decay constant
decay product
decerebrate
decerebration
deciduocellular
    sarcoma, d.
deciduoma
    malignum, d.
deciduomatosis
deciduosarcoma
Declinax
decoagulant
De-Comberol
decomplementize
decontaminate
decontaminating kit
decontamination
Decopac
decubitus
    ulcer, d.
dedifferentiate
dedifferentiation
Deelman effect
deep
    roentgen ray therapy, d.
    -seated tumor, d.
    venous thrombosis, d. (DVT)
    x-ray, d. (DXR)
Deetjen bodies
defense mechanism
defensin
deferoxamine
defibrinate
defibrination syndrome
defibrotide
deficiency
    adenine phosphoribosyl transferase
      d.
    adenosylcobalamin d.
    adenylate kinase d.
    aldolase d.
    antithrombin d.
    cellular immune d.
    debrancher d.
    dihydrofolate reductase d.
    enzyme d.
    erythrocyte hexokinase d.
    erythrocyte pyruvate kinase d.
    folate d.
    folic acid d.
    glucose-6-phosphate
      dehydrogenase (G6PD) d.
    glutamate formiminotransferase d.

    glutathione peroxidase d.
    glutathione reductase d.
    glutathione synthetase d.
    G6PD (glucose-6-phosphate
      dehydrogenase) d.
    hexoamidase d.
    IgA d.
    immune d.
    iron d.
    leukocyte G6PD (glucose-6-
      phosphatase dehydrogenase) d.
    myeloperoxidase d.
    phosphohexose isomerase d.
    protein C d.
    protein S d.
    riboflavin d.
    severe combined immune d. (SCID)
    sphingomyelinase d.
    vitamin d.
deficiency disease
deficiency state
definitive therapy
deftazidime
deglobulinization crisis
deglutition
deglycerolized red cells
Degos
    disease, D.
    syndrome, D.
degradable
    starch microspheres, d. (DSM)
dehiscence
dehydroemetine (Mebadin)
dehydroepiandrosterone (DHEA)
dehydrogenase
    glucose-6-phosphate d. (G6PD)
    lactate d. (LDH)
    lactic d. (LDH)
deionization
deionized
Dejerine syndrome
Deladiol (estradiol)
Delalutin
Delatest (testosterone)
Delatestryl (testosterone)
delayed-type hypersensitivity (DTH)
Delclos
    applicator, D.
    ovoid, D.
    vaginal cylinder, D.
Delestrogen (estradiol)
deletion
    antigenic d.

ADDITIONAL TERMS

deletion—*Continued*
  chromosome d.
  clonal d.
deletion analysis
Delimmun
delirium
delitescence
delomorphic
delomorphous
DeLouche afterloading system
Delphian node
delta
  agent, d.
  -aminolevulinic acid, d.
  antigen, d.
  beta thalassemia, d.
  chain, d.
  hepatitis, d. (hepatitis D)
  OD450, d.
  receptors, d.
deltacortisone
Deltasone
demarcated
  lesion, d.
  margin, d.
demarcation
  surface d.
demasculinization
Dematium
demeclocycline
demented
dementia
4-demethoxydaunorubicin
demilune bodies
demineralization
demineralized bone matrix (DBM)
DeMorgan spots
Demser (metyrosine)
demustardization
demyelinated
demyelinating
Dendrid
dendrite
dendritic
  cancer, d.
  cells, d.
  lesion, d.
dendrodendritic
dendroid
dendrophagocytosis
denervate
denervation
dengue

denial
Denker-Kahler approach
Denonvilliers aponeurosis
de novo
  cancer, d.
  fibrosis, d.
  lesion, d.
  pathway, d.
  protein synthesis, d.
dense deposit disease
density
  bone d.
  calcified d.
  ill-defined d.
  nodular d.
  soft tissue d.
densometer
densometry
dental dam
dentinoblastoma
dentinoma
dentinosteoid
denucleated
Denver
  classification, D.
  pleuroperitoneal shunt, D.
Denys-Leclef phenomenon
deoxyadenosine (dA)
  diphosphate, d. (dADP)
  monophosphate, d. (dAMP)
  triphosphate, d. (dATP)
deoxycoformycin (DCF or pentostatin)
11-deoxycorticosterone (DOC)
deoxycytidine (dC)
  diphosphate, d. (dCDP)
  kinase, d.
  monophosphate, d. (dCMP)
  triphosphate, d. (dCTP)
deoxy-D-glucose
deoxygenated hemoglobin
deoxygenation
deoxyguanosine (dG)
  diphosphate, d. (dGDP)
  monophosphate, d. (dGMP)
  triphosphate, d. (dGTP)
deoxyhemoglobin
2′-deoxy-5-iodouridine
deoxynojirimycin (butyl-DNJ)
deoxyribonuclease (DNase)
deoxyribonucleic acid (DNA)
  complementary d. (cDNA)
  copy d. (cDNA)
  messenger d. (mDNA)

ADDITIONAL TERMS

deoxyribonucleoside
deoxyribonucleotide
deoxynucleotidyl transferase
deoxyribose
deoxyspergualin (DSG)
deoxythymidine (dT)
 diphosphate, d. (dTDP)
 kinase, d.
 monophosphate, d. (dTMP)
 triphosphate, d. (dTTP)
deoxythymidylate
deoxyuridine
 monophosphate, d. (dUMP)
dephosphorylation
depilation
dep Medalone
Depo-Medrol
Depo-Pred 40
Depo-Provera (medroxyprogesterone)
Depotest (testosterone)
Depo-Testadiol
Depo-Testosterone
depot
 medroxyprogesterone acetate, d.
depressed
 bone marrow, d.
 genes, d.
 red cell indices, d.
depression
 bone marrow d.
 gene d.
 mental d.
 situational d.
Dep-Test
Dep-Testosterone
Dep-Testradiol
depth
 dose, d.
 ionization, d.
 penetration, d.
dequalinium chloride
de Quervain thyroiditis
dermabrader
dermabrasion
dermal
 melanocytoma, d.
 nevus, d.
dermatan sulfate
dermatitis
 actinic d.
 atopic d.
 herpetiformis, d.
 precancerous d.

radiation d.
roentgen ray d.
x-ray d.
dermatofibroma
 protuberans, d.
dermatofibrosarcoma
 protuberans, d.
dermatofibrosis
dermatoid
dermatologic
dermatology
dermatomal
dermatome
dermatomycosis
dermatomyoma
dermatomyositis
dermatopathic
dermatopathology
dermatosis
 Bowen precancerous d.
 precancerous d.
dermatosparaxis
dermatotherapy
dermoid
 cancer, d.
 cyst, d.
 tumor, d.
dermoidectomy
dermolipoma
dermolysin
DES (diethylstilbestrol)
 daughter, D. (daughter whose
 mother took DES during
 pregnancy)
desacetyl vinblastine amide (DAVA or
 DVA)
desacetylmethylcolchicine
desamino-D-arginine vasopressin
 (DDAVP)
desciclovir
desensitization
desensitize
desetope
desexualize
desferrithiocin
desiccant
desiccate
desiccated
 lesion, d.
 thyroid, d.
desiccation
 needle, d.
Desiclovir

ADDITIONAL TERMS

designated
> donor, d.
> recipient, d.

designer
> antibodies, d.
> drugs, d.
> genes, d.

deslorelin
desmocyte
desmocytoma
desmoid
> fibromatosis, d.
> lesion, d.
> tumor, d.

desmoma
desmoneoplasm
desmoplakin
> I, d.
> II, d.

desmoplasia
desmoplastic
> fibroma, d.

desmopressin acetate (DDAVP)
desmosome
despeciate
despeciation
despecification
desquamated
desquamation
desquamative
> interstitial pneumonia, d. (DIP)

desquamatory
destruction
destructive
> lesion, d.
> process, d.

detector
> collimated scintillation d.
> crystalline phosphor d.
> radiation d.
> tissue-equivalent d.
> x-ray d.

determinant
> antigenic d.
> conformational d.
> hidden d.
> immunogenic d.
> isoallotypic d.
> isotypic d.
> sequential d.

deterioration
deteriorate
de Toni-Fanconi syndrome

deuterium (D or 2H)
> oxide, d.

deuteron
Deutschlander disease
De Veras beverage
devitalized tissue
dexamethasone (DM)
dexormaplatin
dextran
> -coated charcoal, d.
> sulfate, d.

dextranomer
Dextrarine
dextriferron
Dexulate
dezaquinine
> mesylate, d.

DF (distribution factor)
DFA (direct fluorescent antibody)
DFMO (difluoromethylornithine)
> -MGBG protocol, D.

DFS (disease-free survival)
DFT32 (diisofluorophosphate)
DFV (DDP, 5-fluorouracil, VePesid)
dG (deoxyguanosine)
dGDP (deoxyguanosine diphosphate)
dGMP (deoxyguanosine monophosphate)
dGTP (deoxyguanosine triphosphate)
DHA (dihydroxyacetone)
DHAC (5,6-dihydro-5-azacytidine or azacitidine)
DHAD (dihydroxyanthracenedione or mitoxantrone)
DHAP (dexamethasone, high-dose ara-C, Platinol)
DHAP (dihydroxyacetone phosphate)
DHE (dihematoporphyrin ether)
DHEA (dihydroepiandrosterone)
DHFR (dihydrofolate reductase)
DHL (diffuse histiocytic lymphoma)
dhoti cancer
DHPG (dihydroxypropoxymethylguanine or ganciclovir)
DHPR (dihydropteridine reductase)
diabetes
> adult-onset d.
> brittle d.
> insipidus, d.
> insulin-dependent d. (IDDM)
> mellitus, d.
> noninsulin-dependent d. (NIDDM)

ADDITIONAL TERMS

diacylglycerol (DAG)
Diacyte
  DNA ploidy analysis, D.
  fine-needle aspiration biopsy
    system, D.
diagnostic window
Dialyflex dialysis fluid
dialysance
dialysate
dialysis
  acidosis, d.
  dementia, d.
  disequilibrium, d.
Dialyte Pattern LM
dialyzable
  leukocyte extract, d. (DLE)
dialyze
dialyzed iron
cis-diaminodichlorplatinum (DDP)
diaminodiphenylsulfone
Diamond-Blackfan
  anemia, D.
  syndrome, D.
Dianeal
dianhydrogalactitol (DAG)
Dianon prostate profile and diagraph
diaphonoscope
diaphonoscopy
diarrhea
  cachectic d.
  radiation d.
  watery d.
diarrheal
diarrheogenic
diaschisis
diaspironecrobiosis
diaspironecrosis
DiaTAP vascular access button
diathermy
diatheses (pl. of diathesis)
diathesis (pl. diatheses)
diathetic
diatomic
diatrizoate
  meglumine, d.
  sodium I-125, d.
  sodium I-131, d.
diatrizoic acid
diaziquone (AZQ)
diazomycin
diazo-oxo-norleucine (DON)
dibenzanthracene (DBA)
dibenz-dibutyl anthraquinol

dibenzylchlorethamine
dibromodulcitol (DBD or mitolactol)
dibromomannitol (DBM)
dibutyryl cyclic adenosine
  monophosphate (dbcAMP)
DIC (diffuse intravascular coagulation)
DIC (diffuse intravascular coagulopathy)
DIC (disseminated intravascular
  coagulation)
DIC (disseminated intravascular
  coagulopathy)
dicationic
dichloroformoxime
dichloromethyilene biphosphonate
Diclazuril
Dicopac
Dicorvin
dicumarol
didanosine (ddI or Videx)
5,10-dideaza-tetrahydrofolate
  (DDATHF)
didehydrodideoxythymidine (d4T or
  stavudine)
didemnin B
dideoxyadenosine (ddA)
2′,3-dideoxycytidine (ddC or HIVID)
dideoxyinosine (ddI or didanosine)
dideoxynucleoside
dideoxynucleotide
  sequencing, d.
didox
Didronel (etridonate disodium)
1D-IEF (one-dimensional isoelectric
  focusing)
  gel electrophoresis, 1D.
Diego blood group system
dielectrolysis
dienestrol
dietary therapy
Dieterle method
diethylcarbamazine
diethylenetrimine penta-acetic acid
  (DTPA)
diethyldithiocarbamate (DTC or
  Imuthiol)
diethylpropion hydrochloride
diethylstilbestrol (DES or stilbestrol or
  Stilphostrol)
  daughter, d.
  diphosphate, d.
  dipropionate, d.
dietotherapy
differential

ADDITIONAL TERMS

differential—*Continued*
    count, d.
    ionization chamber, d.
differentiated
    moderately d.
    poorly d.
    well d.
differentiation
diffraction
diffuse
    histiocytic lymphoma, d. (DHL)
    intravascular coagulation, d. (DIC)
    intravascular coagulopathy, d.
      (DIC)
    large-cell lymphoma, d.
    undifferentiated non-Hodgkin
      lymphoma, d. (DUNHL)
diffusiometer
diffusion chamber
difluorodeoxycytidine (gemcitabine)
difluoromethylornithine (DFMO)
Diflucan
digastric muscle
DiGeorge syndrome
digitized video microscopy
DiGuglielmo
    disease, D.
    syndrome, D.
dihematoporphyrin ether (DHE)
dihydro-5-azacytidine (azacitidine or
    DHAC)
dihydrofolate reductase (DHFR)
    deficiency, d.
dihydromorphone
dihydropteridine reductase (DHPR)
    deficiency, d.
dihydrotestosterone
dihydroxyacetone (DHA)
    phosphate, d. (DHAP)
dihydroxyanthracenedione (DHAD)
dihydroxybenzene
dihydroxyphenylalanine
dihydroxypropoxymethylguanine
    (DHPG)
diisopropyl flurophosphate
diktyoma
dilatation
    curettage, d. and (D&C)
    cyst, d.
dilator
Dilaudid
DILE (drug-induced lupus
    erythematosus)
dim cells

Dimenest
dimenhydrinate
Dimenoxadole
dimepheptanol
dimepranol acedoben
dimer
    thymine d.
dimercaprol
dimeric
dimerize
dimethisterone
p-dimethylaminoazobenzene (DAB)
7,12-dimethylbenz(a)anthracene
    (DMBA)
dimethylbusulfan
dimethylhydrazine
dimethyl-L-glutamate
dimethylmyleran
dimethylnitrosamine
dimethylsuccinic acid (DMSA)
dimethyl sulfoxide (DMSO)
dimethyltriazeno imidazole carboxamide
    (DTIC)
DIMOPP (dose-intensified MOPP)
    protocol
dimorphic anemia
DIMP
dimple sign
dimpling
Dinacrin
dinitroaminophenol
dinitrochlorobenzene (DNCB)
dinitrofluorobenzene (DNFB)
dinitrophenol
Dinsed
dinucleotide
Diodoquin
DION 10.1.b antibody
dione
Diopterin
diotyrosine I-125
Dioval (estradiol)
dioxin (TCDD)
DIP (desquamative interstitial
    pneumonia)
dipeptide
dipeptidyl
    carboxypeptidase, d.
    peptidase I, d.
diphe
diphenatol
diphenidol
diphenylchlorarsine (toxic smoke)
diphosgene

ADDITIONAL TERMS

diphosphonate
Diphyllobothrium
    latum, D.
    parvum, D.
diphyllobothrium anemia
Diplogonoporus
    grandis, D.
diploid
diploidy
dipolymerase
dipping
    liver, d. of
    snuff d.
Dirac theory
direct
    agglutination, d.
    bilirubin, d.
    conjugate immunoperoxidase, d.
    Coombs test, d. (DCT)
    fluorescent antibody, d. (DFA)
    spread, d.
    transfusion, d.
dirty
    chest, d.
    lung, d.
disaccharide tripeptide glycerol
    dipalmitoyl
discoid lupus erythematosus (DLE)
disconnection syndrome
discrete
    lesion, d.
    mass, d.
    nodule, d.
disease
    -free survival, d. (DFS)
    -modifying antirheumatic drugs, d.
    (DMARDs)
disfigurement
disintegration series
dismutase
dismutation
disodium clodronate tetrahydrate
Disoxaril
disseminated
    candidiasis, d.
    cytomegalovirus, d.
    disease, d.
    herpes zoster, d.
    histoplasmosis, d.
    intravascular coagulation, d. (DIC)
    intravascular coagulopathy, d.
    (DIC)
    lupus erythematosus, d. (DLE)
    melanoma, d.

Mycobacterium avium complex, d.
    (DMAC)
dissemination
dissociation
    constant, d.
distant metastasis
distributed interval censoring
distribution
    equation, d.
    factor, d. (DF)
disulfide
    bond, d.
    bond bridge, d.
    knot, d.
dithioester
dithymol diiodide
ditiocarb
Dittrich plugs
diuresis
diuretic
diurnal
divalency
divalent
diverting colostomy
divided-stoma colostomy
division cycle
DL (doxorubicin, lomustine)
DLE (dialyzable leukocyte extract)
DLE (discoid lupus erythematosus)
DLE (disseminated lupus
    erythematosus)
D,L-leucovorin
DM (dexamethasone)
DM (double minutes)
DMAC (disseminated Mycobacterium
    avium complex)
DMARDs (disease-modifying
    antirheumatic drugs)
Dmax (maximum dose)
DMBA (7,12-
    dimethylbenz(a)anthracene)
DMSA (dimethylsuccinic acid)
DMSO (dimethyl sulfoxide)
DNA (deoxyribonucleic acid)
    alkylation, D.
    -ALU I family, D.
    amplification, D.
    -A protein, D.
    carcinogen, D.
    chain terminator, D.
    cloning, D.
    deletion, D.
    denaturation, D.
    -directed DNA polymerase, D.

ADDITIONAL TERMS

DNA—*Continued*
-directed polymerase, D.
-directed RNA polymerase, D.
fingerprinting, D.
footprinting, D.
-germ line, D.
gyrase, D.
helicase, D.
histogram, D.
histone, D.
hybridization, D.
intercalators, D
lesion, D.
library, D.
ligase, D.
ligation amplification, D.
methylation, D.
nucleotidylexotransferase, D.
nucleotidyltransferase, D.
-ploidy, D.
polymerase, D.
polymerase alpha, D.
polymerase II holoenzyme, D.
primase, D.
probe, D.
reassociation, D.
repair, D.
replication, D.
restriction enzymes, D.
sequence, D.
sequencing, D.
synthesis, D.
template, D.
transfection assay, D.
tumor virus, D.
DNase (deoxyribonuclease)
footprinting, D.
DNCB (dinitrochlorobenzene)
DNFB (dinitrofluorobenzene)
DNJ (N-butyl-deoxynojirimycin)
DNM (daunomycin)
DNR (daunorubicin)
DNS (dysplastic nevus syndrome)
DOAP (daunorubicin, Oncovin, ara-C,
prednisone)
DOC (11-deoxycorticosterone)
docusate sodium
dog-ear
Dohle
bodies, D.
inclusion bodies, D.
Dolichos biflorus
agglutinin, D. (DBA or lectin DBA)

Dolophine
Domagk method
domain
immunoglobulin d.
Dombrock
blood group system, D.
factor, D.
dominance
dominant
factor, d.
gene, d.
domperidone (Motilium)
DON (diazo-oxo-norleucine)
Donath-Landsteiner
antibody, D.
cold hemolysis, D.
phenomenon, D.
test, D.
donee
Donna factor
Donnan equilibrium
donor
bank, d.
blood, d.
cadaver, d.
marrow, d.
organ, d.
recipient, d.
screening, d.
selection, d.
-specific transfusion, d. (DST)
transfusion, d.
transplant, d.
typing, d.
Donovan bodies
donovanosis
dopa reaction
doper
doping
blood d.
Doppler
effect, D.
imaging, D.
Dorfman classification
dormancy
dormant
Dorno rays
Dorothy Reed cells
dorsal
column stimulation, d.
route entry zone, d.
dosage
boost, d.

ADDITIONAL TERMS

dose
- absorbed d.
- allowable d.
- booster d.
- cumulative d.
- curative d.
- deposition, d.
- depth d.
- doubling d.
- effective d.
- erythema d.
- exit d.
- exponential d.
- exposure d.
- fractional d.
- genetically significant d. (GSD)
- integral absorbed d.
- lethal d.
- maintenance d.
- maximum permissible d. (MPD)
- mean d.
- mean gonad d.
- mean lethal d.
- mean marrow d.
- median tissue culture infective d.
- midplane d.
- nominal single d.
- optimal d.
- oral fractionated d.
- organ d.
- organ tolerance d. (OTD)
- percent depth d.
- permissible d.
- priming d.
- radiation absorbed d. (rad)
- roentgen administered d. (RAD)
- skin d. (SD)
- threshold d.
- threshold erythema d. (TED)
- tissue d.
- tissue tolerance d. (TTD)
- tolerance d.
- toxic d.
- tumor d.
- tumor lethal d. (TLD)

dose and beams
dose calculation
dose delivery
dose distribution
dose-effect curve
dose equivalent (DE)
dose-equivalent radiation
dose fractionation

dose level
dose-limited
dose-limiting
dose modification
dose reciprocity theorem
dose-related toxicity
dose-response curve
dose-survival curve
dose tolerance
dosimeter
- chemical d.
- FBX (ferrous sulfate-benzoic acid-xylenol orange) d.
- pencil d.
- pocket d.
- thermoluminescent d.
- ultraviolet fluorescent d.
- Victoreen d.

dosimetric
dosimetrist
dosimetry
- estimation d.
- pion d.
- radiation d.

dosimetry system 1986 (DS86)
dosis
- curativa, d.
- efficax, d.
- refracta, d.
- tolerata, d.

double
- annihilation escape peak, d.
- -barreled colostomy, d.
- -barreled enterostomy, d.
- -blind study, d.
- -contrast study, d.
- diffusion, d.
- -dose technique, d.
- helix, d.
- -minute chromosome, d.
- minutes, d. (DM)
- photon scan, d.
- -plane interstitial implant, d.
- -stranded DNA, d. (dsDNA)
- -stranded RNA, d. (dsRNA)

doubling
- dose, d.
- time, d. (DT)

dounce glass homogenizer
Dover powder
Dow
- hollow fiber dialyzer, D.
- isoniazid, D.

ADDITIONAL TERMS

dowager's hump
down
   -modulate, d.
   -regulate, d.
Down syndrome
Downey
   cells, D.
   -type lymphocyte, D.
DOX (doxorubicin)
Doxaphene
doxorubicin hydrochloride (Adriamycin
  or DOX or Rubex)
   cardiomyopathy, d.
doxorubinol
doxycycline
DP-AZT
D-penicillamine
Drabkin solution
drainable ostomy pouch
drepanocyte
drepanocytemia
drepanocytic
drepanocytosis
Dresbach
   anemia, D.
   syndrome, D.
Dreser formula
Dreyer and Bennett hypothesis
DREZ (dorsal root entry zone)
   lesion, D.
DR4 human fibrosarcoma cell line
Drolban
dromostanolone propionate
dronabinol (Marinol)
drooling
drop metastases
droplet infection
Drosophila
   melanogaster, D.
drug
   abuse, d.
   abuser, d.
   addict, d.
   addiction, d.
   alopecia, d.
   dependence, d.
   dependent, d.
   -induced, d.
   -induced hemolytic anemia, d.
   -induced lupus erythematosus, d.
   (DILE)
   -induced thrombocytopenia,
   d.

infusion pump, d.
interaction, d.
reaction, d.
receptors, d.
regimen, d.
resistance, d,
-resistant, d.
therapy, d.
toxicity, d.
drugfast
drumstick
dry
   colostomy, d.
   gangrene, d.
   heaves, d.
   mouth, d.
   mucous membranes, d.
Drysdale corpuscles
DS86 (dosimetry system 1986)
dsDNA (double-stranded DNA)
DSG (deoxyspergualin)
DSM (degradable starch microspheres)
dsRNA (double-stranded RNA)
DST (donor-specific transfusion)
dT (deoxythymidine)
DT (doubling time)
D4T (didehydrodideoxythymidine or
  stavudine)
DTC (diethyldithiocarbamate)
DTH (delayed-type hypersensitivity)
DTIC (dacarbazine)
DTIC (dimethyltriazenoimidazole
  carboxamide)
DTIC-ACTD (DTIC, actinomycin D)
DTIC-Dome (dacarbazine)
dTDP (deoxythymidine diphosphate)
dTMP (deoxythymidine monophosphate)
DTPA (diethylenetriamine penta-acetic
  acid)
DTS (donor-specific transfusion)
dTTP (deoxythymidine triphosphate)
dU (deoxyuridine)
dual
   electron beam field, d.
   fluorescence cell sorting, d.
   photon absorptiometer, d.
   photon densitometry, d.
dualistic theory
duazomycin
   A, d. (duazomycin)
   B, d. (Azotomycin)
   C, d. (Ambomycin)
Dubin-Johnson phenomenon

ADDITIONAL TERMS

Dubreuilh melanosis
duck
    embryo vaccine, d.
    virus hepatitis yolk antibody, d.
Ducrey bacillus
duct
    cancer, d.
    carcinoma, d.
    cell carcinoma, d.
    tumor, d.
ductal
    breast carcinoma, d.
    cell carcinoma, d.
Duecollement maneuver
Duffy
    antibody, D.
    antigen, D.
    blood group system, D.
Duhring disease
Duke
    bleeding time, D.
    cell counter, D.
    method, D.
    program, D.
    test, D.
Dukes classification of carcinoma
    A invading mucosa and submucosa
    B invading muscularis
    C spread to regional lymph nodes,
      distant metastasis
Dukes staging
Dukes system
Dulbecco
    modified Eagle medium, D.
    theory, D.
Dulong constant
dumbbell tumor
dummy
    ribbons, d.
    seeds, d.
    source, d.
    spacer, d.
dUMP (deoxyuridine monophosphate)
dumping syndrome
Duncan
    disease, D.
    syndrome, D.
DUNHL (diffuse undifferentiated non-Hodgkin lymphoma)
Dunnet test
duodenectomy
duodenitis
duodenocholecystostomy

duodenocholedochotomy
duodenocolic
duodenocystostomy
duodenoduodenostomy
duodenoenterostomy
duodenogram
duodenohepatic
duodenoileostomy
duodenojejunostomy
duodenopancreatectomy
duodenoscopy
duodenostomy
duodenum
duovirus
DuP 785 (brequinar sodium)
DuP 937
duplex
    -directed, d.
    genetic sequence, d.
    scan, d.
    strand, d.
duplication
DuPont ELISA assay
Dupuytren amputation
dura
dural
Duragen (estradiol)
Duragesic (fentanyl)
Duralutin (hydroxyprogesterone)
Duralone
Dura-Meth
Duramorph
Duran-Reynals factor
Durand-Nicolas-Favre disease
Duratest (testosterone)
Duratestrin
Durathate (testosterone)
Dürck
    granuloma, D.
    node, D.
Durie-Salmon staging
duskiness
dusky
dust
    blood d. of Müller
    bone d.
dust-borne
dust cloud
Dutch speech aid
Dutcher body
DVB (DDP, vindesine, bleomycin)
DVP (daunorubicin, vincristine, prednisone)

ADDITIONAL TERMS

DVPL-ASP (daunorubicin, vincristine, prednisone, L-asparaginase)
DVT (deep venous thrombosis)
DXR (deep x-ray)
D-xylose absorption
dyad
dye
      exclusion assay, d.
      exposure, d.
      laser, d.
      reduction spot test, d.
      treatment, d.
      workers' cancer, d.
dynamic computerized tomography
dynein
dynorphin
dysarthria
dysarthric
dysbetalipoproteinemia
dyschezia
dyscrasia
      blood d.
      plasma cell d's
dyscratic
dysentery
dyserythropoiesis
dyserythropoietic
dysesthesia
dysesthetic
dysfibrogenemia
dysgammaglobulinemia
dysgenesis
dysgerminoma
dysgeusia
dysglobulinemia
dysglycemia
dyshematopoiesis
dyshematopoietic
dyshesion
dyskaryosis
dyskaryotic
dyskeratoma
dyskeratosis
dyslipoproteinemia
dysmyelopoiesis
dysmyelopoietic
dysphagia
dysphagic
dysphasia
dysphasic
dysplasia
dysplastic
      gangliocytoma, d.
      lesion, d.

      nevus, d.
      nevus syndrome, d. (DNS)
dyspnea
dyspneic
dyspoiesis
dyspoietic
dyspraxia
dyspraxic
dysproteinemia
dysprothrombinemia
dysstasia
dysstatic
dysthyreosis
dysthyroidism
dystrophic
dystrophin
dystrophy
dysuria
DZAPO (daunorubicin, azactidine, ara-C, prednisone, Oncovin)

E E (erythrocyte)
         antigen, E.
         rosette, E.
         rosette cell marker, E.
E (erythrocyte)
      rosette cell marker receptor, E.
      rosetting, E.
E antigen
E factor
E11 protein
E47 protein
E rosette
      assay, E.
      formation, E.
      receptor, E.
EA (early antigen)
EA (erythrocyte and antibody)
EA (ethacrynic acid)
EAC (Ehrlich ascites carcinoma)
EAC (erythrocyte, antibody, and complement)
      rosette, E.
      rosette assay, E.
EACA (epsilon-aminocaproic acid)
Eagle minimum essential medium
EAHLG (equine antihuman lymphoblast globulin)
EAHLS (equine antihuman lymphoblast serum)
EAP (etoposide, Adriamycin, Platinol)
Earle salts
early

ADDITIONAL TERMS

antigen, e. (EA)
detection, e.
erythroblast, e.
lesion, e.
Eastern Cooperative Oncology Group
(ECOG)
easy
bruisability, e.
bruising, e.
fatigability, e.
fatigue, e.
eating cell
Eaton
agent, E.
agent pneumonia, E.
Eaton-Lambert syndrome
EB (Epstein-Barr [virus])
EBAP (Eldisine, BCNU, Adriamycin,
prednisone)
EBL (erythroblastic leukemia)
EBNA (Epstein-Barr nuclear
antigen)
Ebola virus
ébranlement
EBRT (electron beam radiation
therapy)
EBT (external beam therapy)
EBV (Epstein-Barr virus)
antibody, E.
genomic sequences, E.
VCA (viral capsid antigen antibody)
test, E.
VCA Ig (viral capsid antigen Ig
antibody) test, E.
ECC (extracorporeal circulation)
ecchondroma
ecchordosis physaliphora
ecchymoma
ecchymosed
ecchymoses (pl. of ecchymosis)
ecchymosis (pl. ecchymoses)
ecchymotic
eccrine
acrospiroma, e.
carcinoma, e.
porocarcinoma, e.
poroma, e.
spiradenoma, e.
ECF (eosinophil chemotactic factor)
ECF-A (eosinophil chemotactic factor of
anaphylaxis)
echinacea
echinocandin
echinococcosis

Echinococcus
alveolaris, E.
granulosus, E.
multilocularis, E.
echinocyte
echinocytosis
echinomycin
echinosis
ECHO (etoposide, cyclophosphamide,
hydroxydaunomycin, Oncovin)
echo
-dense, e.
density, e.
-ranging, e.
time, e. (TE)
ECHO 28 virus
echocyte
echoencephalogram
echoencephalography
echogenic
echogenicity
echogram
echography
echoic
echolucency
echolucent
echotomography
echovirus
28, e.
ECIB (extracorporeal irradiation of
blood)
ECIL (extracorporeal irradiation of
lymph)
Ecker fluid
ECLT (euglobulin clot lysis time)
ECM (extracellular matrix)
protein, E.
ECMO (extracorporeal membrane
oxygenation)
ECOG (Eastern Cooperative Oncology
Group)
scale, E.
E. coli (Escherichia coli)
DNA, E.
-L-ASP, E.
econazole nitrate
ecotaxis
ecouvillon
ecouvillonage
ECS (extracellular-like calcium-free
solution)
ECT (euglobulin clot test)
ectasia
mammary duct e.

ADDITIONAL TERMS

ectatic
ecthyma
    contagious e.
    gangrenosum, e.
ectoantigen
ectocytic
ectoenzyme
ectogenous
ectomesenchymoma
ectomize
ectomy
ectopic
    ACTH syndrome, e.
    hypercalcemia syndrome, e.
    receptor, e.
    tumor, e.
ectoplast
ectoplastic
ED (effective or erythema dose)
EDAM (10-ethyl-deaza-aminopterin or
    10-EdAM)
EDAP (etoposide, dexamethasone,
    ara-C, Platinol)
edathamil
edatrexate
EDB (ethylene dibromide)
EDC (etoposide, doxorubicin, cisplatin)
Edelmann
    anemia, E.
    cell, E.
edema
edematous
Eder-Puestow
    dilator, E.
    wire, E.
Edmondson Grading System (grades I,
    II, etc.)
EDR (effective direct radiation)
edrophonium chloride
EDTA (ethylenediaminetetra-acetic acid)
EEA (end-to-end anastomosis)
    stapler, E.
EEG (electroencephalography)
EF (extended field)
effect
    Bohr e.
    boxcar e.
    Compton e.
    Deelman e.
    Hamburger e.
    radiation e.
    Warburg e.
effective

direct radiation, e. (EDR)
dose, e. (ED)
focal spot, e.
half-life, e. (EHL)
renal blood flow, e. (ERBF)
renal plasma flow, e. (ERPF)
thyroxine ratio, e. (ETR)
effectiveness
    relative biological e. (RBE)
effector
    cells, e.
    -to-target ratio, e.
effeminate
effemination
efficacious
efficacy
efflorescence
efflorescent
effluvium
    anagen e.
    telogen e.
effusion
    malignant e.
    pleural e.
eflornithine (DFMO or Ornidyl)
Efudex (fluorouracil)
Egan technique
EGF (epidermal growth factor)
    receptor, E. (EGF-R)
egg
    -infective dose, e. (EID)
    lecithin, e.
    lipids, e.
    yellow reaction, e.
eggcrate mattress
Eggsact
EGOT (erythrocyte glutamic oxaloacetic
    transaminase)
egress
egression
Egyptian splenomegaly
EHL (effective half-life)
Ehlers-Danlos syndrome
Ehrlich
    anemia, E.
    ascites, E.
    ascites carcinoma, E. (EAC)
    biochemical theory, E.
    diazo reaction, E.
    hemoglobinemic bodies, E.
    neutral stain, E.
    side-chain theory, E.
    unit, E.

ADDITIONAL TERMS

Ehrlichia
    canis, E.
ehrlichiosis
EIA (enzyme immunoassay)
EIA (enzyme-linked immunoassay)
Eichhorst corpuscles
eicosanoid
eicosapentaenoic acid (EPA)
EID (egg-infective dose)
    -negative breast tumor, E.
EID (electroimmunodiffusion)
EID (emergency infusion device)
Eikenella
    corrodens, E.
eiloid tumor
EIN (esophageal intraepithelial
    neoplasia)
Einhorn chemotherapy regimen
einsteinium (Es)
Eissner prostatic cooler
EIT (erythrocyte iron turnover)
EJ-ras oncogene
EL-10 (dehydroepiandrosterone or
    DHEA)
EL1020
elastase
elastin
elastofibroma
elastoid
elastoma
Eldisine (vindesine)
Eldorado 9 cobalt unit
electrocardiogram
electrocardiography
electrocauterization
electrocautery
electrochromatography
electrocoagulation
electroconization
electrocystography
electrodesiccation
electrodialysis
electrodialyzer
electroencephalography (EEG)
electroexcision
electrofulguration
electrogastrogram
electrogastrography
electroimmunoassay
electroimmunodiffusion (EID)
Electrolarynx
    Neovox E.
    Servox E.

Western Electric E.
electrolyte
    balance, e.
    imbalance, e.
electrolytic
electromagnetic
    decay, e.
    field, e. (EMF)
    irradiation, e.
    radiation e.
    spectrum, e.
    waves, e.
electromicroscope
electromicroscopy
electron
    accelerator, e.
    beam, e.
    beam dosimetry, e.
    beam radiation therapy, e. (EBRT)
    boost, e.
    capture, e.
    cascade, e.
    cloud, e.
    -dense, e.
    density, e.
    diffraction analysis, e.
    linear accelerator, e.
    micrography, e.
    microscope, e.
    microscopy, e. (EM)
    multiplier tube, e.
    neutrino, e.
    physics, e.
    -positron pair, e.
    shower, e.
    spin resonance, e. (ESR)
    transfer resonance, e.
    volt, e. (eV)
electronegative element
electronic
    cell counter, e.
    linear accelerator, e.
    voice, e.
electronization
electronmicrography
electro-osmosis
electropathology
electropherogram
electrophile
electrophoresed
electrophoresis
    counter e.
    disc e.

ADDITIONAL TERMS

electrophoresis—*Continued*
  protein e.
  pulsed field gradient e.
electrophoretic
electrophoretogram
electrophysics
electroporation
electropositive element
electroradioimmunoassay (ERIA)
electroradiometer
electroresection
electroscission
electrosection
electrospectrography
electrostatic
electrostimulation
electrosurgery
electrosynthesis
electrotaxis
electrotransfer test
electroultrafiltration
element
  chemical e.
  daughter e.
  parent e.
  radioactive e.
  trace e.
elementary
  body, e.
  particle, e.
  quantum of action, e.
eleoma
ELF (etoposide, leucovorin,
  5-fluorouracil)
Eli
  gene, E.
  strain of HIV-1, E.
ELIEDA (enzyme-linked
  immunoelectrodiffusion assay)
elinguation
Elipten (aminoglutethimide)
ELISA (enzyme-linked immunosorbent
  assay)
Elkind recovery
Elliot B solution
ellipticine
elliptocytary
  anemia, e.
elliptocyte
elliptocytosis
elliptocytotic
  anemia, e.
elongation factor

elsamitrucin (BMY-28090)
Elsberg test
Elspar (L-asparaginase)
ELT (euglobulin lysis time)
eluate
  factor, e.
eluent
elute
Elutek
elution
  membrane e.
elutriate
elutriation
EM (electron microscopy)
emaciated
emaciation
emailloid
eman
emanation
  actinium e.
  radium e.
  thorium e.
emanation treatment
emasculation
ematrophia
Embden-Meyerhof pathway
embechine
embedded
embolectomy
emboli (pl. of embolus)
embolic
embolization
embolize
embolus (pl. emboli)
embryogenesis
embryology
embryoma
embryonal
  adenomyosarcoma, e.
  adenosarcoma, e.
  carcinoma, e.
  carcinosarcoma, e.
  cell, e.
  cell carcinoma, e.
  cyst, e.
  leukemia, e.
  nephroma, e.
  nephromatography, e.
  rhabdomyosarcoma, e.
  sarcoma, e.
  tumor, e.
embryonic
  stem cells, e.

ADDITIONAL TERMS

embutramide
Emcyt (estramustine)
emergency infusion device (EID)
emergent
emeses (pl. of emesis)
emesis (pl. emeses)
emetatrophia
emetic
emetogenic
Emetrol
EMF (electromagnetic field)
EMF (erythrocyte maturation factor)
emigrated cell
emigration
    white cells, e. of
Eminase (anistreplase)
emiocytosis
emission
    electron, e.
EMIT (enzyme-multiplied immunoassay
  technique)
emitter
emotional support system
EMPD (extramammary Paget disease)
empyema
empyesis
empyemic
empyocele
EMT-6 murine mammary tumor
E-MVAC (escalated methotrexate,
  vinblastine, Adriamycin, cisplatin)
E-MVAC (escalated methotrexate,
  vinblastine, Adriamycin,
  cyclophosphamide)
ENA (extractable nuclear antigen)
enameloma
enamthem
ENANB (enterically transmitted non-A,
  non-B) hepatitis
enanthesis
enantiomer
en bloc
    dissection, e.
    resection, e.
    vulvectomy, e.
encapsidation
encapsulated
encapsulation
encephalic
encephalitis
encephalization
encephaloid
encephaloma

encephalon
encephalonarcosis
encephalosepsis
encephalothlipsis
enchondroma
enchondromatosis
enchondromatous
enchondrosarcoma
enchondrosis
encode
encoding
encompass
endemic
    goiter, e.
Endep
endobronchial
endocardial
endocarditis
endocavitary
    irradiation, e.
    radiation therapy, e.
endocellular
endocervical
endocrine
    neoplasia, e.
    system, e.
    therapy, e.
endocrinologic
endocrinology
endocrinopathy
endocrinosis
endocrinotherapy
endocurietherapy
endocyst
endocyte
endocytosis
endodeoxyribonuclease
endodermal
    sinus tumor, e.
endodiascope
endodiascopy
endoenteritis
endoenzyme
endoesophageal
endoexoteric
endogastritis
endogenous
endoglycosidase
endolaryngeal
    brachytherapy mould, e.
Endolimax
    nana, E.
endolysin

ADDITIONAL TERMS

endolysis
endometrectomy
endometrial
    ablation, e.
    biopsy, e.
    carcinoma, e.
    curettage, e.
    curettings, e.
    implant, e.
    lesion, e.
    sampling, e.
endometrioid
endometrioma
endometriosis
endometriotic
    implant, e.
endometritis
    syncytial e.
endometrium
endomitosis
endomitotic
endonuclear
endonuclease
    restriction e.
endopeptidase
endoplasm
endoplasmic
endoplast
endoplastic
endopolyploid
endopolyploidy
endoprosthesis
endoradiography
endorectal ultrasound (ERU)
endoreduplication
endoribonuclease
endorphin
endosalpingoma
endoscope
endoscopic
    ultrasonogram, e. (EUS)
endoscopy
    diagnostic e.
    therapeutic e.
endosmosis
endosmotic
endosteoma
endostoma
endosymbiont
endosymbiosis
endothelial
endothelialization
endothelin

endothelioblastoma
endotheliocyte
endotheliocytosis
endothelioid
endotheliolysin
endotheliolytic
endothelioma
    angiomatosum, e.
    capitis, e.
    cutis, e.
    diffuse e.
    dural e.
    perithelial e.
endotheliomatosis
endotheliomyoma
endotheliosarcoma
endothelium
endotoxemia
endotoxin
endotracheal
Endoxan-Asta (cyclophosphamide)
endpoint
end-sigmoid colostomy
end-stage disease
end-to-end anastomosis (EEA)
enediyne
enema
    air contrast barium e.
    barium e.
    contrast e.
    double contrast e.
    Fleet e.
    nutrient e.
    nutritive e.
    oil retention e.
    soapsuds e.
en face
    irradiation field, e.
Engel alkalimetry
Engerix-B
English yew
Englund method
engraftment
enhancement
enhancer
enhancing
    antibody, e.
    lesion, e.
enilconazole
enisoprost
enkephalin
ENM (extraneural metastases)
en masse

ADDITIONAL TERMS

Enneking staging
enolase
enostosis
ENP (extractable nuclear protein)
en plaque
enpromate
Ensure
Entamoeba
    histolytica, E.
Entera-Flor
enteral
    absorption, e.
    feeding, e.
    nutrition, e.
    solution, e.
enterectomy
enteric
    cyst, e.
    pathogen, e.
enterically transmitted non-A, non-B
  (ENANB) hepatitis
enteritis
enteroanastomosis
Enterobacter
    aerogenes, E.
    agglomerans, E.
    cloacae, E.
    gergoviae, E.
    liquefaciens, E.
    sakazakii, E.
    vermicularis, E.
enterobiliary
enterochromaffin cells
enteroclysis
enterococcemia
enterococci (pl. of enterococcus)
enterococcus (pl. enterococci)
enterocolectomy
enterocolitis
enterocolostomy
enterocutaneous
    fistula, e.
enterocystoma
enteroenterostomy
enterogenous cyst
enterohepatic
enterointestinal
enteromegaly
enteromycosis
enteropathic
enteropathogenic
enteropathy
    gluten e.

    protein-losing e.
enterorrhagia
enterorrhaphy
enteroscope
enteroscopy
enterosepsis
enterostaxis
enterostomal
    therapist, e.
    therapy, e.
enterostomy
    double-barreled e.
    gun-barrel e.
    percutaneous e.
enterotoxigenic
enterotoxin
enterovirus
entostosis
enucleate
enucleation
env (envelope) gene
Envacor test
envelope
    cell e.
    nuclear e.
envelope (env) gene
envelope protein
enviradene
environmental
    antigen, a.
    carcinogen, e.
    radiation, e.
enviroxime
enzymatic
    debridement, e.
    gene amplification, e.
enzyme
    autoagglutination factor, e.
    conjugase, e.
    immunoassay, e. (EIA)
    immunoelectrotransfer, e.
    immunosorbent assay, e. (EIA)
    -linked immunoassay, e. (EIA)
    -linked immunoelectrodiffusion
      assay, e. (ELIEDA)
    -linked immunosorbent assay, e.
      (ELISA)
    marker, e.
    -multiplied immunoassay
      technique, e. (EMIT)
enzymological
enzymolysis
enzymolytic

ADDITIONAL TERMS

enzymopathy
Eos (eosinophils)
eosin
eosinocyte
eosinopenia
eosinophil
　　chemotactic factor, e. (ECF)
　　chemotactic factor of anaphylaxis,
　　　e. (ECF-A)
　　leukocytic infiltrate, e.
　　maturation factor, e.
　　progenitor, e.
　　stimulation promoter, e.
eosinophilia
eosinophilic
　　adenoma, e.
　　erythroblast, e.
　　granulocytosis, e.
　　granuloma, e.
　　index, e.
　　leukemia, e.
　　leukocytes, e.
　　leukocytosis, e.
eosinophilopoiesis
eosinophilopoietic
eosinophilopoietin
eosinophilosis
eosinophilotactic
eosinophilous
eosinotactic
EP (erythropoietin)
EP (etoposide, Platinol)
EPA (eicosapentaenoic acid)
EPA (Environmental Protection Agency)
ependyma
ependymal
ependymoblast
ependymoblastoma
ependymocytoma
ependymoma
ependymopathy
epi (epinephrine)
EPI (epirubicin)
epi-ADR (epinephrine-Adriamycin)
4'-epi-Adriamycin (epirubicin)
EPIblot
　　HIV Western blot test, E.
　　HIV-1 test, E.
epibulbar
epicarcinogen
epicenter
epidemic
epidemiology

epidermal
　　growth factor, e. (EGF)
　　growth factor receptor, e. (EGF-R)
epidermodysplasia
　　verruciformis, e.
epidermoid
epidermoidoma
epidermoma
epidermomycosis
epidermotropism
epididymectomy
epididymis
epididymovasectomy
4'-epidoxorubicin
epiesophageal cancer
epifluorescence
epigastric
epigastrium
epigenesis
epiglottidectomy
epimer
epimerase
epimerite
epimerize
epimestrol
epinephrine
epinephroma
epipodophyllotoxin
　　derivative, e.
epiplosarcomphalocele
epirubicin (EPI)
episarkin
espistasis
epistaxis
epithelia (pl. of epithelium)
epithelial
　　basement membrane, e.
　　cancer, e.
　　dysplasia, e.
　　hyperplasia, e.
　　mesothelioma, e.
　　pearls, e.
　　shedding, e.
　　sloughing, e.
　　thymic-activating factor, e. (ETAF)
　　tumor, e.
epithelialization
epithelialized
epithelioblastoma
epithelioid
　　cells, e.
　　hemangioma, e.
　　leiomyoma, e.

ADDITIONAL TERMS

malignant schwannoma, e.
sarcoma, e.
epitheliolysis
epitheliolytic
epithelioma
  adamantinum, e.
  adenoides cysticum, a.
  basal cell e.
  benign calcifying e.
  calcified e.
  calcifying e.
  calcifying e. of Malherbe
  chorionic e.
  columnar e.
  contagiosum, e.
  cylindrical e.
  deep-seated e.
  diffuse e.
  glandular e.
  Malherbe calcifying e.
  malignant e.
  multiple self-healing squamous e.
  self-healing squamous e.
  suprarenal e.
epitheliomatosis
epitheliomatous
epitheliotoxin
epitheliotropia
epithelite
epithelium (pl. epithelia)
epithelization
epitope
  addition, e.
EPO (erythropoietin)
EPOCH (etoposide, prednisone,
  Oncovin, cyclophosphamide,
  Halotestin)
Epodyl
epoetin
  alfa, e. (Epogen)
  beta, e.
Epogen (epoetin alfa)
epoprostenol
epoxide hydrolase
EPP (erythropoietic protoporphyria)
Eprex (erythropoietin)
epsilon-aminocaproic acid (EACA)
Epstein method
Epstein-Barr
  nasopharyngeal carcinoma, E.
  nuclear antigen, E. (EBNA)
  virus, E. (EBV)
epulis

congenital e.
  fibromatosa, e.
  fissurata, e.
  giant cell e.
  gigantocellularis, e.
  granulomatosa, e.
  newborn, e. of
epulofibroma
epuloid
equally loaded opposed lateral portals
equation
equilibrium
  constant, e.
  dialysis, e.
equilibratory ataxia
equilibrium
equine
  antihuman lymphoblast globulin, e.
    (EAHLG)
  antihuman lymphoblast serum, e.
    (EAHLS)
  encephalomyelitis virus, e.
equivalent
  aluminum e.
  concrete e.
  dose e.
  lead e.
ER (estrogen receptor)
ER (estrogen replacement)
ERA (estrogen receptor assay)
erb A oncogene
erb B oncogene
erb B2 oncogene
ERBF (effective renal blood flow)
Erdheim cystic medial necrosis
erectile
  dysfunction, e.
  function, e.
erection
Ergamisol (levamisole)
ergocalciferol
ergot
ERIA (electroradioimmunoassay)
Erikson stages
Erlangen magnetic colostomy device
Ernst
  radium application, E.
  radium applicator, E.
  radium capsule, E.
  radium tandem, E.
erode
erosion
erosive

ADDITIONAL TERMS

erosive—*Continued*
   balanitis, e.
   duodenitis, e.
   esophagitis, e.
   gastritis, e.
   vulvitis, e.
eroticism
erotism
   anal e.
ERP (estrogen receptor protein)
Erpalfa
ERPF (effective renal plasma flow)
ERT (estrogen replacement therapy)
ERU (endorectal ultrasound)
Erwinase
Erwinia
   L-asparaginase, E. (porton
     asparaginase)
   herbicola, E.
erythema
   gyrate e.
   gyratum, e.
   gyratum repens, e.
   multiforme, e.
   necrolytic migratory e.
   necroticans, e.
   nodosum leprosum, e.
   paraneoplastic e.
   toxic e.
erythema dose (ED)
erythematosus
   discoid lupus e. (DLE)
   systemic lupus e. (SLE)
erythematous
erythemogenic
erythremia
erythremic
   myelosis, e.
erythroblast
   acidophilic e.
   basophilic e.
   definitive e's
   early e.
   eosinophilic e
   intermediate e.
   late e.
   orthochromatic e.
   oxyphilic e.
   polychromatic e.
   primitive e's
erythroblastemia
erythroblastic
   anemia of childhood, e.

   leukemia, e. (EBL)
erythroblastoma
erythroblastomatosis
erythroblastopenia
erythroblastosis
   ABO e.
   fetalis, e.
   neonatorum, e.
   Rh e.
erythroblastosis virus
erythroblastotic
erythrochromia
erythroclasis
erythroclast
erythroclastic
erythrocytapheresis
erythrocyte (E)
   achromic e.
   basophilic e.
   burr e.
   crenated e.
   hemolyzed e.
   hypochromic e.
   immature e.
   macrocytic e.
   Mexican hat e.
   microcytic e.
   normochromic e.
   nucleated e.
   orthochromatic e.
   polychromatic e.
   polychromatophilic e.
   target e.
erythrocyte antibody (EA)
erythrocyte autosensitization
erythrocyte fragility
erythrocyte glutamic oxaloacetic
   transaminase (EGOT)
erythrocyte iron turnover (EIT)
erythrocyte mass
erythrocyte maturation factor (EMF)
erythrocyte mosaicism
erythrocyte protoporphyrin test
erythrocyte sedimentation rate (ESR)
erythrocyte-sensitizing substance
erythrocyte transfusion
erythrocythemia
erythrocytic
   marrow, e.
   series, e.
erythrocytoblast
erythrocytolysin
erythrocytolysis

ADDITIONAL TERMS

erythrocytometer
erythrocytometry
erythrocyto-opsonin
erythrocytopenia
erythrocytophagous
erythrocytophagy
erythrocytopoiesis
erythrocytopoietic
erythrocytorrhexis
erythrocytoschisis
erythrocytosis
   leukemic e.
   megalosplenica, e.
   stress e.
erythrodegenerative
erythroderma
erythrogenesis
   imperfecta, e.
erythrogenic
erythrogone
erythroid
   cells, e.
   hyperplasia, e.
   hypoplasia, e.
   pool, e.
   potentiating activity, e.
erythrokatalysis
erythrokinetics
erythroleukemia
erythroleukoblastosis
erythroleukosis
erythroleukothrombocythemia
erythrolysin
erythrolysis
erythromyeloblastic
   leukemia, e.
erythron
erythroneocytosis
erythronoclastic
erythronormoblastic
erythropathy
erythropenia
erythrophage
erythrophagia
erythrophagocytic
   lymphohistiocytosis, e.
erythrophagocytosis
erythrophagous
erythrophthisis
erythroplakia
   speckled e.
erythroplasia
   Queyrat, e. of

erythropoiesis
erythropoietic
   marrow, e.
   porphyria, e.
   protoporphyria, e. (EPP)
   quantum theory, e.
   stimulating factor, e. (ESF)
   uroporphyrin, e.
erythropoietin (EPO)
erythropyknosis
erythrorrhexis
erythrosedimentation
erythrose
erythrosis
erythrostasis
erythrostatic
Es (einsteinium)
Esbach reagent
Escherichia
   coli, E.
escorcin
ESF (erythropoietic stimulating factor)
ESHAP (etoposide, Solu-Medrol, ara-C,
   Platinol)
eskimoma
esophageal
   bypass, e.
   carcinoma, e.
   dilatation, e.
   intraepithelial neoplasia, e. (EIN)
   speech, e.
   stricture, e.
   varices, e.
esophagectasia
esophagectomy
esophagitis
esophagocardiomyotomy
esophagocologastrostomy
esophagocoloplasty
esophagoduodenostomy
esophagodynia
esophagoenterostomy
esophagoesophagostomy
esophagofundopexy
esophagogastrectomy
esophagogastric
esophagogastroanastomosis
esophagogastroduodenoscopy
esophagogastromyotomy
esophagogastroplasty
esophagogastroscopy
esophagogastrostomy
esophagojejunogastrostomosis

ADDITIONAL TERMS

esophagojejunogastrostomy
esophagojejunoplasty
esophagojejunostomy
esophagolaryngectomy
esophagomalacia
esophagomycosis
esophagomyotomy
esophagopharyngeal
esophagopharyngoscopy
esophagopharynx
esophagoplasty
esophagoplication
esophagosalivary symptom
esophagoscope
esophagoscopy
esophagostenosis
esophagostoma
esophagostomy
esophagotomy
esophagotracheal
esophagram
esophagraphy
esophagus
esorubicin hydrochloride
esperamicin
ESR (electron spin resonance)
ESR (erythrocyte sedimentation rate)
essential
    anemia, e.
    thrombocytopenia, e. (ET)
    thrombocytosis, e.
ester
    phorbol e.
esterapenia
esterase-D
esterified
    estrogens, e.
esthesioneuroblastoma
Estinyl (ethinyl estradiol)
Estlander
    flap, E.
    procedure, E.
Estrace (estradiol)
Estracyst
estradiol
    RIA antiserum, e.
Estradurin (polyestradiol)
Estra-L (estradiol)
estramustine (Emcyt)
Estratab (esterified estrogen)
Estraval (estradiol)
Estren-Damashek
    anemia, E.

familial aplasia, E.
estrinization
estriol
estrogen
    conjugated e's
    esterified e's
estrogen receptor (ER)
estrogen receptor assay (ERA)
estrogen receptor protein (ERP)
estrogen replacement therapy
estrogen window hypothesis
estrogen withdrawal bleeding
estrogenic
estrogenicity
estrogenous
estrone
estrophilin
estropipate
estrostilben
ET (essential thrombocytopenia)
ETAF (epithelial thymic-activating
  factor)
etanidazole (SR-2508)
ethacrynic acid (EA)
ethambutol (Myambutol)
ethanol gelation test
ethinyl estradiol (Estinyl)
ethiodol
ethiofos (amifostine or Ethyol or
  gammafos or WR-2721)
ethionamide
ethmoid
ethmoidal
ethmoidectomy
ethnic
    background, e.
    variation, e.
ethnicity
ethoglucid
ethyl chaulmoograte
10-ethyl-10-deaza-aminopterin
  (edatrexate)
ethylene
    dibromide, e. (EDB)
    vinyl alcohol, e. (EVAL)
ethylenediaminetetra-acetic acid (EDTA)
Ethyol (ethiofos)
etidronate disodium (Didronel)
etidronic acid
etoglucid
etomidate
etoposide (VePesid or VP-16)
etoprine

ADDITIONAL TERMS

ETR (effective thyroxine ratio)
ets oncogene
ets-2 oncogene
Eubacterium
    alactolyticum, E.
    lentum, E.
    limosum, E.
Euglena
    gracilis, E.
euglobulin
    clot lysis time, e. (ECLT)
    clot test, e. (ECT)
    lysis test, e.
    lysis time, e. (ELT)
euglycemia
EU8-induced lymphoma
eukaryotic
    transcription, e.
Eulexin (flutamide)
eumycetoma
eunuch
eunuchism
eunuchoid
euoxic
euploid
euploidy
European
    Kaposi sarcoma, E.
    mistletoe, E.
EUS (endoscopic ultrasonogram)
euthanasia
Euthroid
euthymic
euthyroid
    sick syndrome, e.
euthyroidism
eV (electron volt)
EVA (etoposide, vinblastine,
    Adriamycin)
EVAL (ethylene vinyl alcohol)
Evans
    blue, E. (T-1824)
    classification, E.
    staging of neuroblastoma, E.
    syndrome, E.
eventration
Everone
evidement
evideur
eviscerate
evisceration
evolution
Ewing

sarcoma, E.
tumor, E.
exacerbate
exacerbation
ExacTec meter
exanthem
exarticulation
excavate
excavation
excess antigen
exchange
    plasma e.
    sister chromatid e.
    transfusion, e.
exchanger
Excimer cool laser
excisional
    biopsy, e.
    conization, e.
excited atom
excitometabolic
exclusion
    allelic e.
    isotypic e.
exclusion criteria
excrement
excrementitial
    absorption, e.
excrementitious
excrescence
    fungating e.
excrescent
excreta
exenterate
exenteration
    orbital contents, e. of
    pelvic organs, e. of
exenterative
exeresis
exfoliative
    cytodiagnosis, e.
    cytology, e.
    lesion, e.
existential pain
exit
    dose, e.
    -to-entrance dose penetration, e.
exoantigen
exocolitis
exocrine
exocytosis
exodeoxyribonuclease
exoenzyme

ADDITIONAL TERMS

exoerythrocytic
    plasmodium, e.
exogenous
    antigen cell-bound antibody
        reaction, e.
    antigen-circulating antibody
        reaction, e.
    hemosiderosis, e.
exon
exonuclease
exopeptidase
exophytic
    adenocarcinoma, e.
    carcinoma, e.
    lesion, e.
    mass, e.
    tumor, e.
exoribonuclease
exosmosis
exostoses (pl. of exostosis)
exostosis (pl. exostoses)
exothelioma
expanded
    access protocol, e.
    plasma, e.
expansion chamber
explant
exploratory
    laparotomy, e.
    procedure, e.
    surgery, e.
exponential
    decay, e.
exposure
    acute e.
    air e.
    chronic e.
    fractionation e.
    occupational e.
    protraction e.
    radiation e.
    x-ray e.
exposure dose
exsanguinate
exsanguination
exsanguinotransfusion
extended-field radiation
exteriorization
exteriorize
external beam
    radiation, e.
    therapy, e. (EBT)
externally quenched counter

extirpate
extirpation
extra-adrenal
extracellular
    fluid volume, e.
    -like calcium-free solution, e.
        (ECS)
    matrix, e.
    matrix protein, e.
extracorporeal
    circulation, e.
    irradiation of blood, e. (ECIB)
    irradiation of lymph, e. (ECIL)
    membrane oxygenation, e. (ECMO)
    membrane oxygenator, e. (ECMO)
    photophoresis, e.
extracranial
extractable
    nuclear antigen, e. (ENA)
    nuclear protein, e. (ENP)
extragonadal
    germ cell tumor, e.
extrahepatic
extralymphatic
extramammary Paget disease (EMPD)
extramedullary
    blastic tumor, e.
    disease, e.
    erythropoiesis, e.
    hematopoiesis, e.
    megakaryocytopoiesis, e.
extraneural metastases (EN)
extranodal
extranuclear
extrapleural
extrapolate
extrapolation
    ionization chamber, e.
extraskeletal
    Ewing sarcoma, e.
    chondrosarcoma, e.
    osteosarcoma, e.
extravasation
extrinsic
    clotting reaction, e.
    factor, e.
    pathway, e.
exuberant tissue
exudate
exudation
    cyst, e.
exudative
ex vivo

ADDITIONAL TERMS

T-cell marrow depletion, e.
E-Z-EM Cut biopsy needle

F

f (suffix added to classification indicating known family history)
F19
    antigen, F.
    IgG monoclonal antibody, F.
F31
    antigen, F.
    IgM monoclonal antibody, F.
F antigen
F cell
F factor
F thalassemia
FA (filterable agent)
FA (fluorescent antibody)
Fab (fragment, antigen-binding)
FAB (French/American/British) classification of acute lymphoid leukemia
    M1 myeloblastic with no differentiation
    M2 myeloblastic with differentiation
    M3 promyelocytic
    M4 myelomonocytic
    M5 monocytic
    M6 erythroleukemia
FAB staging
Faber
    anemia, F.
    syndrome, F.
fabism
Fabricius bursa
FAC (5-fluorouracil, Adriamycin, cyclophosphamide)
Facb (fragment, antigen-and-complement-binding)
FAC-BCG (Ftorafur, Adriamycin, cyclophosphamide, bacille Calmette-Guérin)
facial
    moulage, f.
    prosthesis, f.
facies
    cushingoid f.
    moon f.
facioplasty
FAC-LEV (5-fluorouracil, Adriamycin, cyclophosphamide, levamisole)

FAC-M (5-fluorouracil, Adriamycin, cyclophosphamide, methotrexate)
FACP (ftorafur, Adriamycin, cyclophosphamide, Platinol)
FACS (5-fluorouracil, Adriamycin, cyclophosphamide, streptozocin)
FACS (fluorescence-activated cell sorter)
FACScan
facteur thymique serique
factitial proctitis
factor (see below for Factor I through XIII)
    A, f.
    accelerator f.
    acetate replacement f.
    activation f.
    adrenocorticotropic releasing f.
    albumin autoagglutinating f.
    allogeneic effect f. (AEF)
    amino acid trap f.
    angiogenesis f.
    antianemia f.
    antichromotrichia f.
    antigen-specific T-cell helper f.
    antigen-specific T-cell suppressor f.
    antihemophilic f. A
    antihemophilic f. B
    antihemophilic f. C
    antihemorrhagic f.
    anti-intrinsic f.
    antinuclear f. (ANF)
    anti-pernicious anemia f.
    antirachitic f.
    antiscorbutic f.
    atrial natriuretic f.
    autoagglutinating f.
    B, f.
    basophil chemotactic f. (BCF)
    B cell differentiation f's (BCDF)
    B cell growth f's (BCGF)
    Bittner milk f.
    B-lymphocyte stimulatory f's (BSF)
    blastogenic f. (BF)
    blocking f.
    C f.
    C3 nephritic f.
    CAMP f.
    Castle intrinsic f.
    chemotactic f.
    Christmas f.
    chromotrichial f.
    citrovorum f.
    clonal inhibitory f.

ADDITIONAL TERMS

factor—*Continued*
  cloning inhibitory f.
  clotting f.
  coagulation f's (I through XIII)
  coenzyme f.
  colony-inhibiting f.
  colony-stimulating f. (CSF)
  complement chemotactic f.
  conglutinogen activating f. (KAF)
  contact f.
  corticotropin-releasing f.
  coupling f.
  cryoprecipitated antihemophilic f.
  crystal-induced chemotactic f.
    (CCF)
  cytotoxic T-lymphocyte
    differentiation f.
  D, f.
  D deficiency f.
  Day f.
  decay-accelerating f.
  decay-activating f.
  diffusion f.
  Duran-Reynals f.
  E f.
  elongation f.
  eluate f.
  eosinophil chemotactic f. (ECF)
  eosinophil chemotactic f. of
    anaphylaxis (ECF-A)
  epidermal growth f. (EGF)
  epithelial thymic-activating f.
  erythrocyte maturation f. (EMF)
  erythropoietic stimulating f. (ESF)
  extrinsic f.
  F, f.
  fibrin stabilizing f.
  fibroblast growth f. (FGF)
  Fitzgerald f.
  Fitzgerald-Williams-Flaujeac f.
  Flaujeac f.
  Fletcher f.
  follicle-stimulating hormone-
    releasing f.
  gastric antipernicious anemia f.
  genetic f.
  glass f.
  glucose tolerance f.
  glucose trap f.
  glycotropic f.
  Gm f.
  gonadotropin-releasing f.
  granulocyte colony-stimulating f.

  granulocyte-macrophage colony-
    stimulating f.
  growth hormone releasing f.
  growth inhibiting f.
  H, f.
  H deficiency f.
  Hageman f. (HF)
  hepatocyte nuclear f.
  hepatocyte-stimulating f.
  high-molecular-weight neutrophil
    chemotactic f. (HMW-NCF)
  histamine-releasing f.
  host f.
  human antihemophilic f.
  hydrazine-sensitive f.
  hyperglycemic-glycogenolytic f.
  I, f.
  I deficiency f.
  immunoglobulin-binding f. (IBF)
  inhibiting f's
  initiation f.
  insulin-like growth f. (IGF)
  intrinsic f.
  kappa f.
  labile f.
  Lactobacillus casei f.
  Lactobacillus lactis Dorner f.
  Laki-Lorand f.
  LE f.
  lethal f.
  leukocyte inhibitory f. (LIF)
  leukocytosis-promoting f.
  leukopenic f.
  LLD f. (cyanocobalamin)
  luteinizing hormone-releasing f.
  lymph node permeability f. (LNPF)
  lymphocyte activating f. (LAF)
  lymphocyte blastogenic f. (LBF)
  lymphocyte mitogenic f. (LMF)
  lymphocyte transforming f. (LTF)
  lysogenic f.
  macrophage-activating f. (MAF)
  macrophage-chemotactic f. (MCF)
  macrophage colony-stimulating f.
  macrophage cytotoxic f.
  macrophage-derived growth f.
  macrophage growth f. (MGF)
  macrophage-inhibitory f. (MIF)
  macrophage inhibiting f.
  macrophage inhibitory f.
  maturation f.
  melanocyte-stimulating hormone-
    inhibiting f.

ADDITIONAL TERMS

melanocyte-stimulating hormone-
releasing f.
migration inhibiting f.
milk f.
mitogenic f.
mouse mammary tumor f.
necrotizing f.
nephritic f.
nerve growth f.
neutrophil chemotactic f. (NCF)
osteoclast-activating f. (OAF)
osteoclast-stimulating f.
P, f.
P-cell growth f.
Passovoy f.
plasma coagulation f.
plasma immune f.
plasma labile f.
plasma prothrombin conversion f.
plasma thromboplastin f.
platelet f's
platelet activating f. (PAF)
platelet aggregating f.
platelet coagulation f.
platelet-derived growth f. (PDGF)
prolactin-inhibiting f.
prolactin-releasing f.
prothrombin conversion f.
Prower f.
R, f.
radiation protection f. (RPF)
recognition f.
recruitment f.
releasing f's
resistance-inducing f.
resistance transfer f.
Rh (Rhesus) f.
Rhesus (Rh) f.
rheumatoid f. (RF)
risk f.
Romunda f.
S, f.
secretor f.
Simon septic f.
skin reactive f. (SRF)
slow-reacting f. of anaphylaxis
somatotropin-releasing f.
specific macrophage arming f.
(SMAF)
stable f.
Stones f.
Stuart f.
Stuart-Prower f.

sulfation f.
T f.
T-cell growth f.
thymic lymphopoietic f.
thymus-replacing f.
thyroid-stimulating hormone-
releasing f.
thyrotropin-releasing f. (TRF)
trans-acting f.
transfer f. (TF)
transformed mesothelial growth f.
(TMGF)
transforming f.
tumor-angiogenesis f.
tumor necrosis f. (TNF)
V f.
Va f.
von Willebrand f.
W f.
Williams f.
Wills f.
X f.
Xa f.
yeast eluate f.
factor I (fibrinogen)
factor II (prothrombin)
factor III (tissue thromboplastin)
Factor III multimer assay
factor IV (calcium)
factor V (proaccelerin)
factor VI (Factor VI)
factor VII (serum prothrombin
conversion accelerator)
factor VIIa
factor VIII (antihemophilic factor)
factor VIII correctional unit (FECU)
factor IX (plasma thromboplastin)
Factor IX Complex
factor X (Stuart-Prower factor)
factor XI (plasma thromboplastin
antecedent)
factor XII (Hageman factor)
factor XIII (fibrin-stabilizing factor)
Factorate
facultative aerobes
FACVP (5-fluorouracil, Adriamycin,
cyclophosphamide, VP-16)
FAD (flavin adenine dinucleotide)
FADF (fluorescent antibody darkfield)
Fahraeus method
FAIDS (feline AIDS)
falces (pl. of falx)
fallout

ADDITIONAL TERMS

false cord
false-negative
false-positive
    biologic f. (BFP)
falx (pl. falces)
FAM (5-fluorouracil, Adriamycin,
  mitomycin)
FAMA (fluorescent antibody against
  membrane antigen)
FAM-C (5-fluorouracil, Adriamycin,
  methyl-CCNU)
FAM-CF (5-fluorouracil, Adriamycin,
  mitomycin, citrovorum factor)
FAME (5-fluorouracil, Adriamycin,
  MeCCNU)
familial
    adenomatous polyposis, f.
    aggregation, f.
    atypical multiple mole melanoma, f.
    (FAMMM)
    erythroblastic anemia, f.
    erythrophagocytic
    lymphohistiocytosis, f. (FEL)
    immunity, f.
    megaloblastic anemia, f.
    predisposition, f.
FAMMe (5-fluorouracil, Adriamycin,
  mitomycin-C, MeCCNU)
FAMMM (familial atypical multiple mole
  melanoma)
famotin hydrochloride
FAMP (fludarabine monophosphate)
FAM-S (5-fluorouracil, Adriamycin,
  mitomycin-C, streptozotocin)
FAMTX (5-fluorouracil, Adriamycin,
  high-dose methotrexate)
FANA (fluorescent antinuclear antibody)
Fanasil
Fanconi
    anemia, F.
    pancytopenia, F.
    syndrome, F.
fanetizole mesylate
Fansidar (sulfadoxine-pyrimethamine)
Fanzil
FAP (familial adenomatous polyposis)
FAP (5-fluorouracil, Adriamycin,
  Platinol)
Farabeuf amputation
Farber disease
Farber-Dana series
Farr test
Farre tubercles

fascia
fascial
fascicular
    lymphosarcoma, f.
fasciectomy
fasciitis
    infiltrative f.
    necrotizing f.
    nodular f.
    proliferative f.
    pseudosarcomatous f.
Fasciola
    gigantica, F.
    hepatica, F.
fast
    black 2 dye, f.
    black K, Pt dye, f.
    hemoglobin, f.
    neutron, f.
    neutron beam therapy, f.
    pile, f.
    protein liquid chromatography, f.
    (FPLC)
fasting
    blood sugar, f.
    profile, f.
FAT (fluorescent antibody test)
fat necrosis
fate map
fatigability
fatigue
fatty
    liver, f.
    tumor, f.
fauces (pl. of faux)
faucial
    carcinoma, f.
    pillar, f.
faux (pl. fauces)
favism
Favre-Durand-Nicholas disease
fazarabine
FBJ osteosarcoma virus
FBL-3 lymphoma
FBS (fasting blood sugar)
FBX dosimeter
Fc (fragment, crystallizable)
    component, F.
    fragment, F.
    receptor, F.
5-FC (5-fluorocytosine)
FCA (ferritin-conjugated antibody)
FCA (Freund complete adjuvant)

ADDITIONAL TERMS

FCAP (5-fluorouracil, cyclophosphamide, Adriamycin, Platinol)
FCE (5-fluorouracil, cisplatin, etoposide)
fCi (femtocurie)
F-CL (5-fluorouracil, leucovorin calcium)
FCP (5-fluorouracil, cyclophosphamide, prednisone)
Fd (heavy chain portion of Fab fragment)
FDA (Food and Drug Administration)
FDP (fibrin degradation product)
Fe (iron)
FEAU (2-fluoro-5-ethyl-l-B-d-arabinofuranosyluracil)
febrile
    agglutination test, f.
    antigen, f.
    pleiomorphic anemia, f.
FEC (5-fluorouracil, epirubicin, cyclophosphamide)
fecal
    incontinence, f.
    occult blood, f.
fecaloma
fecapentaenes
feces
FECU (factor VIII correctional unit)
FED (5-fluorouracil, etoposide, DDP)
feeding gastrostomy tube
FEGO (Federation of Gynecology and Obstetrics) staging
Feiba VH Immuno
FEL (familial erythrophagocytic lymphohistiocytosis)
Felbamate
feline
    adenovirus, f.
    AIDS, f. (FAIDS)
    leukemia, f.
    leukemia virus, f. (FeLV)
    oncornavirus-associated cell membrane antigen, f. (FOCMA)
Felty syndrome
FeLV (feline leukemia virus)
feminization
feminizing
    ovarian tumor, f.
    testis syndrome, f.
Feminone (ethinyl estradiol)
Femogen
femtocurie (fCi)

femtoliter (fL)
femtomole (fmol)
fenestrated
    tracheostomy tube, f.
fenestration
fenretinide (HPR)
fentanyl
    citrate, f. (Duragesic)
Fenwick disease
Feosol
Feostat
FEP (free erythrocyte protoporphyrin)
Fergon
Fermilab
fermium (Fm)
Fero-Gradumet
Ferrata cell
ferrated
ferredoxin
ferric
    chloride, f.
ferrihemoglobin
ferritin
    -conjugated antibody, f. (FCA)
    -coupled antibody, f.
Ferrizyme
ferrochelatase
ferrocholinate
ferroflocculation
ferrohemoglobin
ferrokinetics
ferroprotein
ferrotherapy
ferrous
    fumarate, f.
    gluconate, f.
    lactate, f.
    sulfate, f.
ferruginous bodies
ferrum
fes oncogene
fetal
    carcinoembryonic antigen, f.
    globin switch, f.
    hemoglobin, f.
    sulfoglycoprotein antigen, f.
fetoglobin
fetomaternal
    transfusion, f.
fetoplacental
    blood, f.
    transfusion, f.
fetoprotein

ADDITIONAL TERMS

fetoprotein—*Continued*
   alpha-f.
Feulgen
   method, F.
   reaction, F.
fever
   induction, f.
   treatment, f.
F-5-fluorouracil deoxyribonucleoside
   (18F-FUDR)
FFP (fresh frozen plasma)
18F-FUDR (F-5-fluorouracil
   deoxyribonucleoside)
FGF (fibroblast growth factor)
fgr oncogene
Fi (fibrinogen) test
FIA (fluorescent immunoassay)
FIA (fluoroimmunoassay)
FIAC (fiacitabine)
fiacitabine (FIAC)
fialuridine (FIAU)
FIAU (fialuridine)
fiber
   carcinogenesis, f.
   -illuminated, f.
fiberbronchoscope
fibercolonoscope
fibergastroscope
fiberoptic
   anoscope, f.
   bronchoscope, f.
   colonoscope, f.
   culdoscope, f.
   cystoscope, f.
   endoscope, f.
   esophagoscope, f.
   gastroscope, f.
   hysteroscope, f.
   laryngoscope, f.
   light, f.
   otoscope, f.
   panendoscope, f.
   proctosigmoidoscope, f.
   sigmoidoscope, f.
fiberoptics
fiberscope
Fibiger method
Fibonacci search scheme
fibremia
fibril
fibrin
   bodies, f.
   clots, f.

   degradation products, f. (FDP)
   glue, f.
   monomers, f.
   split products, f.
   -stabilizing factor, f. (FSF)
   titer test, f.
fibrinase
fibrinocellular
fibrinogen
   breakdown products, f.
   split products, f.
fibrinogenase
fibrinogenemia
fibrinogenesis
fibrinogenic
fibrinogenolysis
fibrinogenolytic
fibrinogenopenia
fibrinogenous
fibrinoid
   change, f.
fibrinokinase
fibrinolysin
fibrinolysis
fibrinolytic
   split products, f.
fibrinopenia
fibrinopeptide
fibrinoplastin
fibrinoplatelet
fibrinopurulent
fibrinoscopy
fibroadenia
fibroadenoma
   giant f. of breast
fibroadenomatous
   hyperplasia of prostate, f.
fibroadenosis
fibroangioma
fibroblast
   growth factor, b. (FGF)
fibroblastic
fibroblastoma
   perineural f.
fibrocarcinoma
fibrocartilaginous
fibrochondroma
fibrocollagenous
fibrocyst
fibrocystic
   disease, f.
   nodules, f.
fibrocyte

ADDITIONAL TERMS

fibrocytogenesis
fibrocytoma
fibrodysplasia
    ossificans progressiva, f.
fibrodysplastic
fibroenchondroma
fibroepithelial
fibroepithelioma
    Pinkus, f. of
    premalignant f.
Fibrogammin
fibroglioma
fibrohemorrhagic
fibrohistiocytic
fibrohistiocytoma
fibroid
    interstitial f.
    uterine f.
fibroid tumor
fibroid uterus
fibroidectomy
fibrolipoma
fibrolipomatous
fibroma (pl. fibromata)
    ameloblastic f.
    aponeurotic f.
    breast, f. of
    cavernosum, f.
    cementifying f.
    chondromyxoid f.
    concentric f.
    cutis, f.
    cystic f.
    desmoplastic f.
    durum, f.
    hard f.
    intracanalicular f.
    intramural f.
    juvenile active ossifying f.
    juvenile aponeurotic f.
    juvenile nasopharyngeal f.
    molle, f.
    mucinosum, f.
    myxomatodes, f.
    nonossifying f.
    nonosteogenic f.
    odontogenic f.
    ossifying f.
    osteogenic f.
    parasitic f.
    pendulum, f.
    recurrent digital f. of childhood
    sarcomatosum, f.

    soft f.
    subserous f.
    telangiectatic f.
    thecocellulare xanthomatodes, f.
    uterine f.
    xanthoma, f.
fibromata (pl. of fibroma)
fibromatogenic
fibromatoid
fibromatosis
    colli, f.
    congenital generalized f.
    gingivae, f.
    gingival f.
    infantile digital f.
    juvenile hyaline f.
    palmar f.
    penile f.
    plantar f.
    Stout f.
    subcutaneous pseudosarcomatous
        f.
    ventriculi, f.
fibromatous
fibromectomy
fibromyoma (pl. fibromyomata)
    uteri, f.
fibromyomata (pl. of fibromyoma)
    uteri, f.
fibromyomectomy
fibromyositis
fibromyxoma
    odontogenic f.
fibromyxosarcoma
fibronectin
fibroneuroma
fibro-odontoma
    ameloblastic f.
fibro-osseous
fibro-osteoma
fibropapilloma
fibroplasia
fibroplastic
fibropolypus
fibropurulent
fibrosarcoma
    FSaIIC, f.
    odontogenic f.
fibrosclerosis
fibroserous
fibrosis
fibrositis
fibrotic

ADDITIONAL TERMS

fibrotic—*Continued*
 changes, f.
fibrous
  dysplasia, f.
  hamartoma, f.
  histocytoma, f.
  mesothelioma, f.
  tumor, f.
  xanthoma, f.
fibrovascular
fibroxanthoma
Fichera treatment
ficin
Ficoll
  -Hypaque, F.
  isokinetic gradient, F.
field
  inverted Y f.
  mantle f.
  radiation f.
field inversion gel electrophoresis
  (FIGE)
Fiessinger-Leroy syndrome
Fiessinger-Leroy-Reiter syndrome
FIGE (field inversion gel
  electrophoresis)
FIGLU (formiminoglutamic acid)
  excretion test, F.
FIGO (Fédération Internationale de
  Gynécologie et Obstétrique)
  staging of endometrial
    adenocarcinoma, F.
filament
  -nonfilament count, f.
  protein, f.
filamentous
filaria
filarial
filariasis
Filatori disease
Filatov disease
filgrastim (Neupogen)
filling defect
film badge
filter
  binding assay, f.
filterable
  agent, f. (FA)
  virus, f.
filtration
  gel f.
  leukapheresis, f.
  roentgen rays, f. of

FIMe (5-fluorouracil, ICRF-159,
  MeCCNU)
finasteride (MK-906)
fine-needle
  aspiration, f. (FNA)
  aspiration biopsy, f. (FNAB)
  aspiration cytology, f. (FNAC)
fingerprint
  genetic f.
fingerprinting
  genetic f.
fingerstick blood sample
Finsen
  bath, F.
  lamp, F.
  light, F.
firefly enzyme
first-set
  phenomenon, f.
  rejection, f.
Fischer rats
FISH (fluoresceinated in situ
  hybridization)
Fisher
  autocytometer, F.
  exact test, F.
Fisher-Race theory
Fishman-Doubilet test
Fisk and Subbarow method
Fisoneb nebulizer
Fisons nebulizer
fission
  atomic f.
  binary f.
  nuclear f.
fission reaction
fissionable
fisting
fistula
fistulous
FITC (fluorescein isothiocyanate)
Fitzgerald factor
Fitzgerald-Williams-Flaujeac factor
fixation
  complement f.
fixative
Fixott-Everett grid
FK-506
fL (femtoliter)
FL (flutamide, leuprolide acetate depot)
FL (flutamide, Luprin)
FL160 antigen
FLAC (5-fluorouracil, leucovorin

ADDITIONAL TERMS

calcium, Adriamycin,
cyclophosphamide)
flap
    skin f.
FLAP (5-fluorouracil, leucovorin
    calcium, Adriamycin, Platinol)
flap amputation
flapless amputation
flapping tremor
flare
flash burn
Flatau-Schilder disease
Flaujeac factor
flavin
    adenine dinucleotide, f. (FAD)
Flavobacterium
    breve, F.
    meningosepticum, F.
    odoratum, F.
flavone
flavoprotein
FLC (Friend leukemia cells)
FLe (5-fluorouracil, levamisole)
fleam
fleck
    blood f's
    tobacco f's
fleckmilz
fleroxacin
Fletcher
    afterloading colpostat, F.
    afterloading tandem, F.
    factor, F.
    loading applicator, F.
    ovoid system, F.
    tandem, F.
Fletcher-Suit
    application, F.
    applicator, F.
    ovoid, F.
    tandem, F.
Fletcher-Suit-Delclos (FSD) applicator
fleurettes
flexible fiberoptic
    bronchoscope, f.
    sigmoidoscope, f.
Flexner-Wintersteiner rosettes
Flex-Strand cable
flip angle
flocculation
floccule
flocculi (pl. of flocculus)
flocculoreaction

flocculus (pl. flocculi)
Flolan
floor of mouth
flora
florentium
florid
flow
    cytometer, f.
    cytometry, f.
    -sorting, f.
flowmeter
floxuridine (FUdR)
FLT (fluorodeoxythymidine or
    fluorothymidine)
flubendazole
fluconazole
flucytosine (Ancobon or 5-FC)
Fludara (fludarabine)
fludarabine
    monophosphate, f. (FAMP)
    phosphate, f. (Fludara)
fludazonium chloride
fludalanine
fludeoxyglucose F-18 injection
fludrocortisone
flumecinol
Fluogen
fluoresce
fluorescein
    conjugated monoclonal antibody, f.
    isothiocyanate, f. (FITC)
fluoresceinated in situ hybridization
    (FISH)
fluorescence
    -activated cell sorter, f. (FACS)
    enhancement, f.
    quenching, f.
fluorescent
    antibody, f. (FA)
    antibody against membrane
      antigen, f. (FAMA)
    antibody darkfield, f. (FADF)
    antibody staining, f.
    antibody test, f. (FAT)
    antinuclear antibody, f. (FANA)
    auramine-rhodamine stain, f.
    immunoassay, f. (FIA)
    screen, f.
    spot test, f.
fluorine F-18
fluorochrome
    -labeled, f.
fluorocyte

ADDITIONAL TERMS

5-fluorocytosine (5-FC)
fluoro-ddC
fluorodeoxythymidine (FLT)
fluorodeoxyuridine (FUdR)
fluorodopa F-18
fluorodopan
2-fluoro-5-ethyl-l-B-d-
arabinofuranosyluracil (FEAU)

fluorography
fluoroimmunoassay (FIA)
fluorometer
fluorometry
fluorophotometry
Fluoroplex (fluorouracil)
fluoropyrimidine
fluoroquinolone
fluoroscope
fluoroscopy
fluorosulfonylbenzoyl 5'-adenosine
    (FSBA)
3'-fluorothymidine (FLT)
fluorouracil (Adrucil or Efudex or
    5-fluorouracil or 5-FU or Fluoroplex)
5-fluorouracil (Adrucil or Efudex or
    Fluoroplex or fluorouracil or 5-FU)
    deoxyribonucleoside, f. (^{18}F-
    FUDR)
fluorouridine
    monophosphate, f, (FUMP)
    triphosphate, f. (FUTP)
5-fluorouridine (5-FUR)
Fluosol
    artificial blood, F.
    -DA/02, F. (green blood)
    -DA 20%, F.
Fluosol/BCNU (Fluosol-DA20, BCNU)
fluoxymesterone (FXM or Halotestin)
fluphenazine
flurocitabine
flush
    carcinoid f.
flushing
flutamide (Eulexin or FLUT)
flux
FLV (Friend leukemia virus)
Fm (fermium)
FMEL (Friend murine erythroleukemia)
FMLP (N-formyl-1-methionyl-1-leucyl-1-
    phenylalanine)
fmol (femtomole)
fmol/mg (femtomoles per milligram)

FMS (5-fluorouracil, mitomycin-C,
    streptozocin)
fms oncogene
FMV (5-fluorouracil, methyl CCNU,
    vincristine)
FNA (fine-needle aspiration)
FNAB (fine-needle aspiration biopsy)
FNAC (fine-needle aspiration cytology)
FNM (5-fluorouracil, Novantrone,
    methotrexate)
FOAM (5-fluorouracil, Oncovin,
    Adriamycin, mitomycin-C)
foam cell
focal
    finding, f.
    lesion, f.
    mass, f.
    spot, f.
    tumor, f.
foci (pl. of focus)
FOCMA (feline oncornavirus-associated
    cell membrane antigen)
focus (pl. foci)
focused
    beam, f.
    grid, f.
folate
    deficiency anemia, f.
    storage, f.
Folex (methotrexate)
folic acid
    antagonist, f.
    deficiency anemia, f.
Folin method
Folin and Wu method
folinic acid (leucovorin)
    rescue, f.
follicle
    -stimulating hormone, f. (FSH)
    -stimulating hormone/releasing
    hormone, f. (FSH/RH)
follicular
    adenocarcinoma, f.
    adenoma, f.
    carcinoma, f.
    dendritic cells, f.
    lymphoma, f.
folliculitis
folliculoma
    lipidique, f.
Folvite
folylpolyglutamate synthetase (FPGS)

ADDITIONAL TERMS

inhibitor, f.
FOM (5-fluorouracil, Oncovin,
    mitomycin-C)
FOMi (5-fluorouracil, Oncovin,
    mitomycin-C)
Fonio solution
Fontana removal of lung cysts
footprinting
foramen (pl. foramina)
    Bochdalek, f. of
    Morgagni, f. of
foramina (pl. of foramen)
Forbes-Albright syndrome
foreign body carcinogenesis
forequarter amputation
formaldehyde
formalin
formiminoglutamic acid (FIGLU)
formycin
formyl-methionyl-leucyl-phenylalanine
Forssman
    antibody, F.
    antigen, F.
Fortaz
fos oncogene
fosarilate
foscarnet
    sodium, f.
Foscavir
fosfonet sodium
fosquidone
fostriecin sodium
fotemustine (S 10036)
Fouchet test
Foulis cells
Fourier transform infrared (FTIR)
    spectroscopic system, F.
Fourneau 309
four-point assay
FPGS (folylpolyglutamate synthetase)
FPLC (fast protein liquid
    chromatography)
fps oncogene
Fr (francium)
FRACON (framycetin, colistin, nystatin)
fraction
    absorbed f.
    filtration f.
    human plasma protein f.
    penetration f.
    plasma protein f.
    scatter f.

fractional
    biopsy, f.
    dilatation and f. curettage
    dose, f.
fractionated
    brachytherapy, f.
    high-dose rate, f.
    radiation, f.
    radiotherapy, r.
fractionation
    dose f.
fractography
fragile X syndrome
fragility
    blood, f. of
    capillary f.
    erythrocyte f.
    mechanical f.
    osmotic f.
fragilocyte
fragilocytosis
fragment
    antigen-binding, f. (FAB)
    antigen-crystallizable, f. (Fc)
    restriction f.
fragmentography
frambesioma
frameshift mutation
framycetin
francium (Fr)
Franklin liver puncture needle
Franseen lung biopsy needle
Fraunfelder technique
FRC (frozen red cells)
freckle
    Hutchinson f.
    melanotic f. of Hutchinson
freckled
free
    -air ionization chamber, f.
    anastomosis, f.
    erythrocyte coproporphyrin, f.
    erythrocyte protoporphyrin, f.
    flap, f.
    -floating cancer cells, f.
    -floating clot, f.
    -induction decay, f.
    radical, f.
    thyroxine index, f. (FTI)
freebasing
Freenseen liver biopsy needle
Frei antigen

ADDITIONAL TERMS

French/American/British (FAB)
   staging of carcinoma, see under
   "FAB"
frequency
   gene f.
   recombination f.
Freich theory
frentizole
fresh frozen plasma (FFP)
Freund
   adjuvant, F.
   complete adjuvant, F. (FCA)
   incomplete adjuvant, F.
   reaction, F.
friability
friable
Friedländer bacillus
   pneumonia, F.
Friend
   leukemia cells, F. (FLC)
   leukemia virus, F. (FLV)
   murine erythroleukemia, F. (FMEL)
frigotherapy
Frischblut reaction
Frost method
frozen
   marrow, f.
   plasma, f.
   red cells, f. (FRC)
   section, f.
fructose
   -1,6-diphosphate, f.
   -6-phosphate, f.
fructosemia
FSaIIC murine fibrosarcoma
FSBA (fluorosulfonylbenzoyl
   5'-adenosine)
FSD (Fletcher-Suit-Delclos) applicator
FSF (fibrin-stabilizing factor)
FSH (follicle-stimulating hormone)
FSH/RH (follicle-stimulating
   hormone/releasing hormone)
FSV (feline fibrosarcoma virus)
FT3 (free triiodothyronine)
FT4 (free thyroxine)
FTI (free thyroxine index)
FTIR (Fourier transform infrared)
   spectroscopic system, F.
Ftorafur (l, 2-tetrahydrofuranyl-
   5-fluorouracil)
5-FU (5-fluorouracil or fluorouracil)
FUdR (floxuridine)
FUdR (fluorodexoyuridine)

FUDR (5-fluorouracil
   deoxyribonucleoside)
Fujinami sarcoma virus
full-blown AIDS
Fuller cells
fulminant
fulminate
fulminating
FUM (5-FU, methotrexate)
fumagillin
fumarylacetoacetase
Fumiron
FUMP (fluorouridine monophosphate)
functional
   cyst, f.
   tumor, f.
functioning tumor
fundi (pl. of fundus)
fundoplication
fundus (pl. fundi)
funduscopy
fundusectomy
fungal
   infection, f.
   septicemia, f.
fungate
fungating
   excrescence, f.
   lesion, f.
   mass, f.
   tumor, f.
fungemia
fungi (pl. of fungus)
Fungilin
Fungizone (AmB or amphotericin B)
fungoid
   lesion, f.
   mass, f.
fungous
   cancer, f.
fungus (pl. fungi)
   ball, f.
5-FUR (5-fluorouridine)
FUra (fluorouracil)
FURAM (Ftorafur, Adriamycin,
   mitomycin-C)
furazolidone
Furoxone
fusidic acid
fusiform
Fusiformis
   necrophorus, F.
fusion

ADDITIONAL TERMS

protein, f.
fusional
Fusobacterium
   gonidiaformans, F.
   mortiferum, f.
   necrophorum, F.
   nucleatum, F.
   plauti-vincentii, F.
   russii, F.
   varium, F.
fusocellular
fusospirillary
fusospirillosis
FUTP (fluorouridine triphosphate)
FUVAC (5-FU, vinblastine, Adriamycin,
   cyclophosphamide)
Fv fragment
FXM (fluoxymesterone)
FXM (Halotestin)

G

G (gauss)
G (histopathologic grade)
   G1 well differentiated
   G2 moderately well differentiated
   G3 poorly differentiated
   G4 undifferentiated
   GX grade cannot be assessed
G250 (IgG antibody)
G band
G banding
G cell
G-myeloma protein
G69l protocol
Ga (gallium)
   57, G.
   66, G.
   67, G.
   68, G.
   citrate, G.
   gamma camera, G.
   scan, G.
   scintigraphy, G.
   uptake, G.
GABA (gamma-aminobutyric acid)
gadolinium (Gd)
   diethylenetriamine-pentaacetate, g.
   (Gd-DTPA)
gadopentetate dimeglumine
gag (group-specific antigen) gene
GAG (glycosaminoglycan)
gag-pol (group-specific antigen-
   polymerase) oncogene

Gaisbock
   disease, G.
   syndrome, G.
galactocele
galactography
galactoma
galactorrhea
galactose
   epimerase, g.
galactosemia
galamustine (G-6-M)
galea
galeal
gallbladder
gallium (Ga)
   66, g.
   67, g.
   68, g.
   72, g.
   gamma camera, g.
   nitrate, g. (GAN)
   scan, g.
   scintigraphy, g.
   uptake, g.
GALT (gut-associated lymphoid tissue)
GaLV (gibbon ape lymphosarcoma virus)
Gamastan
Gambro Lundia Minor
gamete
gametic
gametocyte
gametocytemia
gametogenesis
gametoid cells
Gamimune N
Gamiunen
gamma
   allotype, g.
   aminobutyrate, g.
   -aminobutyric acid, g. (GABA)
   camera, g.
   carboxyglutamic acid, g.
   chain, g.
   chain disease, g.
   counter, g.
   decay, g.
   dose, g.
   -Favre body, g.
   field, g.
   globulin, g.
   -glutamyl carboxypeptidase, g.
   -glutamyl transpeptidase, g. (GGT)
   -glutamyltransferase, g. (GGT)

ADDITIONAL TERMS

gamma—*Continued*
  heavy chain disease, g.
  interferon, g. (IFN-G)
  knife, g.
  -lactone, g.
  photon, g.
  radiation, g.
  radiography, g.
  ray, g.
  ray counter, g.
  ray scanner, g.
  ray spectrometer, g.
  scintillation camera, g.
  teletherapy unit, g.
  thalassemia, g.
  well counter, g.
Gamma
  disease, G.
  nodules, G.
Gamma-Gee
Gamma Knife
Gamma-Med II afterloading system
gammaglobulinopathy
gammagram
gammagraphic
Gammaguard
gammaphos
Gammar
gammopathy
  benign monoclonal g.
  monoclonal g.
Gammune
Gamna-Gandy
  bodies, G.
  nodules, G.
Gamulin Rh
GAN (gallium nitrate)
ganciclovir
  sodium, g.
Gandy-Gamna
  bodies, G.
  nodules, G.
Gandy-Nanta disease
ganglioblast
gangliocyte
gangliocytoma
ganglioglioma
ganglioglioneuroma
ganglioma
ganglion
ganglionated
ganglioneuroblastoma
ganglioneurofibroma

ganglioneuroma
ganglioneuromatosis
ganglionic
ganglioside
gangliosidosis
gangrene
gangrenosis
gangrenous
Ganite
gantry
  rotation alignment, g.
  rotation range, g.
gap
  junction, g.
  repair, g.
Garcin syndrome
Gardner syndrome
Gardner-Diamond syndrome
Gardner-Rasheed sarcoma virus
Gardos phenomenon
gargle
gargling
gargoylism
Garre osteomyelitis
Gartner cyst
gartnerian cyst
gas
  binary g.
  blood g's
  coal g.
  lewisite g.
  lung irritant g.
  mustard g.
  nerve g.
  nose irritant g.
  suffocating g.
  toxic g.
  vesicant g.
  war g's
gas chromatography
gas cyst
gas-liquid chromatography (GLC)
Gasser syndrome
gasserian
gastradenitis
gastrectomy
gastric
  bypass, g.
  cancer, g. (types I, II, III)
  carcinoma, g.
  glomus tumor, g.
  inhibitory polypeptide, g. (GIP)
  lavage, g.

ADDITIONAL TERMS

resection, g.
stapling, g.
stoma, g.
tumor, g.
ulcer, g.
washings, g.
gastricsin
gastrin
    level, g.
    -releasing peptide, g. (GRP)
    -secreting, g.
    -secreting non-beta islet cell tumor,
    g.
    -secreting tumor, g.
Gastrin Immutope kit
gastrinoma
gastritis
    radiation g.
gastroanastomosis
Gastroccult
gastrocolic
gastrocolitis
gastrocolostomy
gastrocolotomy
Gastrocrom
gastrodiaphany
gastroduodenal
gastroduodenectomy
gastroduodenoscopy
gastroduodenostomy
gastroenteritis
gastroenteroanastomosis
gastroenterocolitis
gastroenterocolostomy
gastroenterology (GE)
gastroenteroplasty
gastroenterostomy
gastroenterotomy
gastroesophageal
gastroesophagitis
gastroesophagostomy
gastrofiberscope
gastrogastrostomy
gastrogavage
Gastrografin
gastrohepatic
gastrohepatitis
gastroileac
gastroileostomy
gastrointestinal (GI)
    adenocarcinoma, g.
    anastomosis, g. (GIA)
    bleed, g.

carcinoma, g.
lymphoma, g.
mass, g.
tract, g.
gastrojejunocolic
gastrojejunoesophagostomy
gastrojejunostomy
gastrolienal
gastromegaly
gastromycosis
gastropancreatitis
gastroparalysis
gastroparesis
gastrophotography
gastrophthisis
gastroplication
gastroplasty
GastroPort enteral feeding
gastropylorectomy
gastroscope
    fiberoptic g.
gastroscopic
gastroscopy
gastrosia
gastrosplenic
gastrostaxis
gastrostogavage
gastrostolavage
gastrostoma
gastrostomy
    Beck g.
    Glassman g.
    Janeway g.
    Stamm g.
    Witzel g.
gate control theory
gated
gating
Gaucher
    cells, G.
    disease, G.
    splenomegaly, G.
gauss (G)
gaussian
    distribution, g.
gavage
gay
    bowel infection, g.
    bowel syndrome, g.
    lifestyle, g.
    lymph node syndrome, g. (GLNS)
    -related immunodeficiency, g.
    (GRID)

ADDITIONAL TERMS

Gay gland
gayness
GBIA (Guthrie bacterial inhibition assay)
GBM (glioblastoma multiforme)
GCA (giant-cell arteritis)
GCN-4
G-CSF (granulocyte-colony-stimulating factor)
GCT (giant cell tumor)
Gd (gadolinium)
    -DTPA. g. (gadolinium diethylenetriamine-pentaacetate)
GDP (guanosine diphosphate)
Ge (germanium)
GE (gastroenterology)
Gee-Gee
Geenan cytology brush
Gegenbaur cells
Geiger
    counter, G.
    counter-telescope, G.
Geiger-Klemperer counter
Geiger-Müller counter
gel
    electrophoresis, g.
    filtration, g.
gelatiniform carcinoma
gelatinous
    bone marrow, g.
    carcinoma, g.
    tissue, g.
    tumor, g.
Gelfoam
    cookie, G.
    cube, G.
    pledget, G.
    sheet, G.
    sponge, G.
Gell and Coombs classification
gemastete
gemcitabine
    hydrochloride, g.
gemistocyte
gemistocytic
    astrocyte, g.
    astrocytoma, g.
gemmangioma
gender
    determination, g.
    dysphoria, g.
    orientation, g.
    -specific, g.
gene (oncogene)

Abelson g.
abl g.
adipocyte P2 g.
allelic g's
amorphic g.
ars/trs g.
autosomal g.
BCL2 g.
c-abl g.
c-bic g.
cell interaction (CI) g's
cellular g.
c-fas g.
c-fes g.
c-fgr g.
c-fms g.
CI (cell interaction) g's
cloned g.
c-mos g.
c-myb g.
c-myc g.
codominant g's
complementary g's
c-onc g.
crbB g.
c-src g.
cumulative g's
cyclin g.
dbl g.
DCC g.
derepressed g.
dominant g.
Eli g.
env (envelope) g.
erb-B g.
erb-B2 g.
ets g.
ets-2 g.
expression g.
fgr g.
fms g.
fos g.
fps/fes g.
gag (group-specific antigen) g.
gag-erbA g.
gag-pol g.
glp-1 g.
globin g's
GRO g.
group-specific antigen (gag) g.
H (histocompatibility) g.
Ha-ras g.
hemizygous g.

ADDITIONAL TERMS

HER/neu g.
heterozygous g.
histocompatibility (H) g.
histone g.
HIV-1 nef g.
HO g.
holandric g's
homozygous g.
human SE-B g.
human SE-C g.
ICAM-1 (intercellular adhesion
  molecule 1) g.
Ig (immunoglobulin) g's
immune response (Ir) g's
immune suppressor (Is) g's
immunoglobulin (Ig) g's
inhibiting g.
intercellular adhesion molecule 1
  (ICAM-1) g.
Ir (immune response) g's
Is (immune suppressor) g's
JE g.
Ki-ras g.
kit g.
lck g.
leaky g.
lentiviral g.
lethal g.
Lewis g.
linked g's
liver-specific g.
L-myc g.
major g.
MCC (mutated in colon cancer) g.
mcf-3 g.
MDR1 g.
MDR2 g.
mel g.
met g.
mht g.
modifying g.
mos g.
multidrug-resistance g.
mutant g.
mutS g.
myb g.
myc g.
nef g.
neo g.
neomycin-resistance g.
neu g.
neu/erb-B2 g.
NF1 g.

N-myc g.
N-nyc g.
N-ras g.
nonstructural g's
operator g.
P53 g.
Pck 1 g.
phenylalanine hydroxylase g.
pleiotropic g.
pol (polymerase) g.
polymerase (pol) g.
PR 310 g.
priA g.
priB g.
priC g.
pro (protease) g.
protease (pro) g.
proteolipid g.
raf-1 g.
raf-2 g.
raf/mil g.
ras (rate sarcoma) g.
ras H1 g.
ras K1 g.
ras K2 g.
Rb g.
recessive g.
reciprocal g.
regulator g.
regulatory g.
rel g.
reporter g.
repressed g.
repressor g.
rev g.
rex g.
ros g.
sec 18 g.
secretor g.
sex-conditioned g.
sex-influenced g.
sex-limited g.
sex-linked g.
silent g.
sis g.
ski g.
sor g.
src g.
STOP g.
structural g.
sublethal g.
supplementary g's
suppressor g.

ADDITIONAL TERMS

gene—*Continued*
   syntenic g's
   tas g.
   tat g.
   tat-1 g.
   tax g.
   TcR g.
   TFP3 g.
   topo g.
   transforming g.
   trk g.
   tumor-necrosis factor g.
   tumor-progression g.
   u-fms g.
   V g.
   v-abl g.
   variant surface glycoprotein (VSG) g.
   vbx g.
   v-erbA g.
   v-erbB g.
   v-ets g.
   v-fps g.
   v-Ha-ras g.
   vif g.
   v-Ki-ras g.
   v-kit g.
   v-mil g.
   v-mos g.
   v-myb g.
   v-myc g.
   v-onc g.
   vpr g.
   vpu g.
   v-ras g.
   VSG (variant surface glycoprotein) g.
   v-sis g.
   v-src g.
   wild-type g.
   X-linked g.
   yes g.
   Y-linked g.
gene activation
gene amplification
gene arrangement
gene bank
gene bending
gene block
gene cloning
gene code
gene coding
gene communication

gene complex
gene copy-number
gene deletion
gene designing
gene expression
gene family
gene frequency
gene function
gene fusion
gene inactivation
gene insertion
gene intervention
gene library
gene loci
gene map
gene mapping
gene marker
gene mutation
gene polymorphism
gene pool
gene probe
gene products
gene rearrangement
gene regulation
gene replacement therapy
gene replication
gene repression
gene segment
gene sequence
gene sequencing
gene splicing
gene susceptibility
gene tagging
gene targeting
gene therapy
gene transcription
gene transduction
gene transfer
gene truncation
GeneAmp PCR test
generalized
   disease, g.
   malaise, g.
   malignancy, g.
   metastasis, g.
   Shwartzman reaction, g. (GSR)
   weakness, g.
genesis
genesistasis
genetic
   abnormality, g.
   alteration, g.
   base, g.

ADDITIONAL TERMS

code, g.
counseling, g.
drift, g.
effect, g.
engineering, g.
equilibrium, g.
factor, g.
fingerprinting, g.
immunity, g.
letter, g.
linkage, g.
map, g.
marker, g.
masking tape, g.
molecule, g.
mutation, g.
probe, g.
sequence, g.
switch, g.
tagging, g.
therapy, g.
genetically significant dose (GSD)
Geneticin
geneticist
genetics
    biochemical g.
    molecular g.
Gengou phenomenon
geniocheiloplasty
genital
    carcinoma, g.
    herpes, g.
    neoplasia, g.
    tract, g.
    warts, g.
genitalia
genitography
genitoplasty
genitourinary
    rhabdomyosarcoma, g.
    tract, g.
genocopy
genome
    sequencing, g.
genomic
    clone, g.
    library, g.
    mutation, g.
genotoxic
genotype
genotypic
gentamicin liposome (TLC-G-65)
gentian

blue, g.
violet, g.
Gentran
geophysics
Gerbich
    blood group system, G.
    -negative red cell, G.
germ
    cell, g.
    cell cancer, g.
    cell tumor, g.
    layer tumor, g.
Germanin (suramin sodium)
germanium (Ge)
germinal
    center, g.
    tumor, g.
germinoma
germline
    DNA, g.
    mutation, g.
    theory, g.
Gerota fascia
Gerson
    diet, G.
    method, G.
Gerson-Herrmannsdorfer diet
gerustmark
gestaclone
gestagen
gestational
    trophoblastic neoplasm, g. (GTN)
    tumor, g.
Gesterol (progesterone)
GeV (gigaelectron volt)
Gey solution
GFAP (glial fibrillary acidic protein)
GGT (gamma-glutamyl transferase)
GGT (gamma-glutamyl transpeptidase)
GH (growth hormone)
    -RF, G. (growth hormone-releasing factor)
    -RIH, G. (growth hormone-release-inhibiting hormone)
GH3
Ghajar guide
Ghon
    complex, G.
    focus, G.
    lesion, G.
ghost
    cell, g.
    corpuscle, g.

ADDITIONAL TERMS

ghost—*Continued*
    nodes, g.
GHRF (growth hormone-releasing factor)
GHRH (growth hormone-releasing hormone)
GI (gastrointestinal)
GIA (gastrointestinal anastomosis)
    stapler, G.
Gianotti-Crosti syndrome
giant
    blue nevus, g.
    fibroadenoma, g.
    follicle lymphosarcoma, g.
    follicular lymphoblastoma, g.
    follicular lymphoma, g.
    hairy nevus, g.
    lymph node hyperplasia, g.
    osteoid osteoma, g.
    platelet syndrome, g.
giant cell
    adenocarcinoma, g.
    arteritis, g.
    astrocytoma, g.
    carcinoma, g.
    granuloma, g.
    myeloma, g.
    reparative granuloma, g.
    thyroiditis, g.
    tumor, g.
    xanthoma, g.
Gianturco-Roehm bird's nest vena cava filter
Giardia
    intestinalis, G.
    lamblia, G.
giardiasis
gibbon
    ape lymphosarcoma virus, g. (GaLV)
Gibbs-Donnan equilibrium
Giemsa
    banding technique, G.
    stain, G.
Gierke
    corpuscle, G.
    disease, G.
gigaelectron volt (GeV)
gigantocyte
Gilbert
    phenomenon, G.
    syndrome, G.
Gilchrist mycosis

Gillies flap
Gimenez method
gingiva
gingival
gingivectomy
gingivitis
    acute necrotizing ulcerative g. (ANUG)
    desquamative g.
    gonococcal g.
    herpetic g.
    necrotizing ulcerative g.
    phagedenic g.
    ulceromembranous g.
    Vincent g.
gingivoglossitis
gingivolabial
gingivosis
gingivostomatitis
    herpetic g.
    necrotizing ulcerative g.
ginseng
GIP (gastric inhibitory polypeptide)
gland
glanders
Glandosane
glandular
    cancer, g.
    carcinoma, g.
    hyperplasia, g.
glandulous
glans
    clitoridis, g.
    penis, g.
Glanzmann
    syndrome, G.
    thrombasthenia, G.
glass factor
Glassman gastrostomy
glassy cell
    carcinoma, g.
GLC (gas-liquid chromatography)
Gleason
    grade, G.
    score, G.
    staging, G.
Glenn anastomosis
GLI (glucagon-like immunoreactivity)
glia
Gliadel
glial
    cells, g.
    fibrillary acidic protein, g. (GFAP)

ADDITIONAL TERMS

Glimipride
glioblast
glioblastoma
    multiforme, g. (GBM)
gliocyte
gliocytoma
glioma
    astrocytic g.
    brain stem g.
    endophytum, g.
    ependymal g.
    exophytum, g.
    ganglionic g.
    mixed g.
    nasal g.
    optic g.
    optic chiasm g.
    peripheral g.
    -polyposis syndrome, g.
    pontine g.
    retinae, g.
    sarcomatosum, g.
    telangiectatic g.
gliomatosis
gliomatous
gliomyoma
glioneuroma
gliophagia
gliosarcoma
    retinae, g.
gliosis
glitter cells
GLNS (gay lymph node syndrome)
globe cell
    anemia, g.
globin
    chain, g.
    gene, g.
    mRNA, g.
    pseudogene, g.
globinometer
globulin
    Ac (accelerator) g.
    accelerator (Ac) g.
    alpha g's
    antihemophilic g.
    antihuman g. serum
    antilymphocyte g.
    antithymocyte g.
    beta g's
    corticosteroid-binding g.
    cortisol-binding g.
    gamma g.

    hepatitis B immune g.
    immune g.
    immune human serum g.
    Rho(D) immune g.
    serum g.
    testosterone-estradiol-binding g.
    thyroxine-binding g.
    varicella-zoster immune g. (VZIG)
    X, g.
    zoster-immune g. (ZIG)
glomangioma
glomectomy
glomera (pl. of glomus)
glomerular
    basement membrane, g.
glomerulitis
glomerulonephritis
glomus (pl. glomera)
    body, g.
    jugulare tumor, g.
    tympanicum tumor, g.
glossa
glossagra
glossal
glossalgia
glossectomy
glossitis
glossopathy
glossopharyngeal
glossosteresis
glottic
glottis
Glover serum
glp-1 gene
GLQ223
glucagon
    -like immunoreactivity, g. (GLI)
    stimulation test, g.
glucagonoma
Glucan
glucocerebrosidase
glucocorticoid
glucocorticosteroid
Gluco-Ferrum
Glucometer
glucose
    -6-phosphate dehydrogenase, g.
    (G6PD)
    -6-phosphate isomerase, g. (GPI)
    tolerance test, g.
glucosidase
glucosulfone sodium
glucosylceramidase

ADDITIONAL TERMS

glucosylcerobrosidase
glucosyltransferase
glucuronidase
  beta-g.
glucuronide
glucuronidization
glutamate
  dehydrogenase, g.
  formiminotransferase, g.
glutamate-pyruvic
  anemia, g.
  transaminase, g. (GPT)
glutamic
  -oxaloacetic transaminase, g. (GOT)
  -pyruvic transaminase, g. (GPT)
glutaminase
glutamine
glutamyl transferase (GGT)
glutathione (GSH)
  peroxidase, g.
  reductase, g. (NADPH)
  stability test, g.
  synthetase, g.
  synthetase deficiency, g.
  transferase, g.
glutathionemia
Gluzinski test
glyceraldehyde-3-phosphate
  dehydrogenase (G3PD)
glycerol
  kinase, g.
  -3-phosphate dehydrogenase, g.
glycinamide
  ribonucleotide transformylase, g.
glycogen
glycogenase
glycogenic
glycogenosis
glycohemoglobin
glycol methacrylate
glycolated hemoglobin test
glycolipid
glycolysis
glycolytic
glycopeptide
glycophorin A and C
glycoprotein
  40, g. (GP 41)
  120, g. (GP 120)
  160, g. (GP 160)
glycosaminoglycan (GAG)
glycosylated

hemoglobin, g.
  peptide, g.
glycosylation
glycosylphosphatidylinositol
glycosyltransferase
glycyltryptophan
glycyrrhiza
glycyrrhizin
Gm
  allotype, G.
  antigen, G
  factor, G.
GM (granulocyte-macrophage)
G-6-M (galamustine)
GM-CSA (granulocyte-macrophage
  colony-stimulating activity)
GM-CSF (granulocyte-macrophage
  colony-stimulating factor)
GMK (green monkey kidney)
GMP (guanine monophosphate)
cGMP (cyclic GMP)
GMS (Gomori methenamine silver)
  agonist, G.
GMS (Grocott methenamine silver)
  agonist, G.
gnathoplasty
GnRH (gonadotropin-releasing
  hormone)
goat's milk anemia
Godwin tumor
goiter
  aberrant g.
  adenomatous g.
  Basedow g.
  colloid g.
  congenital g.
  cystic g.
  diffuse g.
  diving g.
  endemic g.
  exophthalmic g.
  fibrous g.   '
  follicular g.
  intrathoracic g.
  iodide g.
  lingual g.
  mediastinal g.
  multinodular g..
  nodular g.
  nontoxic g.
  parenchymatous g.
  retrosternal g.

ADDITIONAL TERMS

retrovascular g.
simple g.
substernal g.
suffocative g.
toxic g.
wandering g.
goitrogen
goitrous
gold
   colloidal g.
   radioactive g.
gold ^{198}Au solution
gold bead-bound avidin
gold seed
gold therapy
Goldie mathematical model
Goldie-Coldman
   hypothesis, G.
   model, G.
Goldstein
   disease, G.
   hematemesis, G.
   rays, G.
Golgi
   apparatus, G.
   complex, G.
   -specific protein, G.
   stack, G.
Gomori
   methenamine silver (GMS)
   reticulin, G.
Gompertz
   curve, G.
   equation, G.
gompertzian
   function, g.
   growth kinetics, g.
   model, g.
gonad
   mean g. dose
   shield, g.
gonadal
   aplasia, g.
   dysfunction, g.
   dysgenesis, g.
gonadectomize
gonadectomy
gonadoblastoma
gonadoinhibitory
gonadotropic
   hormone, g. (GTH)
gonadotropin

human chorionic g. (HCG)
gonadotropin-releasing hormone
   (GnRH)
gonatocele
Gonic
gonioma
gonococcal
gonococci (pl. of gonococcus)
gonococcus (pl. gonococci)
gonorrhea
gonorrheal
gonyoncus
Gonzales
   blood group, G.
   factor, G.
Good
   factor, G.
   syndrome, G.
Goodpasture syndrome
Gordon
   biological test, G.
   elementary body, G.
   encephalopathic agent, G.
Gorlin
   basal cell nevus, G.
   cyst, G.
   syndrome, G.
Gorlin-Chaudhry-Moss syn-
   drome
Gorlin-Goltz syndrome
Gordon
   hemoglobin, G.
   solution, G.
Gore-Tex
   graft, G.
   surgical membrane, G.
   suture, G.
goserelin acetate (ZDX or Zoladex)
GOT (glutamic-oxaloacetic
   transaminase)
Gothlin test
Gott shunt
Gottron papule
Gougerot-Carteaud syndrome
Gougerot-Nulock-Houwer syndrome
gout
gouty
   arthritis, g.
   node, g.
Gower hemoglobin
Gowers solution
GP24/26 antigen

ADDITIONAL TERMS

gp 41 (envelope gene product)
gp 120 (envelope gene product)
gp 160 (envelope gene product)
G3PD (glyceraldehyde-3-phosphate
dehydrogenase)
deficiency, G.
G6PD (glucose-6-phosphate
dehydrogenase)
deficiency, G.
GPI (glucose phosphate isomerase)
GPT (glutamic-pyruvic transaminase)
GR 63178A
grade (G), histopathologic
GX grade cannot be assessed
G1 well differentiated
G2 moderately well differentiated
G3 poorly differentiated
G4 undifferentiated
grading
graft
donor site, g.
rejection, g.
graft-versus-host (GVH)
disease, g. (GVHD)
reaction, g.
graft-versus-leukemia
effect, g.
gram
-amphophilic, g.
atom, g.
-atomic weight, g.
-negative, g.
-positive, g.
-rad, g.
-roentgen, g.
-stained, g.
Gram stain
Gram-Weigart stain
granddaughter cyst
granular cell
myoblastoma, g.
neurofibroma, g.
schwannoma, g.
tumor, g.
granulation
tissue, g.
tumor, g.
granule
granuloblast
granuloblastosis
granulocorpuscle
granulocyte

-colony-stimulating factor, g. (G-
CSF)
-macrophage colony-stimulating
activity, g. (GM-CSA)
-macrophage colony-stimulating
factor, g. (GM-CSF)
macrophage precursor, g.
pool, g.
sarcoma, g.
transfusion, g.
granulocytic
leukemia, g.
sarcoma, g.
granulocytopathy
granulocytopenia
granulocytopoiesis
granulocytopoietic
granulocytosis
granuloma
amebic g.
annulare, g.
apical g.
benign g. of thyroid
beryllium g.
calcified g.
candida g.
candidal g.
caseating g.
cholesterol g.
coccidioidal g.
dental g.
Durck g.
eosinophilic g.
fissuratum, g.
foreign body g.
fungoides, g.
gangraenescens, g.
giant cell reparative g.
gluteale infantum, g.
Hodgkin g.
infectious g.
inguinale, g.
iridis, g.
laryngeal g.
lethal midline g.
lipoid g.
lipophagic g.
Majocchi g.
malarial g.
malignant g.
midline g.
Mignon eosinophilic g.

ADDITIONAL TERMS

monilial g.
multiforme, g.
paracoccidioidal g.
plasma cell g.
pseudopyogenic g.
pudendi, g.
pudens tropicum, g.
pyogenic g.
pyogenicum, g.
reticulohistiocytic g.
silicotic g.
telangiectaticum, g.
trichophytic g.
trichophyticum, g.
venereum, g.
Wegener g.
xanthomatous g.
zirconium g.
granulomatosis
    allergic g.
    benigna, g.
    disciformis progressiva et chronica,
        g.
    eosinophilic g.
    Langerhans cell g.
    lymphomatoid g.
    malignant g.
    siderotica, g.
    Wegener g.
granulomatous
    colitis, g.
    disease, g.
    lesion, g.
    lymphoma, g.
granulomere
granulopenia
granuloplastic
granulopoiesis
granulopoietic
granulopotent
granulosa
    cell, g.
    cell tumor, g.
    -theca cell tumor, g.
grape
    cell, g.
    diet, g.
    mole, g.
Gratiolet radiation
Graves disease
graviton
Gravlee

jet washer, G.
washing, G.
Grawitz tumor
gray (Gy)
    scale imaging, g.
gray platelet syndrome
Graydon factor
Great Ormond Street tracheostomy
Greck ileostomy bag
green
    blood, g. (Fluosol-DA/02)
    cancer, g.
    tea, g.
Greene biopsy needle
Greenfield disease
Greenland-Robbins confidence limits
Greenwald and Lewman method
Greenwood survival formula
Gregerson and Boas test
grenz ray
grid
    Fixott-Everett g.
GRID (gay-related immunodeficiency)
grid therapy
grief
    counseling, g.
    reaction, g.
    therapy, g.
grieve
grieving
Grimelius
    silver, G.
    stain, G.
Griscelli syndrome
griseofulvin
gritty tumor
GRO gene
Grocott methenamine silver (GMS)
groEL protein
Grollman catheter
Groshong catheter
gross
    anatomy, g.
    appearance, g.
    description, g.
    findings, g.
    lesion, g.
    pathology, g.
    tumor, g.
Gross
    cell surface antigen, G.
    leukemia virus, G.

ADDITIONAL TERMS

Gross—*Continued*
  sarcoma virus, G.
Grotthus law
Grotton sign
ground
  -glass appearance, g.
  -itch anemia, g.
  zero, g.
group
  agglutination, g.
  agglutinin, g.
  precipitation, g.
  -specific, g.
  -transfer, g.
grouping
  blood g.
  hapten g.
growth factor
growth hormone (GH)
  -producing tumor, g.
  -releasing factor, g. (GH-RF)
  -release-inhibiting hormone, g.
    (GH-RIH)
GRP (gastrin-releasing peptide)
GSD (genetically significant dose)
GSH (reduced glutathione)
GSSG (oxidized glutathione)
GSR (generalized Shwartzman reaction)
GTH (gonadotropic hormone)
GTM (grade, tumor, metastasis)
  classification, G.
GTN (gestational trophoblastic
  neoplasm)
GTP (guanosine triphosphate)
  cyclohydrolase, G.
guaiac
guaiac'd
guanase
guanidine
  hydrochloride, g.
guanidinemia
guanine
  deaminase, g.
  nucleotide protein, g.
guanosine
  cyclic g. monophosphate (cGMP or
    cyclic GMP)
  derivative, g.
  diphosphate, g. (GDP)
  monophosphate, g. (GMP)
  triphosphate, g. (GTP)
guanylic acid
guanylyl

Gubler tumor
guided
  imagery, g.
  -needle aspiration cytology, g.
guillotine amputation
Guinard treatment
gum bleeding
gumma (pl. gummata)
gummata (pl. of gumma)
gummy tumor
gun-barrel enterostomy
Gun Hill hemoglobin
Gunther disease
Gussenbauer artificial larynx
gut-associated lymphoid tissue (GALT)
Guthrie bacterial inhibition assay
GVH (graft-versus-host)
GVHD (graft-versus-host-disease)
Gy (gray)
gynander
gynandrism
gynandroblastoma
gynandroid
gynecography
gynecologic
gynecological
  cryosurgery, g.
  malignancy, g.
gynecology
gynecomastia
Gynogen (estradiol)
gyrase

H H (host classification/physical
  state of patient)
    H0 (normal activity)
    H1 (symptomatic and
  ambulatory; cares for self)
  H2 (ambulatory more than 50% of
  time; occasionally needs
  assistance)
  H3 (ambulatory 50% or less of
  time; nursing care needed)
  H4 (bedridden; may need
  hospitalization)
H (Hounsfield unit)
H agglutination
H agglutinin
H antigen
H2 antigen
H blood group system
H cells

ADDITIONAL TERMS

H (heavy) chain
H2 complex
H (histocompatibility) gene
H rays
H2 receptor
H unit (Holzknecht unit)
Ha (hahnium)
HA (hepatitis A)
HA Ag (hepatitis A antigen)
HAA (hepatitis-associated antigen)
HAA (hepatitis-associated aplasia)
Haaga biopsy needle
Haagensen
　criteria, H.
　staging of breast carcinoma, H.
　　(stages A, B, C, etc.)
　test, H.
　triple biopsy of breast, H.
Haagensen-Stout
　classification, H.
　criteria, H.
HAb23 antibody
Haber toxicologic principles
HAD (hexamethylmelamine,
　Adriamycin, DDP)
Hadley vaccine
hadron
HAE (hepatic artery embolization)
haema
Haemate P
Haemonetics
　autologous blood recovery system,
　　H.
　bone marrow transplant system, H.
　cell saver, H.
Haemophilus (Hemophilus)
　aegyptius, H.
　ducreyi, H.
　influenzae, H.
　paraphrophilus, H.
　pertussis, H.
　vaginalis, H.
Haering esophageal prosthesis
Hafnia
　alvei, H.
Hagedorn needle
Hagedorn and Jansen method
Hageman factor (HF)
hahnium (Ha)
HAHTG (horse antihuman thymus
　globulin)
HAI (hemagglutination inhibition)
HAI (hepatic artery infusion)

Hailey-Hailey disease
hair-matrix carcinoma
hairy
　cell, h.
　cell leukemia, h. (HCL)
　leukoplakia, h.
　nevus, h.
　sore, h.
haisung
Haitian
　AIDS, H.
　HIV virus, H.
Halbrecht syndrome
Halethazole
half-body irradiation (HBI)
half-life (HL)
　antibody h.
　biological h.
　effective h.
　physical h.
half-time
　plasma iron clearance h.
half-value
　layer, h. (HVL)
　thickness, h.
halo nevus
Halodrin (fluoxymesterone)
halogenated
　thymidine analog, h.
halometer
halometry
Halotestin (fluoxymesterone)
Halsted mastectomy
HAM (hexamethylmelamine,
　Adriamycin, melphalan)
HAM (hexamethylmelamine,
　Adriamycin, methotrexate)
HAM (human albumin microspheres)
Ham test
HAMA (human antimurine antibody)
hamangiopericytoma
hamartoblastoma
hamartoma
hamartomatosis
hamartomatous
Hamburger
　effect, H.
　interchange, H.
　phenomenon, H.
Hammar myoid cells
Hammarsten test
Hammerschlag method
Hammersmith hemoglobin

ADDITIONAL TERMS

HAMP (hexamethylmelamine,
    Adriamycin, methotrexate, Platinol)
Hampson unit
HAN (hyperplastic alveolar nodules)
Hancock amputation
Hand disease
hand-mirror cell leukemia
Hand-Schüller-Christian disease
Hanford Nuclear Reservation
Hanger test
Hankins lucite ovoid
Hanks balanced salt solution
Hanot disease
Hansel stain
Hansen
    bacillus, H.
    disease, H.
haploid
haploidentical
haploidentity
haploidy
haplophase
haplotype
Hapsburg disease
hapten
    -carrier complex, h.
    inhibition test, h.
haptenic
haptoglobin (Hp)
hard
    cancer, h.
    fibroma, h.
    nodule, h.
    ray, h.
    x-ray imaging spectrometer, h.
        (HXIS)
Harding Passey melanoma
Hardy-Weinberg equilibrium
Hardy-Zuckerman
    2 feline sarcoma virus, H.
    4 feline sarcoma virus, H.
C Harlem hemoglobin
Harley disease
Harting bodies
Hartmann
    colostomy, H.
    pouch, H.
    procedure, H.
    solution, H.
Hartmanella
    hyalina, H.
Harvard pump
harvested

harvesting
    bone marrow h.
    peripheral stem cell h. (PSCH)
Harvey sarcoma virus
Hasharon hemoglobin
Hashimoto
    disease, H.
    struma, H.
    thyroiditis, H.
Hassall corpuscles
HAT (heparin-associated
    thrombocytopenia)
HAT (hypoxanthine-aminopterin-
    thymidine)
Hata phenomenon
haupt agglutinin
Hauser program
HAV (hepatitis A virus)
HAVAB EIA test
Hawkins breast localization needle
Hayem
    corpuscles, H.
    solution, H.
Hayem-Widal
    anemia, H.
    syndrome, H.
Haygarth deformities
hazardous
    material, h. (hazmat)
    waste, h.
hazmat (hazardous material)
Hb (hemoglobin)
HB (hepatitis B)
HBA71 antigen
HB Ag (hepatitis B antigen)
HBC (hyperimmune bovine colostrum)
HBcAb (hepatitis B core antibody)
HBeAb (hepatitis B e antibody)
HBeAg (hepatitis B e antigen)
HBI (half-body irradiation)
HBI (hemibody irradiation)
HBI (high serum-bound iron)
HBI fusion protein
HBIg (hepatitis B immune globulin)
HBLV (human B-lymphotrophic virus)
HBO (hyperbaric oxygen)
HbO_2 (oxyhemoglobin)
HBsAb (hepatitis B surface antibody)
HBsAg (hepatitis B surface antigen)
HBV (hepatitis B virus)
HC (hydrocortisone)
4-HC (4-hydroperoxycyclophosphamide
    or Pergamid)

ADDITIONAL TERMS

HCAO (hexamethylmelamine, cyclophosphamide, Adriamycin, Platinol)
H-CAP (hexamethylmelamine, cyclophosphamide, Adriamycin, Platinol)
HCC (hepatocellular carcinoma)
HCD (heavy-chain disease)
hCG (human chorionic gonadotropin)
    -producing tumor, H.
    test, H.
HCL (hairy-cell leukemia)
HCT (hematocrit)
HCV (hepatitis C virus)
HD (Hansen disease)
HD (high dose)
HD (Hodgkin disease)
H2D
    determinant, H.
    gene cluster, H.
HDARA-C (high-dose ara-C)
HDC (high-dose chemotherapy)
HDC (pentostatin)
HDL (high-density lipoprotein)
HDMP (high-dose methylprednisolone)
HDMTX (high-dose methotrexate)
HDMTX/LV (high-dose methotrexate/ with leucovorin rescue)
HDN (hemolytic disease of newborn)
HDPEB (high-dose PEB [Platinol, etoposide, bleomycin])
HD-VAC (high-dose methotrexate plus vinblastine, Adriamycin, cisplatin)
HDZ (hydrazine sulfate)
HE (hereditary elliptocytosis)
H&E (hematoxylin-eosin)
    stain, H.
He (helium)
Heaf
    gun, H.
    test, H.
heaped-up edges
heat
    exchanger, h.
    -shock gene, h.
    -shock proteins, h.
    -stable, h.
    -stable lactic dehydrogenase, h. (HLDH)
HEAT (human erythrocyte agglutination test)
heavy
    -chain, h.

-charged particle therapy, h.
hydrogen, h.
ion accelerator, h.
ion imaging, h.
ion irradiation, h.
ion mammography, h.
ions, h.
metal, h.
-metal screening, h.
particle, h.
particle counter, h.
particle therapy, h.
polypeptide chains, h.
water, h.
heavy chain disease (HCD)
    alpha h.
    gamma h.
    mu h.
Hecht pneumonia
heckle cell
HED (Haut-Einheits-Dosis)
hedaquinium chloride
Hedspa
heelstick hematocrit
Heerfordt disease
Heidenhaim
    cell, H.
    iron hematoxylin stain, H.
Heineke-Mikulicz
    gastroenterostomy, H.
    pyloroplasty, H.
Heinz
    bodies, H.
    body hemolytic anemia, h.
    granules, H.
Heinz-Ehrlich bodies
Hektoen phenomenon
Hektoen, Kretschmer, and Welker protein
HeLa (Henrietta Lacks) cells
Helicobacter
    pylorii, H.
heliotrope erythema
helium (He)
    ion, h.
    -neon, h. (He-He)
    -neon laser, h. (He-Ne laser)
helix
    alpha h.
    double h.
    -loop-helix protein, h.
    Watson-Crick h.
Heller operation

ADDITIONAL TERMS

HELLP (hemolysis, elevated liver
    enzymes, low platelet count)
    syndrome, H.
helmet cell
helminthoma
Helminthosporium
helper
    cells, h.
    -inducer cells, h.
    -suppressor cells, h.
    -suppressor cell ratio, h.
    T-cells, h.
Helsper laryngectomy button
HEM (hereditary erythroblastic
    multinuclearity)
hemachromatosis
hemachrome
hemacytometer
hemacytometry
hemad
hemadsorbent
hemadsorption
hemafacient
hemagglutinating
    antibody, h.
    anti-penicillin antibody, h.
hemagglutination
    indirect h.
    passive h.
    viral h.
hemagglutination inhibition (HAI or HI)
hemagglutination titer
hemagglutinative
hemagglutinin
    cold h.
    warm h.
hemal
hemalum stain
hemanalysis
hemangioameloblastoma
hemangioblastoma
hemangioblastomatosis
hemangioendothelial
hemangioendothelioblastoma
hemangioendothelioma
    benign h.
    malignant h.
hemangioendotheliosarcoma
hemangiofibroma
hemangioma (pl. hemangiomata)
    ameloblastic h.
    arteriovenous h.
    capillary h.

cavernous h.
sclerosing h.
simplex, h.
soap-bubble h.
strawberry h.
sunburst h.
hemangioma-thrombocytopenia
    syndrome
hemangiomata (pl. of hemangioma)
hemangiomatosis
hemangiopericyte
hemangiopericytoma
hemangiosarcoma
hemapheresis
hemartoma
hemarthroses (pl. of hemarthrosis)
hemarthrosis (pl. hemarthroses)
hematal
hematapostema
hematein test
hematemesis
Hematest
hematherapy
hematic
hematin
hematinemia
hematinic
hematinometer
hematinometry
hematoblast
hematocele
    parametric h.
    pelvic h.
    pudendal h.
    retrouterine h.
    scrotal h.
    vaginal h.
hematochezia
hematocrit (HCT)
    large vessel h.
    total body h.
    whole body h.
    Wintrobe h.
hematocrystallin
hematocyanin
hematocyte
hematocytolysis
hematocytometer
hematocytopenia
hematocyturia
hematogen
hematogenic
hematogenous

ADDITIONAL TERMS ■■■

metastases, h.
pathways, h.
spread of cancer, h.
hematoglobin
hematoglobulin
hematogone
hematoid
hematoidin
  crystals, h.
hematologic
hematologist
hematology
hematolymphangioma
hematolysis
hematoma
hematometer
hematometry
hematomole
hematonic
hematopathology
hematopenia
hematophage
hematophagocyte
hematoplastic
hematopneic
  index, h.
hematopoiesis
  extramedullary h.
  megaloblastic h.
hematopoietic
  growth factor, h.
  maturation, h.
  system, h.
hematopoietin
hematoporphyrin
  derivative, h. (HPD)
hematoporphyrinemia
hematospectrophotometer
hematospectroscope
hematospectroscopy
hematospermatocele
hematospherinemia
hematostatic
hematosteon
hematotherapy
hematotoxic
hematotoxicosis
hematotropic
hematoxylin-eosin (HE)
  azure II stain, h.
hematoxyphilic
hematozemia
hematuria

heme
  arginate, h.
  -oxygenase, h.
  pigment, h.
  pocket, h.
  synthesis, h.
  -synthetase, h.
hemendothelioma
hemiallogeneic
hemiangioma
hemiataxia
hemibody
  irradiation, h. (HBI)
hemic
hemicolectomy
hemicorporectomy
hemicraniectomy
hemicraniosis
hemidesmosome
hemigastrectomy
hemiglossectomy
hemihepatectomy
hemilaryngectomy
hemilesion
hemimandibulectomy
hemimaxillectomy
hemin
heminephrectomy
heminephroureterectomy
hemipelvectomy
hemipelvis
hemiplegia
hemiplegic
hemiprostatectomy
hemipylorectomy
hemisection
hemisoantibody
hemisphere
hemispherectomy
hemispheric
hemistrumectomy
hemithorax
hemithyroidectomy
hemizygosity
hemizygous
Hemlock Society
hemoaccess
hemoagglutination
hemoagglutinin
hemoblast
    lymphoid h. of Pappenheim
hemoblastic
hemoblastosis

ADDITIONAL TERMS

hemocatheresis
hemocatheretic
Hemoccult test
hemochromatosis
hemochromatotic
hemochrome
hemochromogen
   hemoglobin h.
hemochromometer
hemoclasia
hemoclasis
hemoclastic
   crisis, h.
hemocoagulin
hemoconcentration
hemoconia
hemoconiosis
hemocrinotherapy
hemocryoscopy
hemocrystallin
HemoCue photometer
hemoculture
hemocyanin
   keyhole-limpet h. (KLH)
hemocyte
hemocytoblast
hemocytoblastic
hemocytoblastoma
hemocytocatheresis
hemocytogenesis
hemocytology
hemocytolysis
hemocytoma
hemocytometer
hemocytometry
hemocytophagia
hemocytophagic
hemocytopoiesis
hemocytopoietic
hemocytotripsis
hemodiagnosis
Hemo-Dial dialysate additive
hemodialysis
hemodialyze
hemodialyzer
hemodilution
hemodynamic
hemodystrophy
Hemofil T
hemofilter
hemofiltration
hemofuscin
hemogenesis

hemoglobin (Hgb)
   A, h.
   A2, h.
   Alc, h.
   acetylated h.
   A/F, h.
   Bart, h.
   C, h.
   C Harlem h.
   carbamate, h.
   carbamoylated h.
   Chesapeake, h.
   Constant Spring, h.
   D, h.
   deoxygenated h.
   E, h.
   embryonic h.
   F (fetal), h.
   fast h's
   fetal (F) h.
   G, h.
   G Philadelphia, h.
   glycosylated h.
   Gower h.
   Gun Hill, h.
   H, h.
   Hammersmith, h.
   Hasharon, h.
   I, h.
   Indianapolis, h.
   intracellular h.
   Kansas, h.
   Kenya, h.
   Köln, h.
   Korle Bu, h.
   Lepore, h.
   M. h.
   mean corpuscular h. (MCH)
   Milwaukee, h.
   muscle h.
   mutant h.
   nitric oxide h.
   Norfolk, h.
   oxidized h.
   oxygenated h.
   Portland, h.
   primitive h.
   pyridoxilated stroma-free h. (SFHb)
   Rainier, h.
   reduced h.
   S. h.
   Saskatoon, h.
   SC, h.

ADDITIONAL TERMS

SD, h.
Seattle, h.
slow h's
SO, h.
Yakima, h.
Zurich, h.
hemoglobin-binding capacity
hemoglobin C-beta thalassemia
hemoglobin C trait
hemoglobin disease
hemoglobin E-beta thalassemia
hemoglobin electrophoresis
hemoglobin hemochromogen
hemoglobin Korle Bu sickle disease
hemoglobin nadir
hemoglobin-oxygen dissociation curve
hemoglobin Q-alpha thalassemia
hemoglobin SC disease
hemoglobin SD sickle disease
hemoglobin SO Arab sickle disease
hemoglobinated
hemoglobinemia
hemoglobinolysis
hemoglobinometer
hemoglobinometry
hemoglobinopathy
hemoglobinopepsia
hemoglobinophilic
hemoglobinous
hemoglobinuria
    epidemic h.
    intermittent h.
    march h.
    paroxysmal cold h. (PCH)
    paroxysmal nocturnal h. (PNH)
    toxic h.
hemoglobinuric
hemogram
hemohistioblast
hemohistioblastic
hemokonia
hemokoniosis
hemolymph
    heteroagglutinin, h.
hemolymphangioma
hemolysate
hemolysin
    alpha h.
    bacterial h.
    beta h.
    heterophile h.
    hot-cold h.
    immune h.

hemolysis
    alpha h.
    beta h.
    contact h.
    Donath-Landsteiner cold h.
    drug-induced h.
    extravascular h.
    fragmentation h.
    gamma h.
    immune h.
    passive h.
    venom h.
hemolytic
    anemia, h.
    complement assay, h.
    crisis, h.
    disease of newborn, h. (HDN)
    icteroanemia, h.
    icterus, h.
    jaundice, h.
    plaque assay, h.
    splenomegaly, h.
    -uremic syndrome, h. (HUS)
hemolytopoiesis
hemolytopoietic
hemolyzable
hemolyzation
hemolyze
hemopathic
hemopathology
hemopathy
hemoperfusion
hemopexin
hemophage
hemophagocyte
hemophagocytic
hemophagocytosis
hemophil
hemophilia
    A, h.
    B, h.
    B Leyden, h.
    C, h.
    classical h.
    Hapsburg h.
    neonatorum, h.
    vascular h.
hemophiliac
hemophilic
hemophilioid
Hemophilus (Haemophilus)
    aegyptius, H.
    ducreyi, H.

ADDITIONAL TERMS

Hemophilus (Haemophilus)—*Continued*
  influenzae, H.
  paraphrophilus, H.
  pertussis, H.
  vaginalis, H.
hemophthisis
hemopoiesis
hemopoietin
hemoprecipitin
hemoproctia
hemoprotein
hemopsonin
hemoptic
hemoptysic
hemoptysis
hemorrhage
hemorrhagenic
hemorrhagic
  anemia, h.
  ascites, h.
  disease of newborn, h.
  fever, h.
  thrombocytopenia, h.
hemorrhagin
hemosiderin
hemosiderosis
  hepatic h.
  pulmonary h.
  transfusion h.
hemosiderotic
hemostased
hemostasis
hemostatic
Hemostix
hemotherapeutics
hemotherapy
hemotoxin
  cobra h.
hemozoin
HEMPAS (hereditary erythroblasic
  multinuclearity with positive acidified
  serum test)
He-Ne (helium-neon)
  laser, H.
Henle
  fibrin, H.
  loop, H.
  trunk, H.
Henoch purpura
Henoch-Schönlein
  purpura, H.
  syndrome, H.
Henry test

Henschke
  colpostat, H.
  ovoid, H.
  tandem, H.
Henschke-Mauch unit
HEPA (high-efficiency particulate air)
heparan sulfate
heparanase
heparin
  drip, h.
  flush, h.
  lock, h. (hep-lock)
  sodium, h.
  sulfate proteoglycan anticoagulant,
    h.
heparinate
heparinemia
heparinize
HepatAmine
hepatectomize
hepatectomy
hepatic
  adenoma, h.
  angiosarcoma, h.
  artery embolization, h. (HAE)
  artery infusion, h. (HAI)
  bed, h.
  carcinoma, h.
  fibrosis, h.
  lobectomy, h.
  lobes, h.
  metastases, h.
  necrosis, h.
  neoplasm, h.
  outflow tract, h.
  parenchyma, h.
  porphyria, h.
  resection, h.
  tumor, h.
  venous web disease, h.
  web dilatation, h.
  zones, h.
hepatides (pl. of hepatitis)
hepatitis (pl. hepatitides)
  A, h. (HA)
  acute parenchymatous h.
  acute viral h.
  amebic h.
  anicteric h.
  autoimmune h.
  B, h. (HB)
  C, h. (formerly called non-A, non-B
    hepatitis)

ADDITIONAL TERMS

cholangiolitic h.
cholangitic h.
cholestatic h.
chronic active h.
chronic aggressive h.
chronic interstitial h.
chronic persistent h.
delta agent h.
drug-induced h.
E, h.
epidemic h.
F, h. (non-A, non-B, non-C
  hepatitis)
familial h.
fulminant h.
giant cell h.
halothane h.
homologous serum h.
infectious h.
inoculation h.
long-incubation h.
lupoid h.
MS-1 h.
MS-2 h.
NANB (non-A, non-B) h. (now
  called hepatitis C)
neonatal h.
neonatal giant cell h.
non-A h.
non-A, non-B (NANB) h. (now
  called hepatitis C)
non-B h.
plasma cell h.
posttransfusion h.
serum h.
short-incubation h.
subacute h.
syphilitic h.
toxic h.
transfusion h.
viral h.
hepatitis A antigen (HAAg)
hepatitis A virus (HAV)
hepatitis-associated antigen (HAA)
hepatitis-associated aplasia (HAA)
hepatitis B antigen (HBAg)
hepatitis B core antibody (HBcAb)
hepatitis B e antibody (HBeAb)
hepatitis B e antigen (HBeAg)
hepatitis B immune globulin (HBIG)
hepatitis B surface antibody (HBsAb)
hepatitis B surface antigen (HBsAg)
hepatitis B virus (HBV)

hepatitis B virus vaccine inactivated
hepatitis C virus (HCV)
hepatization
hepatobiliary
  tree, h.
hepatoblastoma
hepatocarcinogen
hepatocarcinogenesis
hepatocarcinogenic
hepatocarcinoma
hepatocele
hepatocellular
  cancer, h.
  carcinoma, h.
hepatocholangiocarcinoma
hepatocholangioduodenostomy
hepatocholangioenterostomy
hepatocholangiostomy
hepatocirrhosis
hepatocyte
  nuclear factor, h.
  -stimulating factor, h.
hepatoenterostomy
hepatogastric
hepatogenic
hepatogenous
hepatogram
hepatography
hepato-iminodiacetic acid (HIDA)
  scan, h.
hepatolienal
hepatolienography
hepatolienomegaly
hepatolysin
hepatolytic
hepatoma
  malignant h.
hepatomegaly
hepatomelanosis
hepatonecrosis
hepatonephromegaly
  glycogenica, h.
hepatopathy
hepatophage
hepatophlebography
hepatoportal
hepatoportogram
hepatopulmonary
hepatorenal
hepatoscan
hepatoscopy
hepatosplenic
hepatosplenitis

ADDITIONAL TERMS

hepatosplenography
hepatosplenomegaly (HSM)
hepatosplenopathy
hepatostomy
hepatotoxemia
hepatotoxicity
Hep-B-Gammagee
hep-lock (heparin lock)
Heprofile ELISA
hepsulfam
HEPT derivative
heptad
heptapeptide
Heptavax-B
heptoglobin
heptoglobinemia
herbal
    extract, h.
    tea, h.
herbicide
hereditary
    elliptocytosis, h.
    erythroblastic multinuclearity, h.
    (HEM)
    erythroblastic multinuclearity with
    positive acidified serum test, h.
    (HEMPAS)
    hemorrhagic telangiectasia, h.
    nonspherocytic hemolytic anemia,
    h.
    persistence of fetal hemoglobin, h.
    (HPFH)
    plasmathromboplastin component,
    h.
    spherocytosis, h.
heredity
heredofamilial
HER-2 gene
heritable
Herlitz disease
Hermansky-Pudlak syndrome
Hermes-1 epitope
HER-neu oncogene
heroin
heroinism
HERP (human exposure dose/rodent
  potency dose)
Herp-Check
herpes
    anorectal h.
    corneae, h.
    digitalis, h.
    encephalitis, h.

facialis, h.
febrilis, h.
genital h.
genitalis, h.
gestational h.
gestationis, h.
gladiatorum, h.
labialis, h.
McKrae strain h.
menstrualis, h.
ocular h.
ophthalmicus, h.
pharyngeal h.
progenitalis, h.
simian h.
simplex, h.
traumatic h.
wrestler's h.
zoster, h.
zoster auricularis, h.
zoster ophthalmicus, h.
zoster oticus, h.
herpes-like virus (HLV)
herpes simplex virus (HSV)
    types I, II, h. (HSV I, II)
herpes-specific enzyme
herpes whitlow
herpes zoster virus (HZV)
herpesencephalitis
Herpesviridae
Herpesvirus (HV)
    hominis, H.
    saimiri, H.
    simiae, H.
herpesvirus
    McKrae strain h.
herpetic
    gingivostomatitis, h.
    lesion, h.
    proctitis, h.
    sore throat, h.
    whitlow, h.
herpetiform
herpetiformis
Herpex Liquifilm
Herplex (idoxuridine)
Herrick anemia
hertz (Hz)
Herxheimer reaction
Heryng sign
HES (hypereosinophilic syndrome)
Hespan
hesperidin

ADDITIONAL TERMS

hetastarch plasma expander
HETE (hydroxyeicosatetaraenoic acid)
heteradenoma
heteroagglutination
heteroagglutinin
heteroantibody
heteroantigen
heteroautoplasty
heteroblastic
heterocellular
heterochromatin
heterochromatinization
heteroclitic
heterocliticity
heterocycle
heterocyclic
heterocytotropic
heterodimer
heterodimeric
heteroduplex
heterogeneic
heterogeneity
    genetic h.
heterogeneous
    nuclear RNA, h.
heterogenesis
heterogenetic
heterogenote
heterogeny
heterohemagglutination
heterohemagglutinin
heterohemolysin
heterohemolysis
heterohemolytic
heteroimmune
heteroimmunity
heterokaryon
heterokaryosis
heterologous
    antigen, h.
heterology
heterolysin
heterolysis
heterolytic
heterometaplasia
heteronuclear
heterophil
    antibody, h.
    antigen, h.
    hemolysin, h.
heterophilic
    leukocyte, h.
heteroplasia

heteroplastic
heteroploid
heteroploidy
heteropolymer
heteropyknosis
heteropyknotic
heteroserotherapy
heterosexual
heterosexuality
heterotopia
heterotopic
heterotransplant
heterotransplantation
heterotypic
heterotypical
heterozygosis
heterozygosity
heterozygote
heterozygous
    hemoglobinopathy, h.
    thalassemia, h.
Heublein irradiation method
Hewitt criteria
Hexa-CAF (Hexalen, cyclophosphamide,
    Adrucil, Folex)
hexad
Hexadrol
Hexalen (hexamethylmelamine)
hexamethylene bisacetamide (HMBA)
hexamethylmelamine (altretamine or
    Hexalen or Hexastat or HMM or HXM)
Hexastat (hexamethylmelamine)
hexose
    monophosphate shunt, h.
Hey amputation
Heyer-Schulte tissue expander
Heyman capsule
Heymann nephritis
Heyman-Simon capsule
HF (Hageman factor)
Hgb (hemoglobin)
HGG (human gamma globulin)
hGH (human growth hormone)
hGHr (human growth hormone-
    recombinant)
HGP-30
HGPRT (hypoxanthine-guanine
    phosphoribosyltransferase)
H&H (hemoglobin and hematocrit)
HHNC (hyperosmolar hyperglycemic
    nonketotic coma)
HHNK (hyperglycemic hyperosmolar
    nonketotic)

ADDITIONAL TERMS

HHT (homoharringtonine)
HHT (hydroxyhepadecatrienoic acid)
HHV-6 (human herpesvirus-6)
HI (hemagglutination inhibition)
 titer, H.
5-HIAA (5-hydroxy-indoleacetic acid)
hibernoma
HiC-COM (ara-C, citrovorum factor,
 allopurinol, Elliot B solution,
 cyclophosphamide, Oncovin,
 methotrexate)
Hickey-Hare test
Hickman catheter
Hicks-Pitney thromboplastin generation
 test
HICRV (human intracisternal retrovirus)
HIDA (hepato-iminodiacetic acid)
 scan, H.
HIDAC (high-dose ara-C)
hidden determinant
hidradenoma
 eruptivum, h.
hidradenocarcinoma
hidrocystoma
Hieshima coaxial catheter
high
 -density lipoprotein, h. (HDL)
 -dose chemotherapy, h. (HDC)
 -dose radiation therapy, h.
 -dose tolerance, h.
 -efficiency particulate air, h.
 (HEPA)
 -energy linear accelerator, h.
 -energy photons, h.
 LET (linear energy transfer)
 irradiation, h.
 LET (linear energy transfer)
 radiation, h.
 linear energy irradiation, h.
 linear energy transfer (LET), h.
 mobility group, h. (HMG)
 -molecular-weight neutrophil
 chemotactic factor, h. (HMW-
 NCF)
 -performance liquid
 chromatography, h. (HPLC)
 -power field, h. (hpf)
 -resolution darkfield electron
 microscopy, h.
 serum-bound iron, h. (HBI)
 -voltage electrophoresis, h. (HVE)
high-risk
 ATAC, h. (L-asparaginase, ara-C,

 VP-16, anti-J2 26 monoclonal
 antibody, anti-CALLA hybridoma
 antibody)
 behavior, h.
 patient, h.
 population, h.
 sex, h.
hilar
 adenoma, h.
 adenopathy, h.
 dissection, h.
 lymph node, h.
 lymphadenopathy, h.
hilus cell
 tumor, h.
hindquarter amputation
hinge region
Hinton test
Hipputope
Hiroshima atomic bomb explosion
hirsute
hirsuties
hirsutism
hirudin
hirudiniasis
hirudinization
histaminase
histamine
 -fast, h.
 -releasing factor, h. (HRF)
Histerone (testosterone)
histidine loading test
histidinemia
histioblast
histiocyte
histiocytic
 cells, h.
 leukemia, h.
 lymphoma, h.
 medullary reticulosis, h. (HMR)
histiocytoma
 fibrous h.
 lipoid h.
histiocytomatosis
histiocytosis
 sinus h.
 X, h.
histioma
histo (histology)
histoblast
histochemical
histochemistry
histochemotherapy

ADDITIONAL TERMS

histochromatosis
histoclastic
histocompatibility
    antigens, h.
    complex, h.
    genes, h.
    locus, h.
histocompatible
histocyte
histocytic
histodiagnosis
histodifferentiation
histofluorescence
histogenesis
histohematogenous
histoid
histoincompatibility
histoincompatible
histologic
    diagnosis, h.
    grading, h.
    lesion, h.
histologically
    benign, h.
    malignant, h.
    significant, h.
histology
histolysis
histolytic
histoma
histometaplastic
histone
    gene, h.
    nucleinate, h.
histopathologic
histopathology
histophysiology
Histoplasma
    capsulatum, H.
    capsulatum polysaccharide
      antigen, H. (HPA)
    duboisii, H.
    farciminosus, H.
histoplasmic
histoplasmin
histoplasmoma
histoplasmosis
histothrombin
histotope
histotoxic
    anoxia, h.
histrelin
histotropic

HIV (human immunodeficiency virus)
    -1, H.
    -2, H.
    AC1e vaccine, H.
    -Ag, H. (HIV antigen)
    -associated, H.
    -associated thrombocytopenia, H.
    bands, H.
    dementia, H.
    -1 Eli strain, H.
    -1 ELISA, H.
    embryopathy, H.
    encephalopathy, H.
    envelope protein, H.
    Immunogen, H.
    -induced, H.
    -infected macrophage, H.
    -1 nef gene, H.
    p24 antigen, H.
    proviral clone pHXBc2, H.
    -1 specific primer pair, H. (SK38-39)
    transmission, H.
    wasting syndrome, H.
HIVAGEN test
HIVID (ddC or dideoxycytidine)
HIVIG (anti-HIV immune serum globulin)
HK (heat-killed)
H2K
    determinant, H.
    locus, H.
HKLM (heat-killed Listeria monocytogenes)
HL (half-life)
HL-60 cell
HLA (human leukocyte antigens)
    -A, H.
    -B antigen, H.
    -B8, H.
    -B27, H.
    -C antigen, H.
    -C8, H.
    -compatible, H.
    -D antigen, H.
    -DR, H.
    -DR 1, H.
    -DR 2, H.
    -DR 5, H.
    -identical, H.
    -L antigen, H.
    -linked disease, H.
    -matched, H.

ADDITIONAL TERMS

HLA —*Continued*
-matching, H.
-mismatched, H.
-nonidentical marrow, H.
-transgenic mice, H.
-typing, H.
HLA (human lymphocyte antigens)
HLDH (heat-stable lactic
dehydrogenase)
HLV (herpes-like virus)
HMA-CMV (human monoclonal
antibody to cytomegalovirus)
HMBA (hexamethylene bisacetamide)
HMD (oxymetholone)
HMFG-2 (human milk fat globule
antigen-2)
HMG (high-mobility group)
HMM (hexamethylmelamine)
HMTX (high-dose methotrexate)
HMW-NCF (high molecular weight-
neutrophil chemotactic factor)
HN2 (mechlorethamine)
HN2 (nitrogen mustard)
Ho (holmium)
HO gene
HOAP-BLEO (hydroxydaunomycin,
Oncovin, ara-C, prednisone, bleomycin)
hoarse voice
hoarseness
hobnail
appearance, h.
cells, h.
liver, h.
Hochenegg operation
hockey-stick effect
Hockin lucite ovoid
Hodgkin
cells, H.
disease, H.
granuloma, H.
lymphoma, H.
sarcoma, H.
HOE 602
HOE-BAY 964
Hoechst 33342
cells, H.
dye diffusion, H.
Hoerr rule
Hofbauer cells
Hoffmeister series
Hogness box
holandric genes
holistic

medicine, h.
therapy, h.
Hollande solution
Holliday junction
Hollinghead antigen
hollow fiber dialyzer
Holman-Miller sign
holmium (Ho)
laser, h.
holoantigen
Holtzman rats
Holzknecht
chromoradiometer, H.
unit, H.
home O_2 (home oxygen)
home oxygen (home O_2)
homeobox (HOX)
cluster, h.
homeotherapy
homeotransplant
homeotransplantation
Homer-Wright rosettes
homing receptor
homobody
homocycle
homocyclic
homocytotropic antibody
homocysteine
homodimer
homodimeric
homogenic
homogeneity
homogeneous
homogenously staining region (HSR)
homograft
homoharringtonine (HHT)
homologous
analogue, h.
antigen, h.
blood, h.
chromosome, h.
graft, h.
series, h.
homologue
homology
region, h.
unit, h.
homolysin
homolysis
homonuclear
homophil
homophilic
homophobe

ADDITIONAL TERMS

homophobia
homoplastic
homoplasty
homopolymer
homopolymeric
homosexual
    intercourse, h.
    panic, h.
homosexuality
homotransplantation
homotypic
homovanillic acid (HVA)
homozygosity
homozygote
homozygous
    genes, h.
    hemoglobin S disease, h.
    typing cells, h. (HTC)
honeycomb lung
honeycombing
Hood stoma stent
hooded anode
Hoogsteen binding mode
hook
    barbed h.
    localization h.
    wire h.
hooked
hookworm anemia
HOP (hydroxydaunomycin, Oncovin,
    prednisone)
Hoppe-Seyler test
Hormodendrum
hormonagogue
hormonal
    imbalance, h.
    manipulation, h.
    receptors, h.
    therapy, h.
hormone
    assay, h.
    profile, h.
    tan, h.
    therapy, h.
hormonogenesis
hormonogenic
hormonopoiesis
hormonopoietic
hormonoprivia
hormonotherapy
hormonotropic
horn cell
horse

antihuman thymus globulin, h.
    (HAHTG)
cell test, h.
red blood cells, h. (HRBC)
serum, h.
horseradish peroxidase
Hortega cell
    tumor, H.
HOS (human osteogenic sarcoma)
hospice
host
    cell, h.
    defenses, h.
    factors, h.
    immunocompromise, h.
    lesion, h.
    mechanism, h.
    performance scale, h.
    -related factor, h.
    response, h.
    -specific, h.
    target site, h.
    vector system, h.
hot
    atom, h.
    biopsy, h.
    -cold hemolysin, h.
    cone, h.
    conization, h.
    gangrene, h.
    knife, h.
    lesion, h.
    nodule, h.
    spot, h.
    water circulating suit, h.
Hounsfield
    scale, H.
    unit, H. (HU)
hourglass tumor
Houston valve
Howel-Evans syndrome
Howell
    bodies, H.
    method, H.
    test, H.
Howell-Jolly bodies
HOX (homeobox)
    cluster, H.
Hoxley method
Hoxsey treatment
Ho-YAG (holmium-yttrium-aluminum-
    garnet)
    laser, H.

ADDITIONAL TERMS

Hp (haptoglobin)
HPA (Histoplasma capsulatum polysaccharide antigen)
HPA-23 (antimonium tungstate)
HPD (hematoporphyrin derivative)
hpf (high-power field)
HPFH (hereditary persistence of fetal hemoglobin)
HPL (human placental lactogen)
   -producing tumor, H.
HPLC (high-performance liquid chromatography)
HPMPC
HPR (fenretinide)
HPV (human papillomavirus)
   -16, H.
   E6 protein, H.
H-ras gene
H-ras 1 gene
HRBC (horse red blood cells)
HRF (histamine-releasing factor)
Hryniuk dose-intensity hypothesis
HSA (human serum albumin)
HSM (hepatosplenomegaly)
hsp (heat shock protein)
HSR (homogeneously staining region)
HSV (herpes simplex virus)
   -1 antibody, H.
   -2 antibody, H.
HTACS (human thyroid adenylate cyclase stimulators)
HTC (homozygous typing cells)
HT1080/DR4 human fibrosarcoma cell line
H.T. Factorate
HTLA (human T-lymphocyte antigen)
HTLV (human T-cell leukemia virus)
   -I, H.
   -II, H.
   -III, H.
   provirus, H.
HTLV (human T-cell lymphoma virus)
   -I, H.
   -II, H.
   -III, H.
   provirus, H.
HTLV (human T-cell lymphotrophic virus)
   -I, H.
   -II, H.
   -III, H.
   provirus, H.
5-HT3 receptors

HTSH (human thyroid-stimulating hormone)
   EIA test, H.
   RIABead test, H.
HU (Hounsfield unit)
HU (hydroxyurea)
Hu antigen
Hubbard E meter
Huber needle
Huebener-Thomsen-Friedenreich phenomenon
Huggins operation
HuIFN (human interferon)
Huldshinsky radiation
human
   adenovirus, h.
   albumin, h.
   albumin microspheres, h. (HAM)
   AML cell line, h.
   antihemophilic factor, h.
   antimurine antibody, h. (HAMA)
   B-lymphotropic virus, H. (HBLV)
   chorionic gonadotropin, h. (HCG)
   chromosome, h.
   erythrocyte agglutination test, h. (HEAT)
   exposure dose–rodent potency dose, h. (HERP)
   factor IX, h.
   gamma globulin, h. (HGG)
   genome, h.
   genome project, h.
   growth hormone, h. (hGH)
   growth hormone-recombinant, h. (hGRr)
   herpesvirus-6, h. (HHV-6)
   immunodeficiency virus, h. (HIV)
   interferon, h. (HuIFN)
   intracisternal retrovirus, h. (HICRV)
   leukocyte antigens, h. (HLA)
   leukocyte interferon milieu, h.
   lymphocyte antigens, h. (HLA)
   lymphocyte transformation, h.
   milk fat globule antigen-2, h. (HMFG-2)
   monoclonal antibody to cytomegalovirus, h. (HMA-CMV)
   murine xenograft, h.
   osteogenic sarcoma, h. (HOS)
   papillomavirus, h. (HPV)
   papillomavirus E6 protein, h.
   peripheral lymphocyte, h.

ADDITIONAL TERMS

pharmacy, h.
placental lactogen, h. (HPL)
recombinant beta interferon, h.
 (Betaseron)
serum albumin, h. (HSA)
skin peroxidase, labeled antibody
 immunofluorescence test, h.
T-cell leukemia virus, h. (HTLV)
T-cell lymphadenotrophic virus, h.
T-cell lymphocyte antigen, h.
 (HTLA)
T-cell lymphoma virus, h. (HTLV)
T-cell lymphotrophic virus, h.
 (HTLV)
thymus antiserum, h. (HUTHAS)
thymus antilymphocyte antigen, h.
 (HTLA)
thyroid adenylate cyclase
 stimulators, h. (HTACS)
T-lymphotropic retrovirus, h.
tumor clonogenic assay, h.
tumor colony-forming assay, h.
umbilical vein, h.
humanized
 antibodies, h.
Humate-P
Humatin
Humatrope
humor therapy
humoral
 antibody, h.
 hypercalcemia of malignancy, h.
 immune response, h.
 immunity, h.
hungry-bone syndrome
Hunner interstitial cystitis
Hunt Limo-Basto pouch
Hunter
 disease, H.
 glossitis, H.
Hurler
 disease, H.
 syndrome, H.
Hurthle cell
 adenoma, H.
 carcinoma, H.
 neoplasia, H.
 tumor, H.
HUS (hemolytic-uremic syndrome)
Hutch-1 epitope
Hutchinson
 freckle, H. (lentigo maligna)
 Fred H. Cancer Center

melanotic freckle of H.
 type, H.
Hutchinson-Boeck granulomatosis
HUTHAS (human thymus antiserum)
Hutter tumor
HV (Herpesvirus)
HVA (homovanillic acid)
HVL (half-value layer)
HXIS (hard x-ray imaging spectrometer)
HXM (hexamethylmelamine)
hyaline
 carcinoma, h.
 fibromatosis, h.
 leukocyte, h.
 membrane disease, h.
hyalinization
hyaloenchondroma
hyalomere
hyaloserositis
hyaluronic acid
hyaluronidase
Hy antigen
H-Y antigen
Hyate
Hyazyme
HYB-24 antibody
hybrid
 antibody, h.
 cell, h.
hybridization
 DNA h.
hybridoma
 antibody, h.
 cell, h.
hybridons
hycamptamine
hycanthone
Hyclone
hydatid
 cyst, h.
 fremitus, h.
 mole, h.
 pregnancy, h.
hydatidiform
 mole, h.
hydatidocele
hydatidoma
hydatidostomy
hydradenoma
hydrazine
 -sensitive factor, h.
 sulfate, h. (HDZ)
Hydrazone

ADDITIONAL TERMS

Hydrea (hydroxyurea)
hydrocarbon
  carcinogenic h.
hydrocortisone (HC)
Hydrocortone
hydrocystadenoma
Hydro-D
hydrogen (H)
  bomb, h.
  cyanide, h.
  ion, h.
  peroxide, h.
  sulfide, h.
hydroma
hydrolase
hydro-lyase
hydrolysate
hydromyoma
4-hydroperoxycyclophosphamide (4-HC
  or Pergamid)
hydroperoxyeicosatetraenoic acid
hydrophagocytosis
hydrophobic protein
hydrosarcocele
hydroxocobalamin
hydroxyapatite
hydroxychloroquine sulfate
hydroxycorticosteroid
hydroxydaunomycin
hydroxydaunorubicin
hydroxyeicosatetaraenoic acid (HETE)
hydroxyester
hydroxyheptadecatrienoic acid (HHT)
5-hydroxy-indoleacetic acid (5-HIAA)
hydroxyl
hydroxylamine
hydroxylase
hydroxylation
hydroxymethylglutaryl-CoA lyase
hydroxynaphthoquinone (566-C80)
hydroxyperoxycyclophosphamide
4-hydroxyphenylpyruvate dioxygenase
hydroxyprogesterone (Duralutin or Hy-
  Gestrone or Hylutin)
  caproate, h.
  hexanoate, h.
hydroxystilbamidine isethionate
hydroxyurea (HU or Hydrea)
Hy-Gestrone (hydroxyprogesterone)
hygroma
  colli, h.
  cystic h.
  subdural h.

hyloma
Hylutin (hydroxyprogesterone)
hyper IgE
Hyperab
hyperadenosis
hyperadrenalism
hyperal (hyperalimentation)
hyperaldosteronemia
hyperaldosteronism
hyperalimentation
  parenteral h.
hyperalphalipoproteinemia
hyperamylasemia
hyperbaric oxygen (HBO)
  chamber, h.
  drenching, h.
  therapy, h.
hyper-beta-alaninemia
hyperbetalipoproteinemia
hyperbilirubinemia
hyperblastosis
hypercalcemia
hypercarotenemia
hypercellular
hypercellularity
hyperchromatic
hypercoagulable
  state, h.
hypercoagulability
hypercortisolism
hypercythemia
hypercytosis
hyperdense
hyperdiploid
hyperdiploidy
hyperemesis
hyperemia
hyperemic
hypereosinophilia
hypereosinophilic
  syndrome, h. (HES)
hyperepinephrinemia
hypererythrocythemia
hyperesthesia
hyperesthetic
hyperestrogenemia
hyperferremia
hyperfibrinogenemia
Hyperforat
hyperfractionation
hypergammaglobulinemia
  monoclonal h.
hyperglobulinemia

ADDITIONAL TERMS

hyperglycemia
hyperglycemic
    hyperosmolar nonketotic, h.
    (HHNK)
hypergonadotropic
hyperhemoglobinemia
Hyper-Hep
hyperheparinemia
hyperhistaminemia
hypericin (St. John's wort or VIMRxyn)
Hypericum triquetrifolium turra
hyperimmune
    bovine colostrum, h. (HBC)
hyperimmunity
hyperimmunoglobulin
hyperimmunoglobulinemia
    E syndrome, h.
hyperinfection
hyperkalemia
hyperkeratosis
hyperkeratotic
hyperleukocytosis
hyperlipemia
hyperlipidemia
hyperlipoproteinemia
hyperlithemia
hyperlymphocytosis
hypermagnesemia
hypermelanosis
hypermetabolism
hypermetaplasia
hypermorph
hypernatremia
hyperneocytosis
hypernephroid
    carcinoma, h.
    tumor, h.
hypernephroma
    halo sign, h.
hypernitremia
hypernormocytosis
hyperon
hyperorthocytosis
hyperosmolality
hyperosmolar
    hyperglycemic nonketotic coma, h.
    (HHNC)
hyperosmolarity
hyperostosis
hyperparathyroidism
hyperphenylalaninemia
hyperphosphatemia
hyperphosphorylation

hyperpigmentation
hyperpigmented
    mole, h.
hyperpituitarism
hyperplasia
hyperplastic
    alveolar nodules, h. (HAN)
hyperploid
hyperploidy
hyperpolypeptidemia
hyperprolactinemia
hyperpyrexia
hyperpyrexial
hypersegmented
hyperskeocytosis
hypersplenic
    anemia, h.
hypersplenism
hypersusceptibility
hyperthermia
hyperthermic
hyperthrombinemia
hyperthyroidism
hyperthyroidosis
hyperthyroxinemia
    familial dysalbuminemic h.
hypertonia
    polycythaemica, h.
hypertonic
hypertrichosis
hypertriglyceridemia
hypertrophied
hypertrophy
hyperuricemia
hyperviscosity
hypervolemia
hyphomycetoma
hypnosis
hypnotic
hypoadrenalism
hypoaeration
hypoalbuminemia
hypoaldosteronemia
hypoaldosteronism
hypoalimentation
hypoaminoacidemia
hypobetalipoproteinemia
hypobilirubinemia
hypocalcemia
hypocellular
hypocellularity
hypocenter
hypochromasia

ADDITIONAL TERMS

hypochromatic
hypochromatism
hypochromemia
   idiopathic h.
hypochromia
hypochromic
   erythrocyte, h.
   microcytic anemia, h.
hypochrosis
hypocoagulability
hypocoagulable
hypocomplementemia
hypocomplementemic
hypocycloidal tomography
hypocythemia
hypocytosis
hypodense
hypodiploid
hypoechoic
hypoelectrolytemia
hypoeosinophilia
hypoestrogenemia
hypoferremia
hypoferric
   anemia, h.
hypoferrism
hypofibrinogenemia
hypogammaglobulinemia
hypoglucagonemia
hypoglycemia
hypoglycemic
hypoglycemosis
hypogonadism
hypogranulocytosis
hypohepatia
hypohyloma
hypokalemia
hypokalemic
   alkalosis, h.
hypoleydigism
hypolipoproteinemia
hypolymphemia
hypomagnesemia
hypomelanosis
   idiopathic guttate h.
   Ito, h. of
hypomorph
hypomotility
hyponatremia
hyponeocytosis
hypo-orthocytosis
hypo-osmolality
hypo-osmolarity

hypopancreatism
hypoparathyreosis
hypoparathyroidism
hypoperfusion
hypophosphatemia
hypophysectomize
hypophysectomy
hypophysioprivic
hypophysis
hypophysitis
hypopigmentation
   -immunodeficiency disease, h.
hypopituitarism
hypoplasia
hypoplastic
   anemia, h.
   bone marrow, h.
   thrombocytopenia, h.
hypopotassemia
hypoproaccelerinemia
hypoproconvertinemia
hypoproteinemia
hypoprothrombinemia
hyposarca
hyposegmentation
hyposkeocytosis
hyposplenism
hyposthenia
hyposthenic
hypothalamic
hypothalamus
hypothermia
hypothermic
   perfusion, h.
hypothesis
   Dreyer and Bennett h.
   Goldie-Coldman h.
   Hryniuk dose-intensity h.
   lattice h.
   Makeham h.
   methyl FH4 trap h.
   Norton-Simon h.
   one gene-one enzyme h.
   one gene-one polypeptide h.
   unitarian h.
   wobble h.
hypothesize
hypothetical
hypothrombinemia
hypothyroid
hypothyroidism
hypothyroid
hypothyroidea

ADDITIONAL TERMS

hypothyroidism
hypotonia
hypotonic
hypovascular tumor
hypoventilation
hypovolemia
hypovolemic
hypoxanthine
-guanine
phosphoribosyltransferase, h.
(HGPRT)
hypoxemia
hypoxia
anemic h.
histotoxic h.
hypoxic h.
stagnant h.
hypoxic
hypoxidosis
HypRho-D
Hyprogest (hydroxyprogesterone)
Hyproval (hydroxyprogesterone)
Hyproxon (hydroxyprogesterone)
hypsodiploid
hypsodiploidy
hysterectomize
hysterectomy
hysterocarcinoma
hysterogram
hysteromyoma
hysteromyomectomy
hystero-oophorectomy
hysterosalpingectomy
hysterosalpingo-oophorectomy
hysteroscope
hysteroscopy
Hysteroser
hysterotrachelectomy
Hyzyd
Hz (hertz)
HZV (herpes zoster virus)

I (iodine)
123 labeled amines, I.
123 MIBG, I.
(metaiodobenzylguanidine)
125, I.
125 isotope, I.
125 seed, I.
130, I.
131, I. (radioactive iodine)
131 human serum albumin, I.

131 implantation, I.
131 irradiation, I.
131 isotope, I.
131 labeled hippuran, I.
131 labeled M195, I.
131 MIBG, I.
(metaiodobenzylguanidine)
13l labeled OKB7, I.
132, I. (radioactive iodine)
I antigen
I blood group system
I cell
disease, I.
I deficiency factor
I factor
I invariant
Ia (immune-associated)
antigens, I.
IA (immune adherence)
IAHA (immune adherence
hemagglutination assay)
iatrogenesis
iatrogenic
anemia, i.
thyroidism, i.
IBC (iron-binding capacity)
IBD (inflammatory bowel disease)
IBF (immunoglobulin-binding factor)
IBL (immunoblastic lymphadenopathy)
IBM blood cell processor
IBSCSG (International Breast Cancer
Study Group)
IC (immune complex)
ICA (islet cell antibodies)
ICAM (intercellular adhesion molecule)
-1 gene, I.
ICD-O (International Classification of
Diseases for Oncology)
ice
bag, i.
cap, i.
pack, i.
turban, i.
ICE (ifosfamide, carboplatin, etoposide)
ICE (immunoglobulin-complexed
enzyme)
disorders, I.
ICH (intracranial hemorrhage)
ICP (intracranial pressure)
ICRF-159 (razoxane)
ICRF-187
ICS (intracellular-like, calcium-bearing
crystalloid solution)

ADDITIONAL TERMS

ICSH (interstitial cell-stimulating hormone)
ICT (indirect Coombs test)
icteric
icteroanemia
icterogenic
icterohemoglobinuria
icterohemolytic anemia, i.
icterohepatitis
icteroid
icterus
    chronic familial i.
    congenital familial i.
    congenital hemolytic i.
    gravis, i.
    gravis neonatorum, i.
    hemolytic i.
    neonatorum, i.
    nonobstructive i.
    nuclear i.
    obstructive i.
    praecox, i.
ID (intermediate dose)
Id (inhibitor of differentiation) protein
IDA (idarubicin)
Idamycin (idarubicin hydrochloride)
idarubicin hydrochloride (IDA or Idamycin)
IDAV (immunodeficiency-associated virus)
IDD (insulin-dependent diabetes)
IDDM (insulin-dependent diabetes mellitus)
identical plane dose
idioagglutinin
idioheteroagglutinin
idioheterolysin
idioisoagglutinin
idioisolysin
idiolysin
idiopathic
    hypochromic anemia, i.
    megakaryocytic aplasia, i.
    multiple pigmented sarcoma, i.
    pulmonary hemosiderosis, i. (IPH)
    thrombocytopenic purpura, i. (ITP)
idiotope
idiotype
    -anti-idiotype network, i.
idiotypic
    antigen, i.
    variant, i.

idiovariation
L-iditol dehydrogenase
IDL (intermediate-density lipoprotein)
IDMTX (intermediate-dose methotrexate)
idoxuridine (IDU)
IDS (immunity deficiency state)
IDTP (immunodeficient thrombocytopenic purpura)
IDU (idoxuridine)
iduronate-2-sulfatase
L-iduronidase
IDX (4'-iodo-4'-deoxydoxorubicin)
IEOP (immunoelectro-osmophoresis)
IEP (immunoelectrophoresis)
IF (immunofluorescence)
IFA (indirect fluorescent antibody)
IFC (intermittent-flow centrifugation) pheresis, I.
Ifex (ifosfamide)
IFF (ifosfamide)
IFLrA (recombinant interferon alpha)
IFM (ifosfamide)
IFN (interferon)
IFN-A (interferon-alpha)
IFN-A2a (interferon alpha-2a)
IFN-A2b (interferon alpha-2b)
IFN-An
IFN-beta
IFN-G (gamma interferon)
IFNrA (recombinant interferon alpha)
IFOS (ifosfamide)
ifosfamide (Ifex or IFOS or IFX)
IFT (immunofluorescence test)
    human skin peroxidase-labeled antibody I.
    human parathyroid gland I.
    mammalian spinal cord I.
    unfixed human adrenal cortex I.
    unfixed human hyperplastic thyroid tissue I.
    unfixed human salivary gland I.
IFX (ifosfamide)
Ig (immunoglobulin)
    gene assembly, I.
    marker, I.
    mosaicism, I.
    -synthesizing B-cell lymphoma, I.
IgA (immunoglobulin A)
IgD (immunoglobulin D)
IgE (immunoglobulin E)
    receptors, I.
IgG (immunoglobulin G)

ADDITIONAL TERMS

IgG1 antibody
IgG2a antibody (Immurait)
IgG3 antibody
IgG4 antibody
IgM (immunoglobulin M)
IgY (immunoglobulin Y)
IGT (immunization via gene transfer)
IH (infectious hepatitis)
IHA (indirect hemagglutination)
IHBTD (incompatible hemolytic blood
   transfusion disease)
IHSA (iodinated human serum albumin)
Ii
   antigen, I.
   blood group system, I.
IIF (indirect immunofluorescence)
IIFA (indirect immunofluorescent
   antibody)
Il (illinium)
IL (interleukin)
   IL-1 (interleukin-1)
   IL-1A (interleukin-1-alpha)
   IL-1B (interleukin-1-beta)
   IL-2 through IL-9 (interleukin-2
      through interleukin-9)
ILC (incipient lethal concentration)
ILD (interstitial lung disorders)
ileitis
ileoanal
ileoascending colostomy
ileocecal
ileocecostomy
ileocolitis
ileocolostomy
ileocystoplasty
ileocystostomy
ileoileostomy
ileoproctostomy
ileorectal
ileorectosigmoidoscopy
ileosigmoid
   colostomy, i.
ileosigmoidostomy
ileostomy
   appliance, i.
   bag, i.
   effluent, i.
   stoma, i.
ileotransverse colostomy
ileotransversostomy
ileum
ileus
   adynamic i.

dynamic i.
mechanical i.
iliac
   crest, i.
ilioinguinal
iliopelvic
iliopsoas
ill-defined
   lesion, i.
   mass, i.
illinium (Il)
Illinois needle
illudin S
ilmofosine
Iloprost
Ilotycin
IM (infectious mononucleosis)
IMAA (iodinated macroaggregated
   albumin)
image
   analyzer, i.
   enhancement, i.
   intensifier, i.
imagery
imaging
IMC (internal mammary chain)
IMED infusion pump
Imerslund syndrome
Imerslund-Graesbeck syndrome
IMF (Ifex, Mesnex, Folex,
   5-fluorouracil)
Imferon
imidazole carboxamide (dacarbazine)
5-iminodaunorubicin
imipenem-cilastatin
immortalization
Immther
immune
   acquired i. deficiency syndrome
      (AIDS)
   adherence, i.
   adherence hemagglutination assay,
      i. (IAHA)
   agglutinin, i.
   antibody, i.
   -associated (Ia) antigens, i.
   body, i.
   clearance, i.
   competence, i.
   complex, i. (IC)
   complex disease, i.
   compromise, i.
   conglutinin, i.

ADDITIONAL TERMS

immune —*Continued*
  cytolysis, i.
  cytotoxicity, i.
  deficiency, i.
  deposit, i.
  deviation, i.
  gamma globulin, i. (leukoglobulin)
  globulin, i.
  hemolysis, i.
  hemolytic anemia, i.
  incompetence, i.
  markers, i.
  modulation, i.
  modulator, i.
  neutropenia, i.
  phenotype, i.
  reaction, i.
  response, i.
  response (Ir) genes, i.
  rosetting, i.
  self-tolerance, i.
  serum globulin, i. (ISG)
  suppression, i.
  suppressor (Is) genes, i.
  surveillance, i.
  system, i.
  system modulator, i. (IMREG-1)
  thrombocytopenia, i.
  thrombocytopenic purpura, i. (ITP)
immunekorper
Immuneron
Immunex CRP
immunifacient
immunifaction
immunity
  acquired i.
  active i.
  adoptive i.
  antibacterial i.
  antitoxic i.
  antiviral i.
  artificial i.
  athreptic i.
  cell-mediated i. (CMI)
  cellular i.
  community i.
  concomitant i.
  congenital i.
  cross i.
  familial i.
  genetic i.
  herd i.
  humoral i.

  infection i.
  inherent i.
  inherited i.
  innate i.
  intrauterine i.
  local i.
  maternal i.
  native i.
  natural i.
  nonspecific i.
  passive i.
  species i.
  specific i.
  T cell-mediated i. (TCMI)
  tissue i.
immunity deficiency state (IDS)
immunization
  passive i.
  via gene transfer, i. (IGT)
immunize
immunizing unit (IU)
immunoadhesin
immunoadjuvant
immunoadsorbent
immunoadsorption
immunoanatomy
immunoassay
  enzyme i. (EIA)
  enzyme-multiplied i. technique
    (EMIT)
immunobead
  -binding assay, i.
immunobiology
immunoblast
immunoblastic
  lymphadenopathy, i.
  sarcoma of B cells, i.
  sarcoma of T cells, i.
immunoblot
  analysis, i.
  technique, i.
  test, i.
immunoblotting
immunochemical
immunochemistry
immunochemotherapeutic
immunochemotherapy
immunocompetence
immunocompetent
immunocomplex
immunocompromised
immunoconglutinin
immunoconjugate

ADDITIONAL TERMS

immunoconjugation
immunocyte
immunocytic
    amyloidosis, i.
immunocytoadherence
immunocytochemistry
immunodeficiency
    AIDS-related i.
    antibody i.
    cellular i.
    combined i.
    common variable i.
    common variable unclassifiable i.
    gay-related i.
    HIV-related i.
    hyper-IgM, i. with
    severe combined i. (SCID)
    short-limbed dwarfism, i. with
    thymoma, i. with
    X-linked hyper-IgM i.
immunodeficient
    thrombocytopenic purpura, i.
    (IDTP)
immunodepressed
immunodepression
immunodepressive
immunodeviation
immunodiagnosis
immunodiagnostic
immunodiffusion
    radial i. (RID)
immunodominance
immunodominant
immunoelectro-osmophoresis (IEOP)
immunoelectrophoresis (IEP)
    counter-i.
    countercurrent i.
    crossed i.
    Laurell technique i.
    radio-i.
    rocket i.
    two-dimensional i.
immunoelectrophoretic
immunoelectrotransfer
immunoferritin
immunofiltration
immunofixation
    agar, i. in (Agar-IF)
    electrophoresis, i.
immunofluorescence (IF)
    assay, i.
    microscopy, i.
    stain, i.

    test, i. (IFT)
immunofluorescent
    flow cytometry, i.
immunogen
immunogenetic
immunogenetics
immunogenic
    determinant, i.
immunogenicity
immunoglobulin (Ig)
    gamma A, i. (IgA)
    B-cell i.
    cytoplasmic i.
    gamma D, i. (IgD)
    gamma E, i. (IgE)
    gamma G, i. (IgG)
    gamma M, i. (IgM)
    gamma Y, i. (IgY)
    membrane i.
    monoclonal i.
    secretory i. A
    thyroid-binding inhibitory i's (TBII)
    thyroid-stimulating i's (TSI)
    TSH-binding inhibitory i's (TBII)
immunoglobulin alpha chain
immunoglobulin-binding factor (IBF)
immunoglobulin class
immunoglobulin class switching
immunoglobulin-complexed enzymatic
    (ICE) disorders
immunoglobulin conjugates
immunoglobulin delta chain
immunoglobulin domains
immunoglobulin epsilon chain
immunoglobulin fold
immunoglobulin gamma chain
immunoglobulin genes
immunoglobulin gene rearrangement
immunoglobulin kappa chain
immunoglobulin lambda chain
immunoglobulin light chain
immunoglobulin mu chain
immunoglobulin subclass
immunoglobulin superfamily
immunoglobulinopathy
immunogold
    staining, i.
    technique, i.
immunohematology
immunohistochemical
immunohistochemistry
immunohistofluorescence
immunohistologic

ADDITIONAL TERMS

immunoincompetence
immunoincompetent
immunologic
    competence, i.
    diseases, i.
    enhancement, i.
    homeostasis, i.
    imbalance, i.
    mechanism, i.
    memory, i.
    suppression, i.
    surveillance, i.
    tolerance, i.
    typing, i.
immunological
    surveillance, i.
immunologically
    incompetent cell, i.
    privileged sites, i.
immunologist
immunology
immunomodulating
immunomodulation
immunomodulator
immunomodulatory
immunopathogenesis
immunopathologic
immunopathology
immunoperoxidase
    biotin-avidin-peroxidase i.
    direct conjugate i.
    indirect conjugate i.
    labeled antigen i.
    PAP (peroxidase-antiperoxidase) i.
immunophenotype
immunophenotyping
immunophilin
immunophysiology
immunopotency
immunopotentiation
immunopotentiator
immunoprecipitate
immunoprecipitation
immunoprobe
immunoproliferation
immunoproliferative
    small-intestinal disease, i. (IPSID)
immunoprophylactic
immunoprophylaxis
immunoprotein
immunoradioassay (IRA)
immunoradiometric
    assay, i. (IRMA)

immunoradiometry
immunoreactant
    glucagon i's
immunoreaction
immunoreactive (IR)
    glucagon, i. (IRG)
    human growth hormone, i.
    (IRhGH)
    parathyroid hormone, i. (iPTH)
    substance P, i. (ISP)
immunoreactivity
    glucagon-like i.
immunoregulation
immunoregulatory
immunoresponsiveness
immunorestorative
immunoselection
immunoselective
immunosorbent
immunostained
immunostimulant
immunostimulation
immunostimulatory
immunosuppressant
immunosuppressed
immunosuppression
immunosuppressive
immunosurgery
immunosurveillance
immunotherapy
immunotoxicology
immunotoxin
immunotransfusion
immunovar
ImmuRAID (CEA-Tc 99m)
Immurait (IgG2a monoclonal antibody)
Imodium
IMP (inosine monophosphate)
Impact
implant
    breast i.
    cesium i.
    endometrial i.
    gold seed i.
    interstitial i.
    intracavitary i.
    iridium i.
    metastatic i.
    penile i.
    radiation i.
    radioactive i.
    radioactive gold i.
    radioactive iodine i.

ADDITIONAL TERMS

radioactive iridium i.
radium i.
radon i.
implant radiation
implantable
implantation
   interstitial i.
   radioactive isotope, i.
   radium, i. of
impotence
impotent
IMREG-1 (immune system modulator)
Imudon (pegademase bovine)
Imuran
Imuthiol
ImuVert
IMVP-16 (ifosfamide, methotrexate, VP-16)
In (indium)
   111 DTPA, I.
   111-IgG, I. (indium-111 labeled human nonspecific immunoglobulin G)
   111-labeled leukocytes, I.
   111-labeled white blood cells, I.
   111 scan, I.
inactivation
inactivator
inanition
in ano
inappetance
inappropriate
   polycythemia, i.
   syndrome of i. antidiuretic hormone (SIADH)
Inapsine
incidence
incipient
inclusion
incoagulability
incoagulable
incompatibility
   ABO i.
incompatible
   hemolytic blood transfusion disease, i. (IHBTD)
incontinence
incontinent
increased uptake
increment
incremental
   dose, i.
incrementally

incurable
IND (investigational new drug)
indanedione
indenization
index (pl. indices)
   antitryptic i.
   Arneth i.
   biochemical racial i.
   body mass i.
   Broders i.
   centromeric i.
   chemotherapeutic i.
   erythrocyte i's
   Mentzer i.
   mitotic i.
   nucleoplasmic i.
   opsonic i.
   phagocytic i.
   proliferative i.
   stimulation i. (SI)
   therapeutic i.
Indian
   apple, I.
   flap, I.
Indianapolis hemoglobin
indicanemia
indices (pl. of index)
indirect
   agglutination, i.
   conjugate immunoperoxidase, i.
   Coombs test, i. (ICT)
   fluorescent antibody, i. (IFA)
   hemagglutination, i. (IHA)
   immunofluorescence, i. (IIF)
   immunofluorescent antibody, i. (IIFA)
   radioimmunoassay, i. (IRIA)
   transfusion, i.
indium (In)
   64 scan, i.
   111-labeled human nonspecific immunoglobulin G, i. (111In-IgG)
   111 leukocyte scintigraphy scan, i.
   111 leukocyte scanning, i.
   111 leukocytoscan, i.
   111 oxine, i.
   113m, i.
   114, i.
   bone marrow imaging, i.
   chlorides in 113m injection, i.
   tumor imaging, i.
indolaceturia
indole carbinol

ADDITIONAL TERMS

indolent
  lesion, i.
  myeloma, i.
  myoma, i.
  radiation-induced rectal ulcer, i.
  tumor, i.
indomethacin
induced enzyme
inducer cells
inducible enzyme
induction
  accelerator, i.
  chemotherapy, i.
  therapy, i.
  time, i.
indurated
induration
industrial
  carcinogens, i.
  exposure, i.
in extremis
infantile
  embryonal carcinoma, i.
  fibromatosis, i.
  genetic agranulocytosis, i.
  malignant histiocytosis, i.
  myofibromatosis, i.
  nephroblastoma, i.
  sex-linked
    hypogammaglobulinemia, i.
infectious
  hemolytic anemia, i.
  hepatitis, i. (IF)
  lymphocytosis, i.
  mononucleosis, i.
infective
infiltrate
infiltration
infiltrating
  adenocarcinoma, i.
  ductal adenocarcinoma, i.
  ductal cell carcinoma, i.
  glioma, i.
  lobular carcinoma, i.
  papillary carcinoma, i.
  tumor, i.
  tumor borders, i.
inflammatory
  bowel disease, i. (IBD)
  carcinoma, i.
  lesion, i.
  mass, i.
  process, i.

response, i.
infratentorial
  glioblastoma multiforme, i.
Infumorph
infundibuloma
Infusaid
  chemotherapy pump, I.
  implantable drug delivery system, I.
infuse
Infuse-a-port
infusion
  bone marrow, i.
  chemotherapy, i.
  device, i.
  drip, i.
  pump, i.
inguinal
  adenopathy, i.
  lymphadenectomy, i.
  node dissection, i.
INH (inhibitor)
INH (isoniazid)
INH (isonicotine hydrazine)
inhibition
  allogenic i.
  hemagglutination i.
inhibitive
inhibitor (INH)
  alpha-1 protease i.
  membrane attack complex i. (MAC INH)
  monoamine oxidase i. (MAOI)
inhibitory syndrome
inhomogeneity
inhomogeneous
Injectio Trichosanthin
initiation
  factor, i.
  therapy, i. of
initiator
^{111}In labeled IgG
inlay graft
innidiation
innocent bystander
inomyxoma
inoneuroma
inoperable
  cancer, i.
  malignancy, i.
  patient, i.
  tumor, i.
inosine
  monophosphate, i. (IMP)

ADDITIONAL TERMS

phosphorylase, i.
pranobex, i. (isoprinosine)
inosinic acid
inosiplex methisoprinol (isoprinosine)
Inovision video microscope
Inpersol
INPX
Inrad fine-needle prostate aspiration
 kit
insect vector
insecticide
inserted gene
inserter
insertion
 radioactive material, i. of
 radium, i. of
 tandem, i.
insertional
 activation, i.
 mutagenesis, i.
 mutation, i.
insidious
in situ
 carcinoma, i.
 hybridization, i.
insorption
inspissated
inspissation
instillation
instillational therapy
insulin
 -dependent diabetes, i. (IDD)
 -dependent diabetes mellitus, i.
 (IDDM)
 -like growth factors, i.
insulinoma
insuloma
Integra PBS Pageblot
integral absorbed dose
integrase
integrated provirus
integrating ionization chamber
integrin
 family, i.
integumentary barrier
intensification
intensimeter
intensionometer
intentional transoperative hemodilution
intercalate
intercalating
intercalation
intercalator

intercellular
 adhesion molecule, i. (ICAM)
 adhesion molecule 1 gene, i.
 (ICAM-1 gene)
interchain linker
intercostal
intercricothyrotomy
interdigitating cells
interferon (IFN)
 a, i. (IFN-a)
 alfa-2a, i. (IFN-A2a) (Roferon-A)
 alfa-2b, i. (IFN-A2b) (Intron-A)
 alfa-n1, i. (Wellferon)
 alfa-n3, i. (Alferon LDO or Alferon
 N)
 b, i. (IFN-b)
 epithelial i.
 fibroblast i.
 fibroepithelial i.
 gamma 1b, i.
 immune i.
 leukocyte i.
 type I i.
 type II i.
 y, i.
interferon-stimulated response element
interfollicular
 cells, i.
inter-heavy-chain disulfide loop
interilioabdominal amputation
interinnominoabdominal amputation
interlesional therapy
interleukin (IL)
 -1, i. (IL-1)
 -2, i. (IL-2)
 -3, i. (IL-3)
 -4, i. (IL-4)
 -5, i. (IL-5)
 -6, i. (IL-6)
 -7, i. (IL-7)
 -8, i. (IL-8)
 -9, i. (IL-9)
intermediate-density lipoprotein (IDL)
intermedullary
intermittent-flow centrifugation (IFC)
 pheresis, i.
internal
 mammary chain, i. (IMC)
 radiation hazard, i.
Internal Breast Cancer Study Group
 (IBCSG)
internalization
International

ADDITIONAL TERMS

International—*Continued*
  Classification of Diseases for
    Oncology, I. (ICD-O)
  Federation of Gynecology and
    Obstetrics (Fédération
    Internationale de Gynécologie et
    Obstétrique), I. (FEGO/FIGO)
  Society of Pediatric Oncology
    (Société Internationale
    d'Oncologie Pédiatrique), I.
    (SIOP)
internucleosomal
interpelviabdominal amputation
interphase
Interpore
interpose
interposition
interscapulothoracic amputation
interstice
interstitial
  application, i.
  brachytherapy, i.
  fluid, i.
  hyperthermia, i.
  implant, i.
  implantation, i.
  irradiation, i.
  lung disorders, i. (ILD)
  irradiation, i.
  plasma cell pneumonia, i.
  pneumonitis, i.
  radiation therapy, i.
  radiotherapy, i.
interstitium
intertropical anemia
intervening sequence
interventional
  chemotherapy, i.
  radiation therapy, i.
  radiology, i.
  technique, i.
intestinal
  anastomosis, i.
  bypass, i.
  contents, i.
  flora, i.
  intussusception, i.
  obstruction, i.
intestine
in toto
intra-abdominal
intra-arterial
  infusion, i.

  isotopic therapy, i.
intra-axial
  brain tumor, i.
intracanalicular fibroma
intracarotid
intracavernous injection
intracavitary
  application, i.
  applicator, i.
  brachytherapy, i.
  cesium therapy, i.
  gold seeds, i.
  implantation, i.
  irradiation, i.
  radiation therapy, i.
  radiotherapy, i.
  radium insertion, i.
intracellular
  immunization, i.
intracerebral
intra-chain disulfide loop
intracranial
  hemorrhage, i. (ICH)
  lesion, i.
  metastasis, i.
  neoplasm, i.
  pressure, i. (ICP)
  pressure monitor, i. (ICPM)
  pressure TeleSensor, i.
  tumor, i.
intractable
  disease, i.
  pain, i.
  vomiting, i.
intradiploic
intraductal
  carcinoma, i.
intradural
intraepidermal
intraepithelial
intraerythrocytic
intragastric
intragenic
intrahepatic
intralesional
  Velban therapy, i.
intraleukocytic
intraluminal
  brachytherapy, i.
  filling defect, i.
  intubation, i.
  mass, i.
  radiation therapy, i.

ADDITIONAL TERMS

intramammary
intramedullary
intraneoplastic
in trans
^{113m}In-transferrin
intranuclear
intraocular
Intra-Op autotransfusion system
intraoperative
    electron beam therapy, i. (IOEBT)
    radiation therapy, i. (IORT)
    radiotherapy, i. (IORT)
intraoral
    cone irradiation, i.
intraorbital
intraosseous
intraperitoneal
    belly bath, i.
    chemotherapy, i.
    phosphorus therapy, i.
    radioimmunoconjugate, i.
    scan, i.
    washings, i.
intrapleural
    chemotherapy, i.
    pneumonolysis, i.
intrapulmonary
intraspinal
intrathecal (IT)
    chemotherapy, i.
    instillation, i.
    nerve block anesthesia, i.
intrathoracic
intratumor
intrauterine
    immunity, i.
    radium application, i.
    transfusion, i.
intravaginal
    cylinder, i.
    implant, i.
intravasation
intravascular
    consumption coagulopathy, i.
    (IVCC)
intravenation
intravenous (I.V. when written alone, IV
in combination)
    chemotherapy, i.
    drug abuse, i. (IVDA)
    drug abuser, i. (IVDA)
    drug user, i. (IVDU)
    fluids, i.

gamma globulin, i. (IVIG)
hyperalimentation, i. (IVH)
piggyback, i. (IVPB)
pyelogram, i. (IVP)
thiotepa, i.
intravesical
intrinsic
    clotting reaction, i.
    factor, i.
    pathway, i.
introgression
intron
    -exon lariat, i.
Intron
    A, I. (interferon alfa-2b)
    C, I.
intubate
intubation
intussusception
Inv
    allotype, I.
    group antigen, I.
invariant chain
invasion
invasive
    carcinoma, i.
    lesion, i.
    procedure, i.
    tumor, i.
invasiveness
inversion-recovery technique
inverted-Y
    field, i.
    radiation, i.
investigational
    new drug, i. (IND)
    window, i.
in vitro
    clonogenic assay, i.
    correlations, i.
    kinetics, i.
    transcription assay, i.
in vivo
    adhesive platelet, i.
    correlations, i.
    frozen section binding assay, i.
    multicellular system, i.
    purging, i.
    translation, i.
involucre
involucrum
INVOS 2100 test
Io (ionium)

ADDITIONAL TERMS

Iodamoeba
  buetschlii, I.
iodide
  peroxidase, i.
  sodium I 125 solution.
iodinated
  I 125 fibrinogen, i.
  I 125 serum albumin, i.
  I 131 aggregated albumin (human),
    i.
  I 131 serum albumin (human), i.
  human serum albumin, i. (IHSA)
  macroaggregated albumin, i.
    (IMAA)
iodination
iodine (I)
  123, I.
  125, I.
  131, I.
  131 MIGB scintigraphy, I.
  132, I.
  butanol-extractable i. (BEI)
  protein-bound i.
  radioactive i.
iodine chelate
iodine implant
iodine isotope seed
iodine-labeled amines
iodine thyroid scan
iodipamide sodium I 131
iodize
iodoacetamide
iodocholesterol
iododeoxyuridine (IUDR)
5-iodo-2'-deoxyuridine (IDU)
iodohippurate
iodophilia
  extracellular i.
  intracellular i.
iodoquinol
iodotherapy
iodothyroglobulin
Iodotope oral solution
iodotyrosine deiodinase
IOEBT (intraoperative electron beam
  therapy)
iomethin
  I 125, i.
  I 131, i.
ion
  counter, i.
  exchange resin, i.
  flux, i.

laser, i.
ionic
  charge, i.
ionium (Io)
ionization
  avalanche i.
  radioactive i.
ionization chamber
ionize
ionizing
  particle, i.
  radiation, i.
ionogen
ionogenic
ionograph
ionography
ionometer
ionometry
ionophore
ionotherapy
iontophoresis
iontophoretic
iontoquantimeter
iontoradiometer
iontotherapy
IORT (intraoperative radiation therapy)
  applicator system, I.
  electron boost, I.
iothiouracil
Inv allotype
IPH (idiopathic pulmonary
  hemosiderosis)
iphosphamide (IPP)
IPMicro-ELISA test
ipomeanol
IPP (isopropyl pyrrolizine)
iproclozide
iproniazid
iproplatin (CHIP)
IPSID (immunoproliferative small
  intestinal disease)
ipsilateral
IPTG (isopropylthiogalactoside)
iPTH (immunoreactive parathyroid
  hormone)
Ir (immune response)
  gene, I.
Ir (iridium)
  192, I. (Iriditope)
  192 ribbon, I.
  192 wire implant, I.
  194, I.
IR (immunoreactive)

ADDITIONAL TERMS

IRA (immunoradioassay)
IRG (immunoreactive glucagon)
IRhGH (immunoreactive human growth
  hormone)
IRIA (indirect radioimmunoassay)
iridectomy
iridium (Ir)
    192, i. (Iriditope)
    194, i.
    afterloading tube, i.
    eye plaque, i.
    implant, i.
    isodose display, i.
    192 loaded stent, i.
    needle holder, i.
    ribbon, i.
    seeds, i.
    wire implant, i.
iridocyclectomy
Irish node
iritis
IRMA (immunoradiometric assay)
iron (Fe)
    assay, i.
    -binding capacity, i. (IBC)
    -binding protein, i.
    choline citrate, i.
    clearance, i.
    deficiency, i.
    deficiency anemia, i. (IDA)
    -deficient, i.
    deposition, i.
    dextran, i.
    loading, i.
    metabolism, i.
    overload, i.
    plasma, i.
    sequestration, i.
    storage disease, i.
    stores, i.
    supplementation, i.
    turnover, i.
    uptake, i.
irradiable
irradiance
irradiate
irradiated
    blood, i.
    bone, i.
    bone marrow, i.
    cells, i.
irradiating
irradiation

charged-particle i.
heavy ion i.
hemibody i.
interstitial i.
Medinger-Craver i.
total body i.
ultraviolet blood i. (UBI)
whole-body i.
irradiation cataract
irradiation change
irradiation cystitis
irradiation damage
irradiation effect
irradiation field
irradiation gastritis
irradiation menses
irradiation sterilization
irradiation stomatitis
irradiation therapy
irradiation time
irradiator
irreversibly sickled cell (ISC)
irrigoradioscopy
Irvine viable organ-tissue transport
  system (IVOTTS)
Is (immune suppressor)
    gene, I.
isamine blue
ISC (irreversibly sickled cell)
Iscador
ischemia
ischemic
iscom
ISFET (ion-specific field-effect
  transducer)
ISG (immune serum globulin)
islet
    cell, i.
    cell antibodies, i. (ICA)
    cell carcinoma, i.
    cell tumor, i.
    Langerhans, i. of
    tumor, i.
isoagglutination
isoagglutinin
isoagglutinogen
isoallele
isoallotypic
    determinant, i.
isoamyl nitrite
isoanaphylaxis
isoantibody
isoantigen

ADDITIONAL TERMS

isobar
isobaric
isobologram
    equation, i.
    technique, i.
isocellular
isochromosome
isocitrate dehydrogenase (NADP)
isocomplement
isoconazole
isocyclic
isocytosis
isodense
isodose
    curve, i.
    distribution, i.
isoechoic
isoeffect
isoenzyme
    Regan i.
isoform
isogeneic
isograft
isohemagglutination
isohemagglutinin
isohemolysin
isohemolysis
isohydric
isohypercytosis
isohypocytosis
isoimmune
    hemolytic anemia, i.
isoimmunization
    Rh (Rhesus) i.
isointense
isolated heat perfusion
isolation
    hypothermic perfusion, i.
isoleucine
isoleukoagglutinin
isolysin
isolysis
isomer
isomerase
isomeric
    decay, i.
isoniazid (INH)
isonicotine hydrazine (INH)
isonicotinic acid hydrazide
isonicotinyl hydrazide
isonormocytosis
isonuclear
isophil

    antibody, i.
    antigen, i.
isoplastic
isoprecipitin
isoprinosine (inosine pranobex or
    inosiplex methisoprinol)
isopropyl pyrrolizine (IPP)
isopropylthiogalactoside (IPTG)
Isospora
    belli, I.
isosporiasis
isosulfan blue
isoteric
isothromboagglutinin
isotonic
    saline, i.
    solution, i.
isotope
    radioactive i.
    stable i.
isotope bone scan
isotope colloid imaging
isotope dilution mass spectrometry
isotope effect
isotope labeling
isotope therapy
isotopic
isotopology
isotretinoin (Accutane)
isotype
isotypic
    determinant, i.
    variation, i.
isovaleric
    acidemia, i.
isozyme
ISP (immunoreactive substance P)
Issels combination therapy
IT (intrathecal)
itazigrel
IT MTX (intrathecal methotrexate)
ITP (idiopathic thrombocytopenic
    purpura)
itraconazole (Sporanox)
Itrumil
IU (immunizing unit)
IUdR (halogenated thymidine analogue)
IUdR (idoxuridine)
IUdR (iododeoxyuridine)
I.V. (intravenous)
    piggyback, I.
    push, I.
IVAC volumetric infusion pump

ADDITIONAL TERMS

IVAP (in vivo adhesive platelet)
IVCC (intravascular consumption
coagulopathy)
IVDA (intravenous drug abuse)
IVDA (intravenous drug abuser)
IVDU (intravenous drug user)
IVHI (intravenous hyperalimentation)
IVIG (intravenous gamma globulin)
IVOTTS (Irvine viable organ-tissue
transport system)
IVP (intravenous pyelogram)
IVPB (intravenous piggyback)
Ivy
    bleeding time, I.
    method, I.
Iwanoff cysts
Izonid tablets

J J (joining)
    chain, J.
    region, J.
    J (joule)
J (joining) chain
Ja antigen
Jaboulay amputation
Jaccoud arthritis
jacket cancer
Jackson staging
Jackson-Parker classification
Jacob ulcer
Jacobson nerve
Jadassohn-Tieche nevus
Jaffe regimen
Jaksch
    anemia, J.
    disease, J.
JAMG (juvenile autoimmune myasthenia
gravis)
Jamshidi
    liver biopsy needle, J.
    muscle biopsy needle, J.
Jamshidi-Kormed bone marrow biopsy
needle
Jansky classification
Jansky-Bielschowsky syndrome
Janssen R82913
Jarisch-Herxheimer reaction
Jarrow
jaundice
    acholuric j.
    anhepatic j.
    anhepatogenous j.

black j.
Budd j.
catarrhal j.
cholestatic j.
epidemic j.
hemorrhagic j.
hepatocellular j.
hepatogenic j.
hepatogenous j.
homologous serum j.
human serum j.
infectious j.
infective j.
latent j.
leptospiral j.
malignant j.
obstructive j.
occult j.
spirochetal j.
toxic j.
jaundiced
JC virus
    antigen, J.
JCML (juvenile chronic myelogenous
leukemia)
Jectofer
jejeunal
jejunectomy
jejunocecostomy
jejunocolostomy
jejunoileal
jejunoileostomy
jejunoileum
jejunojejunostomy
jejunostomy
Jenner method
jennerization
Jensen
    sarcoma, J.
    tumor, J.
Jerne plaque
    assay, J.
jet
    injection, j.
    nebulizer, j.
Jevity isotonic liquid nutrition
Jewett classification of bladder
carcinoma
    O noninfiltrating
    A infiltrating submucosa
    B invading muscle
    C involvement of surrounding tissues
    D distant involvement

ADDITIONAL TERMS

Jewett-Marshall-Strong staging
system
Jewett-Strong staging system
JIB (jejunoileal bypass)
Jitter test
Job syndrome
Jobbins factor
jodbasedow (hyperthyroidism)
JODM (juvenile-onset diabetes
mellitus)
joining (J)
chain, j.
region, j.
Jolly
bodies, J.
test, J.
Jonckheer statistic
Jones and Campbell staging system
Jones criteria
Jones-Mote reaction
Josephs-Diamond-Blackfan syndrome
joule (J)
Joule equivalent
JRA (juvenile rheumatoid arthritis)
jugular
chain, j.
node, j.
jugulodigastric
node, j.
juice
cancer j.
Junin virus
Jurkat cell line
juvenile
angiofibroma, j.
aponeurotic fibroma, j.
cell, j.
chronic myelogenous leukemia, j.
(JCML)
melanoma, j.
-onset diabetes mellitus, j. (JODM)
Paget disease, j.
pernicious anemia, j.
pilocytic astrocytoma, j.
polyposis, j.
rheumatoid arthritis, j. (JRA)
juxtacortical
chondrosarcoma, j.
osteosarcoma, j.
juxtaglomerular
cell tumor, j.
juxtaposition
juxtapyloric

juxtaregional lymph node
juxtaspinal
juxtavesical

Kk K (killer)
cell, K.
T-cell, K.
K (potassium)
K antigen
K (killer) cell
K factor
K-meson
K-particle
K-Tube
Kabikinase
KAF (conglutinogen activating factor)
Kahler disease
kala-azar infection
kalemia
kaliemia
kaliopenia
kalium
kallikrein
plasma k.
tissue k.
kallikrein-inhibiting unit (KIU)
kallikreinogen
Kallzyne
kang cancer
kangri
burn cancer, k.
cancer, k.
kaolin partial thromboplastin time
(KPTT)
kaon
Kaplan-Meier
method, K.
product limit estimate, K.
survival curve, K.
Kaposi
sarcoma, K. (KS)
sarcoma, K. (European type)
varicelliform eruption, K. (KVE)
kappa
-deleting element, k.
granules, k.
light chain, k.
receptor, k.
Karadanzic flap
karaya
adhesive, k.
powder, k.

ADDITIONAL TERMS

ring, k.
seal, k.
Karnofsky
   index, K.
   performance status, K.
   rating scale, K. (grades l through
     100)
   score, K.
Karnowsky fluid
Karpas T-cells
Karr method
karyochromatophil
karyochrome
karyocyte
karyogenesis
karyogenic
karyokinesis
karyoklasis
karyoklastic
karyolobism
karyolymph
karyolysis
karyolytic
karyomegaly
karyomitosis
karyomitotic
karyomorphism
karyon
karyophage
karyoplasm
karyopyknosis
karyopyknotic
   index, k. (KI)
karyorrhectic
karyorrhexis
karyosome
karyostasis
karyotheca
karyotype
karyotyping
Kasabach-Merritt syndrome
kasai syndrome
Kashin-Beck disease
Kast syndrome
Katayama test
Kaufman pneumonia
Kauffmann-White scheme
Kawasaki disease
Kayser disease
Kaznelson syndrome
kb (kilobase)
K-B (Kleihauer-Betke)
   stain, K.

test, K.
kbp (kilobase pair)
kCi (kilocurie)
KCl (potassium chloride)
kd (kilodalton)
32-kd membrane protein
kDNA (kinetoplast DNA)
Ke (Kern)
   antigen, K.
   isotypic determinant, K.
   marker, K.
Keashy tumor
keego cigarette
Keflin
Kefzol
Kekule formula
kelectome
Kell
   antibody, K.
   antigen, K.
   blood antibody type, K.
   blood group system, K.
Kell-Cellano blood group system
Kellgren disease
Kelly malignancy index
keloid
Kempson grading system
Kemron
Kendall compound B
Kennedy syndrome
Kenya hemoglobin
Keofeed feeding tube
keratectomy
keratin
keratinocyte
keratitis
keratoacanthoma
keratoma (pl. keratomata)
keratomalacia
keratomata (pl. of keratoma)
keratopathy
keratosis
   actinic k.
   arsenic k.
   arsenical k.
   blennorrhagica, k.
   follicularis, k.
   linguae, k.
   obturans, k.
   roentgen k.
   seborrheic k.
   seborrheica, k.
   senile k.

ADDITIONAL TERMS

keratosis—*Continued*
 senilis, k.
 solar k.
 stucco k.
 tar k.
keratotic
kerion
kerma (kinetic energy released in
  material)
Kern (Ke)
 antibody, K.
 antigen, K.
 blood group system, K.
 plasma relation theory, K.
Kernohan grading, grades I through IV
ketamine
kethoxal
ketoacidemia
ketoacidosis
ketoconazole
ketone
 bodies, k.
 threshold, k.
ketonemia
ketonization
ketoplasia
ketosis
ketosteroid (17-KS)
Ketostix
ketotic
Kety-Schmidt method
keV (kiloelectron volt)
keyhole-limpet hemocyanin (KLH)
KFAB (kidney-fixing antibody)
KGC (Keflin, gentamicin, carbenicillin)
KG-1 (Koeffler Golde-1) cell line
KI (karyopyknotic index)
KI (potassium iodide)
Ki-67 (immunophenotypic marker)
 antigen, K.
kicksorter
Kidd
 antigen, K.
 antibody type, K.
 blood group system, K.
kidney
 -fixing antibody, k. (KFAB)
 function test, k.
 transplantation, k.
Kidrolase
Kiel classification of non-Hodgkin
 lymphoma

Kienbock unit
killed
 HIV, k.
 virus, k.
killer (K)
 cells, k.
 T cells, k.
kilobase (kb)
 pair, k. (kbp)
kilocurie (kCi)
kilodalton (kd)
kiloelectron volt (keV)
kilounit
kilovolt (kV)
 peak, k. (kVp)
Kimmelstiel-Wilson syndrome
Kim-Ray Greenfield vena cava filter
Kimura disease
Kin-Air flotation mattress
kinase
kinesin
kinetic
kinetics
 cellular k.
kinetocyte
kinetoplast
 DNA, k. (kDNA)
kinetoplastic
King-Armstrong units
kinin
kininase
 plasma k.
kininogen
Kinnier Wilson disease
Kinyoun stain
Ki-ras oncogene
Kirsten sarcoma virus
kit
 oncogene, k.
 ligand, k.
kitasamycin
Kitzmiller test
KIU (kallikrein-inhibiting unit)
KL growth factor
Klacid
Klatskin
 cholangiocarcinoma, K.
 liver biopsy needle, K.
 tumor, K.
Klebs disease
Klebsiella
 friedlanderi, K.

ADDITIONAL TERMS

oxytoca, K.
ozaenae, K.
pneumoniae, K.
pneumoniae ozaenae, K.
pneumoniae rhinoscleromatis, K.
rhinoscleromatis, K.
Kleihauer test
Kleihauer-Betke (K-B)
stain, K.
test, K.
Klein reaction
Kleinschmidt technique
Klenow fragment
KLH (keyhole-limpet hemocyanin)
carrier, K.
Klinefelter syndrome
Klippel-Trenaunay syndrome
Klippel-Trenaunay-Weber syndrome
Km
allotype, K.
allotypic determinant, K.
antigen, K.
Kneipp cure
kneippism
Knops antigen
knuckle
bowel, k. of
colon, k. of
Knudson hypothesis
Koate-HS
Kobert test
Koch
ileostomy, K.
phenomenon, K.
treatment, K.
Kock
pouch, K.
reservoir, K.
Koeffler Golde-1 (KG-1) cell line
Koeppe nodule
koha
koilocyte
koilocytotic atypia
koilonychia
Kold Kap
Kolmogorov-Smirnov statistic
Köln hemoglobin
Konakion
Konyne-HT
Kopans needle
Koranyi
sign, K.

treatment, K.
Kormed disposable liver biopsy needle
Kostmann
infantile agranulocytosis, K.
neutropenia, K.
syndrome, K.
Kow generator
Kowa MDS
Kowarsky test
Kpn I family
KPTT (kaolin partial thromboplastin
time)
Kr (krypton)
Kraske operation
K-ras oncogene
K-ras 2 oncogene
kraurosis
vulvae, k.
Krebs cycle
krebiozen
Krebs leukocyte index
Krompecher
carcinoma, K.
tumor, K.
Krönlein operation
Krukenberg tumor
Kruppel gene product
Kruskal-Wallis
method, K.
test, K.
krypton (Kr)
laser, k.
KS (Kaposi sarcoma)
17-KS (ketosteroid)
KUB (kidneys, ureters, bladder)
Kübler-Ross staging
Kulchitzky cell
carcinoma, K.
tumor, K.
Kundrat lymphosarcoma
Kunkel syndrome
Kupffer cell
sarcoma, K.
Kushner-Tandatnick curette
Kussmaul respiration
Kustner
law, K.
sign, K.
kV (kilovolt)
KVE (Kaposi varicelliform eruption)
Kveim
antigen, K.

ADDITIONAL TERMS

Kveim—*Continued*
   reaction, K.
   test, K.
KVO (keep vein open) type I.V.
kVp (kilovolt peak)
kwashiorkor

L   L (grading of lymphatic invasion)
   L0 (no evidence of lymphatic
   invasion)
   L1 (evidence of invasion of
superficial lymphatics)
   L2 (evidence of invasion of deep
   lymphatics)
   LX (lymphatic invasion cannot be
   assessed)
L-229
L-697,661
L cell
L (light) chain
   disease, L.
L (light) polypeptides
La (lanthanum)
LA (latex agglutination)
LA (lymphocyte-activating)
LAA (leukemia-associated antigen)
LAA (leukocyte ascorbic acid)
LABC (locally advanced breast
   carcinoma)
label
   cohort l.
   radioactive l.
labeled
   antigen immunoperoxidase, l.
   atom, l.
   leukocytes, l.
   red blood cells, l.
labeling
   index, l.
labrocyte
La Bross spot test
lactalbumin
lactamase
   beta-l.
lactase
lactate
   dehydrogenase, l. (LDH)
lactic
   acid, l.
   acidosis, l.
Lactobacillus
   casei, L.

lactis Dorner factor, L.
lactocele
lactoferrin
lactoglobulin
lactoside
   ceramide, l.
lactosyl ceramidase
lactulose
lacuna (pl. lacunae)
lacunae (pl. of lacuna)
lacunar cell
ladakamycin (5-azacitidine)
L.A.E. 20 (estradiol)
Laennec
   cirrhosis, L.
   thrombus, L.
Laetrile
LAF (lymphocyte-activating factor)
lagging-strand synthesis
Lahey staging system
LAHV (leukocyte-associated
   herpesvirus)
LAI (leukocyte adherence inhibition)
LAIA (leukemia-associated inhibitory
   activity)
LAIF (leukocyte adherence inhibition
   factor)
LAK (lymphokine-activated killer) cells
laked
Laki-Lorand factor (LLF)
laking
laky blood
LAL (limulus amebocyte lysate)
   assay, L.
Lallemand bodies
Lallemand-Trousseau bodies
LAM (L-asparaginase, methotrexate)
LAM (lymphocyte adhesion molecule)
lambda
   bacteriophage, l.
   light chain, l.
   particle, l.
   phage vectors, l.
laminagram
laminagraphy
laminar air flow
laminin
   -elastin binding protein, l.
lampbrush chromosomes
Lamprene (clofazamine)
Lancefield
   classification, L.
   precipitation test, L.

ADDITIONAL TERMS

Landeker-Steinberg light
Landry Vein Light Venoscope
Landsteiner
    blood group system, L.
    classification, L.
Landsteiner-Weiner antigen
Lane operation
Langerhans
    cell, L.
    cell granulomatosis, L.
    granules, L.
    islet, L.
langerhansian adenoma
Langhans giant cells
Laniazid
lanthanic
lanthanum (La)
Lanvis (thioguanine)
LAP (leucine aminopeptidase)
LAP (leukocyte alkaline phosphatase)
laparectomy
laparocolectomy
laparocolostomy
laparocystectomy
laparoenterostomy
laparogastrostomy
laparohepatotomy
laparohysterectomy
laparohystero-oophorectomy
laparohysterosalpingo-oophorectomy
laparoiliotomy
laparomyomectomy
laparonephrectomy
laparosalpingectomy
laparosalpingo-oophorectomy
laparoscope
laparoscopy
laparosplenectomy
laparotomy
LAPOCA (L-asparaginase, prednisone,
    Oncovin, cytarabine, Adriamycin)
LARC (leukocyte automatic recognition
    computer)
large
    granular lymphocytes, l. (LGLs)
    intestinal cancer, l.
    loop excision of transformation
        zone, l. (LLETZ)
    undifferentiated cells, l. (LUCs)
large-cell
    adenocarcinoma, l.
    carcinoma, l.
    lung carcinoma, l. (LCLC)

    lymphoma, l.
Lariam
lariat
Larrey operation
laryngeal
laryngectomee
laryngectomize
laryngectomy
larynges (pl. of larynx)
laryngitis
laryngocele
laryngogram
laryngography
laryngopharyngeal
laryngopharyngectomy
laryngopharyngography
laryngopharyngoesophagectomy
laryngopharyngeal
laryngopharynx
laryngoplasty
laryngophthisis
laryngoscleroma
laryngoscope
laryngoscopy
    direct l.
    indirect l.
    mirror l.
    suspension l.
laryngostat
laryngostenosis
laryngostomy
laryngostroboscope
laryngotome
laryngotomy
laryngotracheal
laryngotracheitis
laryngotracheobronchoscopy
laryngotracheoscopy
laryngotracheotomy
laryngovestibulitis
laryngoxerosis
larynx (pl. larynges)
    artificial l.
LAS (lymphadenopathy-associated
    syndrome)
LAS (lymphadenopathy syndrome)
lasalocid
laser (light amplification by stimulated
    emission of radiation)
    argon l.
    carbon dioxide l.
    dye l.
    He-Ne (helium-neon) l.

ADDITIONAL TERMS

laser —*Continued*
  helium-neon (He-Ne) l.
  ion l.
  krypton l.
  Nd:YAG (neodymium:yttrium-
  aluminum-garnet) l.
  neodymium:yttrium-aluminum-
  garnet (Nd:YAG) l.
laser ablation
laser conization
laser photoablation
laser radiation
laser therapy
laser vaporization
Laserflo blood perfusion monitor
LaserSonics
  EndoBlade, L.
  Nd-YAG LaserBlade, L.
  SurgiBlade, L.
Lasertek YAG laser
L-ASP (asparaginase)
L-asparaginase (Elspar or L-ASP)
  -E. coli, L.
  -Erwinia, L.
lassitude
latency
  -associated transcript, l.
latent
  iron-binding capacity, l. (LIBC)
latentiation
lateral-opposed fields
latex
  agglutination test, l.
  condom, l.
  dam, l.
  fixation test, l.
  flocculation test, l.
  particle agglutination, l. (LPA)
  slide agglutination, l.
Latham bowl
Latino virus
LATS (long-acting thyroid stimulator)
LATS-p (long-acting thyroid stimulator
  protector)
lattice
  hypothesis, l.
  theory, l.
laudanum
laughter therapy
Launois syndrome
Lauren classification
Laurell rocket immunoelectrophoresis

LAV (lymphadenopathy-associated
  virus)
  /HTLV-III, L.
law
  Dulong and Petit, l. of
  Gibbs-Donnan l.
lawn plate
Lawrence pouch
lawrencium (Lw)
lazar
lazy leukocyte syndrome (LLS)
LBF (lymphocyte blastogenic factor)
LBL (lymphoblastic lymphoma)
L-buthionine sulfoximine (BSO)
LCAT (lecithin-cholesterol
  acyltransferase)
L-CF (leucovorin-citrovorum factor)
LCIS (lobular carcinoma in situ)
lck gene
LCL (lymphocytic leukemia)
LCL (lymphocytic lymphosarcoma)
LCLC (large-cell lung carcinoma)
LCM (lymphocytic choriomeningitis)
LCMV (lymphocytic choriomeningitis
  virus)
LCR (vincristine)
LCT (liquid crystal thermogram)
L-cycloserine
LD (lethal dose)
LD (lymphocyte-defined)
  antigens, L.
LDH (lactate dehydrogenase)
LDL (low-density lipoproteins)
L-dopa (levodopa)
Le
  b antigen, L.
  b substance, L.
  c antigen, L.
  x antigen, L.
LE (lupus erythematosus)
  antigen, L.
  cell, L.
  cell prep, L.
  factor, L.
lead
  apron, l.
  blocks, l.
  gloves, l.
  gonad shield, l.
  mask, l.
  shield, l.
  poisoning, l.

ADDITIONAL TERMS

League of Nations staging
leakage radiation
leaky gene
least squares regression
leather bottle stomach
LEC-CAM (lectin cell adhesion molecules)
lecithin
-cholesterol acyltransferase, l. (LCAT)
lecithinase
lecithinemia
lecithoprotein
lectin
binding, l.
cell adhesion molecules, l. (LEC-CAM)
DBA, l. (Dolichos biflorus agglutinin)
Leder stain
Lederer anemia
LeDuc-Camey ileocystoplasty
Lee-White
clotting time, L.
method, L.
LEEP (loop electrosurgical excision procedure)
left shift
Legionella
bozmanii, L.
dumoffii, L.
feeleii, L.
gormanii, L.
jordanis, L.
longbeachae, L.
micdadei, L.
pittsburgensis, L.
pneumophilia, L.
wadsworthii, L.
Legionella direct immunofluorescent antibody
Legionellaceae
legionellosis
legionnaires disease
Leiner disease
leiomyoblastoma
leiomyofibroma
leiomyoma
bizarre l.
cutis, l.
epithelioid l.
uteri, l.

vascular l.
leiomyomatosis
intramural l.
peritonealis disseminata, l.
leiomyosarcoma
Leishman
chrome cells, L.
stain, L.
Leishman-Donovan body
Leishmania
donovani, L.
leishmanial
leishmaniasis
leishmanin test
Leksell stereotactic device
LEL (lowest effective level)
lemmoblast
lemmocyte
LEMMON (lymphoma, Ewing sarcoma, melanoma, medulloblastoma, oat cell sarcoma, neuroblastoma)
group, L.
Lenard rays
Lennert lymphoma
lentectomy
lenticular carcinoma
lentiform
lentigenes (pl. of lentigo)
lentiginous
lentigo (pl. lentigines)
maligna, l. (Hutchinson freckle)
maligna melanoma, l. (LMM)
nevoid l.
senile l.
senilis, l.
simplex, l.
solar l.
lentil
agglutinin binding, l.
lectin affinity chromatography, l.
lentinan
Lentinus edodes
lentiviral
lentivirus
Leonard unit
leopard syndrome
lepidoma
endothelial l.
Lepore
hemoglobin, L.
trait, L.
lepra

ADDITIONAL TERMS

lepra —*Continued*
  cell, l.
  reaction, l.
leproma
lepromatous
    leprosy, l.
lepromin
    skin test, l.
leprosy
leprotic
leprous
leptocyte
leptocytosis
leptomeningeal
leptomeninges (pl. of leptomeninx)
leptomeningioma
leptomeninx (pl. leptomeninges)
leptomeningeal cyst
lepton
leptoscope
Lesch-Nyhan syndrome
Leser-Trelat
    lesion, L.
    sign, L.
lesion
    annular l.
    apple-core l.
    cavitary l.
    coin l.
    cold l.
    discrete l.
    fungating l.
    gross l.
    histologic l.
    hot l.
    indiscriminate l.
    mass l.
    metastatic l.
    multifocal l.
    necrotic l.
    neoplastic l.
    precancerous l.
    space-occupying l.
    stellate l.
LET (linear energy transfer)
lethal
    dose, l. (LD)
    equivalent, l.
    factor, l.
    gene, l.
    mutant, l.
lethality
lethargic

lethargy
Letrazuril
Letterer-Siwe disease
Leu (leucine)
    Leu 1 cells
    Leu 2 cells
    Leu 2+ cells
    Leu + 2a+ cells
    Leu 3 cells
    Leu 7 cells
    Leu 11 cells
    Leu-M1 stain
leucine (Leu)
    aminomutase, l.
    aminopeptidase, l. (LAP)
    zipper, l.
leucocyte
leucocytosis
Leucomax (GM-CSF or molgramostim)
leucovorin
    calcium, l. (Wellcovorin)
    rescue, l.
leucyl-tRNA synthetase
leukanakmesis
leukapheresis
leukemia
    acute granulocytic l.
    acute lymphoblastic l. (ALL)
    acute lymphocytic l. (ALL)
    acute megakaryoblastic l.
    acute megakaryocytic l.
    acute monoblastic l. (AMOL)
    acute monocytic l. (AMOL)
    acute monomyelocytic l.
    acute myeloblastic l. (AML)
    acute myelocytic l. (AML)
    acute myelogenous l. (AML)
    acute myeloid l.
    acute myelomonoblastic l.
      (AMMOL)
    acute myelomonocytic l. (AMMOL)
    acute nonlymphoblastic l.
    acute nonlymphocytic l. (ANLL)
    acute nonlymphoid l. (ANLL)
    acute progranulocytic l.
    acute promyelocytic l.
    acute unclassifiable l. (AUL)
    acute undifferentiated l.
    adult T-cell l.
    aleukemic l.
    aleukocythemic l.
    basophilic l.
    B-cell l.

ADDITIONAL TERMS

B-cell acute lymphoblastic l.
bilineage l.
biphenotypic l.
blast cell l.
blastic l.
Burkitt-type acute lymphoblastic l.
chronic basophilic l. (CBL)
chronic eosophilic l. (CEL)
chronic granulocytic l. (CGL)
chronic lymphocytic l. (CLL)
chronic monocytic l.
chronic myelocytic l. (CML)
chronic myelogenous l. (CML)
chronic myelomonocytic l.
common acute lymphoblastic l.
compound l.
congenital l.
cutis, l.
embryonal l.
eosinophilic l.
feline l.
granulocytic l.
Gross l.
hairy-cell l. (HCL)
hand-mirror cell l.
hemoblastic l.
hemocytoblastic l.
histiocytic l.
hypergranular promyelocytic l.
juvenile chronic granulocytic l.
L1210 l.
leukopenic l.
lymphatic l.
lymphoblastic l.
lymphocytic l.
lymphogenous l.
lymphoid l.
lymphoidocytic l.
lymphosarcoma cell l.
mast cell l.
mature cell l.
megakaryoblastic l
megakaryocytic l.
micromyeloblastic l.
mixed cell l.
monoblastic l.
monocytic l.
myeloblastic l.
myelocytic l.
myelogenic l.
myelogenous l.
myeloid l.
myeloid granulocytic l.

myelomonocytic l.
Naegeli l.
neonatal l.
neutrophilic l.
non-B cell l.
non-T cell l.
nonlymphocytic l.
null-cell l.
null-cell lymphoblastic l.
peripheral stem cell l.
plasma cell l. (PCL)
plasmacytic l.
polylymphocytic l.
polymorphocytic l.
pre-B cell acute lymphoblastic l.
pre-B cell acute lymphocytic l.
pre-T cell acute lymphoblastic l.
pre-T cell acute lymphocytic l.
prolymphocytic l. (PLL)
promyelocytic l.
Rauscher l.
reticuloendothelial cell l.
reticulum cell l.
Rieder cell l.
Schilling l.
Schwartz l.
secondary l.
smoldering l.
splenomedullary l.
splenomyelogenous l.
stem cell l.
subleukemic l.
T-cell l.
T-cell chronic lymphocytic l.
T-cell-derived non-Hodgkin l.
T-cell lymphoblastic l.
thrombocytic l.
undifferentiated cell l.
leukemia-associated inhibitory activity,
   l. (LAIA or LIA)
leukemia erythrocytosis
leukemia line
leukemia-lymphoma syndrome
leukemia virus
leukemic
   cells, l.
   infiltration, l.
   phase, l.
   reticuloendotheliosis, l.
leukemid
leukemogen
leukemogenesis
leukemogenic

ADDITIONAL TERMS

leukemoid
leukencephalitis
Leukeran (chlorambucil)
leukexosis
leukin
Leukine (GM-CSF or sargramostim)
leukoagglutinin
leukoblast
  granular l.
leukoblastosis
leukocidin
  Neisser-Wechsberg l.
  Panton-Valentine (P-V) l.
leukoclastic
  vasculitis, l.
leukocoria
leukocrit
leukocytal
leukocyte
  acidophilic l.
  adherence inhibition l.
  agranular l.
  basophilic l.
  cryopreserved l.
  endothelial l.
  eosinophilic l.
  granular l's
  heterophilic l's
  hyaline l.
  lymphoid l.
  mast l.
  motile l.
  neutrophilic l.
  nongranular l's
  nonmotile l.
  passenger l.
  polymorphonuclear basophilic l.
  polymorphonuclear eosinophilic l.
  polynuclear neutrophilic l.
  transitional l.
  Türk irritation l.
leukocyte acid phosphatase stain
leukocyte adherence inhibition (LAI)
leukocyte adherence inhibition factor
  (LAIF)
leukocyte adhesion deficiency
leukocyte agglutinin
leukocyte alkaline phosphatase (LAP)
leukocyte alloantibodies
leukocyte antigens
leukocyte ascorbic acid (LAA)
leukocyte-associated herpesvirus
  (LAHV)

leukocyte automatic recognition
  computer (LARC)
leukocyte count nadir
leukocyte diapedesis
leukocyte differential count
leukocyte esterase
leukocyte fraction
leukocyte G6PD deficiency
leukocyte inhibitory factor (LIF)
leukocyte interferon
leukocyte margination
leukocyte migration inhibition assay
leukocyte nuclear hyposegmentation
leukocyte-poor red blood cells
leukocythemia
leukocytic
  cream, l.
  crystals, l.
  infiltrate, l.
  marrow, l.
  pyrogen, l.
leukocytoblast
leukocytoclastic
  angiitis, l.
leukocytogenesis
leukocytoid
leukocytology
leukocytolysin
leukocytolysis
  venom l.
leukocytolytic
  serum, l.
leukocytoma
leukocytopenia
leukocytophagy
leukocytoplania
leukocytopoiesis
leukocytopoietic
leukocytosis
  absolute l.
  agonal l.
  basophilic l.
  eosinophilic l.
  mononuclear l.
  neutrophilic l.
  pathologic l.
  physiologic l.
  pure l.
  relative l.
  terminal l.
  toxic l.
leukocytosis-promoting factor (LPF)
leukocytotactic

ADDITIONAL TERMS

leukocytotaxis
leukocytotherapy
leukocytotoxic
leukocytotoxicity
leukocytotoxin
leukocytotropic
leukocyturia
leukodepletion
leukoderivative
leukoderma
leukodermatous
leukodiagnosis
leukodystrophy
leukoedema
leukencephalitis
leukencephalopathy
   necrotizing l.
   progressive multifocal l.
leukencephaly
leukoerythroblastic
   anemia, l.
leukoerythroblastosis
leukoerythrogenetic
leukoglobulin (immune gamma
  globulin)
leukogram
leukokeratosis
leukokinesis
leukokinetic
leukokinetics
leukokinin
leukokoria
leukokraurosis
leukolymphosarcoma
leukolysin
leukolysis
leukolytic
leukoma
   adherent l.
leukomaine
leukomainemia
leukomatous
leukomonocyte
leukomyelitis
leukomyoma
leukon
leukonecrosis
leukopathia
leukopedesis
leukopenia
   basophil l.
   basophilic l.
   congenital l.

   malignant l.
   pernicious l.
leukopenic
leukophagocytosis
leukopheresis
leukoplakia
   buccalis, l.
   glottic l.
   hairy l.
   lingualis, l.
   oral l.
   speckled l.
   vulvae, l.
leukopoiesis
leukopoietic
leukopoietin
leuko-poor red cells
leukoprecipitin
leukosarcoma
leukosarcomatosis
leukosarcomatous
leukoscope
leukosis
   acute l.
   avian l.
   lymphoid l.
   myeloblastic l.
   myelocytic l.
   skin l.
leukostasis
leukotactic
leukotaxine
leukotaxis
leukothrombin
leukotome
leukotomy
leukotoxic
leukotoxicity
leukotoxin
Leukotrap red cell storage system
leukotriene
leukovirus
leuprolide acetate (LEUP or Lupron)
leurocristine
levamisole hydrochloride (Ergamisol or
  LEV)
Levay factor
levcycloserine
LeVeen
   shunt, L.
   valve, L.
Levin tube
levocarnitine

ADDITIONAL TERMS

Levo-Dromoran
levofuraltadone
Levoid
levorphanol
Levothroid
levothyroxine (L-thyroxine)
   sodium, l.
Levoxine
Lewandowsky nevus
Lewis
   antibodies, L.
   blood group system, L.
   gene, L.
   group antigen, L.
   lung carcinoma, L.
   phenomenon, L.
   substance, L.
Lewis-Langmuir
   atom, L.
   theory, L.
Lewis-Tanner procedure
lewisite
Lewisohn method
Leydig cell
   tumor, L.
Leydig-Sertoli cell tumor
LFS (Li-Fraumeni syndrome)
LFT (liver function test)
LGLs (large granular leukocytes)
LGV (lymphogranuloma venereum)
LH (luteinizing hormone)
Lhermitte sign
Lhermitte-Duclos disease
LHRH (luteinizing hormone-releasing
   hormone)
LIA (leukemia-associated inhibitory
   activity)
Liacopoulos phenomenon
LIBC (latent iron-binding
   capacity)
Libowitz metal
Lich-Gregoire repair
lichen
   fibromucinoidosus, l.
   myxedematosus, l.
   planus, l.
lichenification
lichenoid
Lichtheim plaques
licorice
L-iditol dehydrogenase
lidofenin
L-iduronidase

lien
lienal
lienectomy
lienography
LIF (leukocyte inhibitory factor)
life island
Li-Fraumeni syndrome (LFS)
LIFT (lymphocyte immunofluorescence
   test)
ligand
   antibody-bound l.
   bound l.
   free l.
   labeled l.
   radiolabeled l.
   unlabeled l.
ligand-binding
   assay, l.
ligase
light
   actinic l.
   black l.
   coherent l.
   cold l.
   Finsen l.
   Landeker-Steinberg l.
   Minin l.
   Simpson l.
   ultraviolet l.
light-activated
light-activation
light chain (L-chain)
light polypeptide chains
Light Talker
Lignac-Fanconi disease
Lillie hematoxylin
limulus amebocyte lysate (LAL)
   assay, l.
LINAC (linear accelerator)
Linac knife surgery
Lindau tumor
lineage
linear
   accelerator, l.
   amputation, l.
   array, l.
   array scanner, l.
   attenuation coefficient, l.
   coefficient, l.
   energy transfer, l. (LET)
   grid, l.
   iridium wire, l.
   phased array, l.

ADDITIONAL TERMS

regression analysis, l.
ribbon array, l.
linearization
linearize
lingulectomy
linitis
  plastica, l.
linkage
  analysis, l.
  disequilibrium, l.
  map, l.
linker
  insertion, l.
  regions, l.
Linson electronic cell counter
Lintro-scan mammography
Lioresal
liothyronine
  iodine 124, l.
  iodine 131, l.
liotrix
LIP (lymphoid interstitial pneumonia)
LIP/PLH (lymphoid interstitial pneumonia/pulmonary lymphoid hyperplasia)
liparocele
lipid
  -associated sialic acid, l.
  -bound sialic acid, l.
  cell tumor, l.
  histiocytosis, l.
  panel, l.
lipoadenoma
lipoblastoma
lipoblastomatosis
lipochondroma
lipofibroma
lipogenic
lipogranuloma
lipogranulomatosis
Lipo-Hepin
lipoid
  histiocytoma, l.
  nephrosis, l.
  ovarian tumor, l.
lipoma
  annulare colli, l.
  arborescens, l.
  capsulare, l.
  cavernosum, l.
  cystic l.
  diffuse l.
  diffusum renis, l.

dolorosa, l.
fetal fat cell l.
fibrosum, l.
intradural l.
myxomatodes, l.
nevoid l.
ossificans, l.
petrificans, l.
petrificum ossificans, l.
pleiomorphic l.
sarcomatodes, l.
spindle cell l.
telangiectatic l.
telangiectodes, l.
lipomatoid
lipomatosis
  atrophicans, l.
  congenital l. of pancreas
  diffuse l.
  dolorosa, l.
  gigantea, l.
  nodular circumscribed l.
  renal l.
  replacement l. of kidney
  symmetrical l.
lipomatous
lipomeningocele
lipomyohemangioma
lipomyoma
lipomyxoma
lipophilic
  cation, l.
lipophilicity
lipopolysaccharide (LPS)
lipoprotein
  beta l.
  high-density l. (HDL)
  intermediate-density l. (IDL)
  low-density l. (LDL)
  serum l.
lipoproteinemia
liposarcoma
  myxoid l.
  pleomorphic l.
  round-cell l.
liposomal
  daunorubicin, l.
  gentamicin, l.
liposome
  -encapsulated amphotericin-B, l.
Liposyn II, III
lipotropin
  beta-l.

ADDITIONAL TERMS

lipoxygenase
   pathway, l.
Lipschütz bodies
Liquaemin Sodium
liquefaction
liquefactive
liquefying
liquid nitrogen
Lisfranc amputation
Listeria
   monocytogenes, L.
Listerine
listeriosis
lithium
   carbonate, l.
   -carmine stain, l.
littoral cells
liver
   bed, l.
   biopsy, l.
   cell adenoma, l.
   damage, l.
   extract, l.
   failure, l.
   flap, l.
   function test, l. (LFT)
   Lactobacillus casei factor, l.
   metastases, l.
   scan, l.
   solution, l.
   span, l.
   -specific gene, l.
   transplant, l.
   tumor, l.
Lizar operation
LKS (liver, kidneys, spleen)
LLD (Lactobacillus lactis Dorner)
   factor, L.
LLETZ (large loop excision of
   transformation zone)
L-leucovorin
L1210 leukemia
LLF (Laki-Lorand factor)
LL-2-I-131
LLS (lazy leukocyte syndrome)
LLUMC (Loma Linda University Medical
   Center)
   proton accelerator, L.
L-17M
L-176M
LM427 (ansamycin)
LMF (Leukeran, methotrexate,
   5-fluorouracil)

LMF (lymphocyte mitogenic factor)
LMM (lentigo maligna melanoma)
LN2 lymphocyte marker
LNPF (lymph node permeability factor)
loading
   applicator, l.
   dose, l.
lobe
lobectomy
   sleeve l.
lobi (pl. of lobus)
lobotomy
lobular
   carcinoma in situ, l. (LCIS)
   mass, l.
lobulated
   tumor mass, l.
lobule
lobuli (pl. of lobulus)
lobulus (pl. lobuli)
lobus (pl. lobi)
local
   disease, l.
   excision, l.
   immunity, l.
   involvement, l.
   irradiation, l.
   metastases, l.
   radiation therapy, l.
   recurrence, l.
   regional control, l.
   spread, l.
   therapy, l.
localization
   needle l.
   tumor l.
localized
   cancer, l.
   lesion, l.
   mass, l.
   myeloma, l.
   radiotherapy, l.
   tumor, l.
loci (pl. of locus)
locoregional
loculated
   ascites, l.
   effusion, l.
locus (pl. loci)
   HLA l.
   major histocompatibility l.
locus activation region
locus-specific

ADDITIONAL TERMS

Loevit cell
Löffler
    eosinophilia, L.
    pneumonia, L.
    syndrome, L.
L-ofloxacin
logarithm
logarithmic
    response, l.
log
    -kill concept, l.
    -linear method, l.
    -rank testing, l.
Logan procedure
Loma Linda University Medical Center
    (LLUMC)
    proton accelerator, L.
lometrexol sodium
Lomidine
Lomotil
lomustine (CCNU or CeeNu)
long
    -acting thyroid stimulator, l.
      (LATS)
    -acting thyroid stimulator
      protector, l. (LATS-p)
    open reading frame, l. (LORF)
    terminal repeats, l. (LTR)
longiradiate
lonidamine (AF 1890)
look-locker technique
loop
    colostomy, c.
    electrosurgical excision procedure,
      l. (LEEP)
loopogram
loperamide hydrochloride
LORF (long open reading frame)
Lortat-Jacob approach
Los Alamos test site
Lossen rule
Louisiana pneumonia
Love Canal
low
    -density lipoproteins, l. (LDL)
    -energy radiation, l.
    -power field, l. (lpf)
    zone tolerance, l.
lowest effective level (LEL)
LOX cell line
loxoribine (RWJ 21757)
lozenge
LPA (latex particle agglutination)

L-PAM (L-phenylalanine mustard or
    melphalan)
LPC (lysophosphatidylcholine)
LPC-1 plasma cell tumor
LPE (lysophosphatidylethanolamine)
LPF (leukocytosis-promoting factor)
LPF (lymphocytosis-promoting factor)
lpf (low-power field)
L-phase variant
L-phenylalanine mustard (L-PAM or
    melphalan)
LPS (lipopolysaccharide)
LSA2L2 chemotherapy
L-sarcolysin
LSH (lymphocyte-stimulating hormone)
L-tetramizole
LTF (lymphocyte transforming factor)
LTH (luteotropic hormone)
L-thyroxine (levothyroxine)
LTR (long terminal repeats)
lubricin
LUCs (large undifferentiated cells)
lucency
lucent
    defect, l.
Lucey-Driscoll syndrome
Lucifer yellow dye
luciferase
luciferin
Lucio phenomenon
lucite
    applicator, l.
    ovoid, l.
lucotherapy
Lucrin
Ludwig Group
Lugol
    solution, L.
    stain, L.
Luke antigen
Lukes-Butler classification
Lukes-Collins classification of non-
    Hodgkin lymphoma
lump
lumpectomize
lumpectomy
Lunderquist wire
lung
    biopsy, l.
    brushings, l.
    cancer, l.
    carcinoma, l.
    metastasis, l.

ADDITIONAL TERMS

lung—*Continued*
  scan, l.
  washings, l.
Lungaggregate reagent
lupoid
  hepatitis, l.
Lupron (leuprolide)
Lupron Depot
lupus
  chilblain l.
  drug-induced l.
  erythematosus, l. (LE)
  hypertrophicus, l.
  neonatal l.
  nephritis, l.
  pernio, l.
lupus band test
lutein
  cyst, l.
luteinizing hormone (LH)
  -releasing hormone, l. (LHRH)
luteoma
luteotropic hormone (LTH)
Lutheran
  antibody, L.
  antigen, L.
  blood group system, L.
Lutz-Splendore-Almeida disease
LV (leucovorin)
L-VAM (Lupron, Velban, Adriamycin, Mutamycin)
LVVP (Leukeran, vinblastine, vincristine, prednisone)
Lw (lawrencium)
LX (lymphatic invasion cannot be assessed)
LY186641
Ly antigen
Ly 1-2+ T cells
Lyb antigens
lycopene
lycopenemia
Lye stricture
Lygidakis procedure
Lyl B cell
lym-1 monoclonal antibody
Lyme
  arthritis, L.
  borreliosis, L.
  disease, L.
  titer, L.
lymph
  cell, l.
  follicle, l.

  gland, l.
  nodule, l.
  sinus, l.
  spaces, l.
lymph node
  chain, l.
  classification, l.
  dissection, l.
  imaging, l.
  involvement, l.
  irradiation, l.
  metastasis, l.
  permeability factor, l. (LNPF)
  resection, l.
  sampling, l.
lymphaden
lymphadenectasis
lymphadenectomy
lymphadenhypertrophy
lymphadenia
  ossea, l.
lymphadenitis
  mesenteric l.
  nonbacterial regional l.
  tuberculoid l.
  tuberculous l.
lymphadenocele
lymphadenocyst
lymphadenogram
lymphadenography
lymphadenoid
lymphadenoleukopoiesis
lymphadenoma
  malignant l.
  multiple l.
lymphadenomatosis
  general l. of bones
lymphadenopathy
  angioimmunoblastic l.
  angioimmunoblastic l. with dysproteinemia (AILD)
  axillary l.
  dermatopathic l.
  giant follicular l.
  hilar l.
  immunoblastic l.
  mediastinal l.
  mesenteric l.
  tuberculous l.
lymphadenopathy-associated syndrome (LAS)
lymphadenopathy-associated virus (LAV)
lymphadenopathy syndrome (LAS)

ADDITIONAL TERMS

lymphadenosis
  aleukemic l.
  benigna cutis, l.
lymphadenotomy
lymphadenovarix
lymphagogue
lymphangial
lymphangiectasia
lymphangiectasis
lymphangiectomy
lymphangiitis
lymphangioadenography
lymphangioendothelioblastoma
lymphangioendothelioma
lymphangiofibroma
lymphangiogram (LAG)
lymphangiography
lymphangiology
lymphangioma
  capillary l.
  cavernosum, l.
  cavernous l.
  circumscriptum, l.
  colonic l.
  cystic l.
  cysticum, l.
  fissural l.
  intrasplenic l.
  mediastinal l.
  simple l.
  simplex, l.
lymphangiomyomatosis
lymphangiosarcoma
lymphangiotomy
lymphangitic
  carcinomatosis, l.
  metastasis, l.
  spread, l.
lymphangitis
lymphapheresis
lymphatic
  blockade, l.
  chain, l.
  invasion, l.
  involvement, l.
  leukemia, l.
  mesh, l.
  metastasis, l.
  nodules, l.
  spread, l.
  system, l.
  tissue, l.
lymphaticostomy
lymphatism

lymphatitis
lymphatogenous
lymphatology
lymphatolysis
lymphatolytic
Lymphazurin
lymphectasia
lymphedema
lymphendothelioma
lymphepithelioma
lymphization
lymphnoditis
lymphoblast
lymphoblastic
  leukemia, l.
  lymphoma, l. (LBL)
  lymphosarcoma, l.
lymphoblastoma
lymphoblastomatosis
lymphoblastosis
lymphocele
lymphocerastism
lymphocytapheresis
lymphocyte
  activated l.
  amplifier T-l.
  atypical l.
  B (thymus-independent) l's
  CD4-positive l.
  cytotoxic T l's (CTL)
  killer l.
  large granular l's
  null l.
  reticular l.
  Rieder l.
  T (thymus-dependent) l's
  thymus-dependent (T) l's
  thymus-independent (B) l's
lymphocyte-activating factor (LAF)
lymphocyte-adhesion molecule (LAM)
lymphocyte blastogenic factor (LBF)
lymphocyte count
lymphocyte-defined (LD)
lymphocyte-depleted
lymphocyte depletion
lymphocyte doubling time
lymphocyte homing receptor
lymphocyte immunofluorescence test
  (LIFT)
lymphocyte migration
lymphocyte mitogenic factor (LMF)
lymphocyte proliferation assay
lymphocyte recirculation
lymphocyte-stimulating hormone (LSH)

ADDITIONAL TERMS

lymphocyte subset
lymphocyte transforming factor (LTF)
lymphocythemia
lymphocytic
    choriomeningitis, l. (LCM)
    choriomeningitis virus, l. (LCMV)
    interstitial pneumonitis, l. (LIP)
    leukemia, l. (LCL)
    lymphocytosis, l.
    lymphoma, l.
    lymphosarcoma, l. (LCL)
    thyroiditis, l.
lymphocytoblast
lymphocytoma
    cutis, l.
lymphocytomatosis
lymphocytomatous
lymphocytopenia
lymphocytopheresis
lymphocytopoiesis
lymphocytopoietic
lymphocytorrhexis
lymphocytosis
    acute infectious l.
    B-cell l.
lymphocytosis-promoting factor (LPF)
lymphocytotic
lymphocytotoxicity
lymphocytotoxin
lymphocytotropic
lymphoendothelioma
lymphoepithelial
lymphoepithelioma
lymphogenesis
lymphogenous
lymphoglandula
lymphogonia
lymphogram
lymphogranuloma
    inguinale, l.
    malignum, l.
    venereum, l. (LGV)
    venereum antigen, l.
lymphogranulomatosis
    benign l.
    cutis, l.
    inguinalis, l.
    maligna, l.
lymphography
lymphohistiocytic
lymphohistiocytosis
    familial erythrophagocytic l.
lymphohistioplasmacytic

    tissue, l.
lymphoid
    cell, l.
    depletion, l.
    granulomatosis, l.
    hemoblast of Pappenheim, l.
    hyperplasia, l.
    interstitial pneumonia, l. (LIP)
    interstitial pneumonia/pulmonary
        lymphoid hyperplasia, l. (LIP/
        PLH)
    irradiation, l.
    leukemia, l.
    leukosis, l.
    mass, l.
    neoplasm, l.
    stroma, l.
    system, l.
    tissue, l.
lymphoidectomy
lymphoidocyte
lymphoidocytic
lymphokentric
lymphokine
    -activated killer (LAK) cells, l.
lymphokinesis
lymphology
lympholysis
    cell-mediated l. (CML)
lympholytic
lymphoma
    adult T-cell l.
    adult T-cell leukemia/l.
    African l.
    allogeneic l.
    alveolar l.
    autologous l.
    B-cell l.
    Burkitt l.
    Burkitt-like l.
    centroblastic/centrocytic l.
    clasmocytic l.
    colorectal l.
    composite l.
    convoluted T-cell l.
    cutaneous T-cell l.
    cutis, l.
    Darmstruck l.
    diffuse l.
    diffuse histiocytic l.
    diffuse large-cell l.
    diffuse lymphocytic l.
    disseminated l.

ADDITIONAL TERMS

EU8-induced l.
extranodal l.
follicular l.
follicular center cell l.
gastric l.
giant follicle l.
giant follicular l.
granulomatous l.
histiocytic l.
Hodgkin l.
immunoblastic l.
large-cell l.
Lennert l.
lymphoblastic l.
lymphocytic l.
lymphoplasmacytoid l.
malignant l.
mantle zone l.
Mediterranean l.
mixed cell l.
mixed lymphocytic/histiocytic l.
nodular l.
non-Burkitt pleomorphic l.
noncleaved follicular center cell l.
non-Hodgkin l. (NHL)
plasmacytoid lymphocytic l.
pleomorphic l.
poorly differentiated lymphocytic l.
retroperitoneal l.
Sézary l.
small B-cell l.
small-cell lymphocytic l.
small lymphocytic T-cell l.
stem cell l.
T-cell l's
U (undifferentiated) cell l.
undifferentiated l.
UR2AV-induced l.
well-differentiated lymphocytic l.
YC8 l.
lymphoma implant
lymphomatoid
   granulomatosis, l.
   papulosis, l.
lymphomatosis
   granulomatosa, l.
   neural l.
   ocular l.
lymphomatous
   infiltrate, l.
lymphomyxoma
lymphonodus
lymphopathia

venereum, l.
lymphopathy
lymphopenia
lymphopenic
   agammaglobulinemia, l.
lymphoplasia
   cutaneous l.
lymphoplasm
lymphoplasmapheresis
lymphoplasmocytosis
lymphopoiesis
lymphopoietic
lymphoproliferation
lymphoproliferative
lymphoprotease
lymphoreticular
   disorders, l.
   system, l.
lymphoreticulosis
lymphosarcoma
   fascicular l.
   gibbon ape l.
   Kundrat l.
   lymphoblastic l.
   lymphocytic l.
   sclerosing l.
lymphosarcoma cell leukemia
lymphosarcomatosis
lymphosarcomatous
   nodule, l.
lymphoscintigram
lymphoscintigraphy
lymphotaxis
lymphotoxemia
lymphotoxin
lymphotrophy
lymphotrophic
lymphs (lymphocytes)
LYOfoam dressing
Lyon
   hypothesis, L.
   phenomenon, L.
lyonization
lyonized
lyophilization
lyophilize
Lypho-Med
lysate
lysemia
lysin
lysine
   acetylsalicylate, l.
   dehydrogenase, l.

ADDITIONAL TERMS

lysine—*Continued*
-ketoglutarate reductase, l.
lysis
Lysodren (mitotane)
lysogen
lysogenesis
lysogenic
lysogeny
lysokinase
lysolecithin
lysophosphatide
lysophosphatidylcholine (LPC)
lysophosphatidylethanolamine (LPE)
lysosomal
lysosome
lysozyme
lysyl
    bradykinin, l.
    oxidase, l.
Lyt antigen
lytic
    degeneration, l.
    lesion, l.
    molecule, l.
    necrosis, l.
lyzozymuria

Mm (m) (suffix used to indicate
multiple tumors, written
within parentheses)
M (grading of distant
metastasis)

M
    M0 (no distant metastasis)
    M1 (distant metastasis)
    MX (presence of distant metastasis
    cannot be assessed)
M antigen
M344 antigen
M-cell
M-component
M factor
M hemoglobin
M period
M phase
M-protein
Ma (masurium)
MAA (macroaggregated albumin)
MAb (monoclonal antibody)
MABOP (Mustargen, Adriamycin,
    bleomycin, Oncovin, prednisone)
MAC (membrane attack complex)

-INH, M. (membrane attack
    complex-inhibitor)
MAC (methotrexate, actinomycin D,
    cyclophosphamide)
MAC (methotrexate, Adriamycin,
    cyclophosphamide)
MAC (mitomycin-C, Adriamycin,
    cyclophosphamide)
MAC (Mycobacterium avium complex)
-MAI, M. (Mycobacterium avium
    complex-Mycobacterium avium-
    intracellulare)
macaque
MACC (methotrexate, Adriamycin,
    cyclophosphamide, CCNU)
MacConkey agar
macerate
maceration
Mach
    front, M.
    stem, M.
Machado test
Machado-Guerreiro test
Mache unit (Mu)
MACHO (methotrexate, asparaginase,
    cyclophosphamide,
    hydroxydaunomycin, Oncovin)
Machupo virus
MACI (membrane attack complex-
    inhibitor)
Mackenzie amputation
MACOP-B (methotrexate, Adriamycin,
    cyclophosphamide, Oncovin,
    prednisone, bleomycin, with
    leucovorin)
macradenous
Macrisalb ^{131}I injection
macroadenoma
macroaggregated albumin (MAA)
macroaggregates of radioiodinated
    albumin (MARIA)
macroamylase
macroamylasemia
macroangiopathic
macroangiopathy
macrobiotic
    diet, m.
macroblast
    Naegeli, m. of
macrocytase
macrocyte
macrocythemia

ADDITIONAL TERMS

macrocytic
  anemia, m.
  indices, m.
macrocytosis
Macrodex
macroelement
macroflora
macroglia
macroglobulin
macroglobulinemia
  Waldenström m.
macroleukoblast
macrolide
macrolymphocyte
macrolymphocytosis
macromethod of Wintrobe
macromolecular
macromolecule
macromonocyte
macromyeloblast
macronodular
macronormoblast
macronucleus
macro-ovalocyte
macrophage
  alveolar m.
  armed m's
  fixed m.
  foamy m.
  free m.
  inflammatory m.
macrophage-activating factor (MAF)
macrophage agglutination factor
  (MAggF)
macrophage chemotactic factor (MCF)
macrophage colony-stimulating factor
  (M-CSF)
macrophage cytotoxic factor
macrophage-derived growth factor
macrophage electrophoretic mobility
  (MEM)
macrophage-inhibiting factor (MIF)
macrophage-inhibitory factor (MIF)
macrophage migration inhibiting factor
  (MMIF)
macrophage proliferation
macrophage surface receptor
macrophagocyte
macrophysics
macropolycyte
macroprolactinoma
macropromyelocyte

macroradiography
macroreticulocyte
Macroscan-131
macroscopic
macroscopy
Macrotec kit
macrothrombocyte
macula (pl. maculae)
maculae (pl. of macula)
macular
MAD (MeCCNU, Adriamycin)
Madagascan periwinkle plant
MADDOC (mechlorethamine,
  Adriamycin, dacarbazine, DDP,
  Oncovin, cyclophosphamide)
Madelung
  disease, M.
  neck, M.
Madigan prostatectomy
Madin-Darby canine kidney cells
madreporic coral
Madura foot
maduramicin
maduromycosis
maedivirus
MAF (macrophage-activating factor)
mafenide
Maffucci syndrome
mafosfamide
3M afterloading system
MAggF (macrophage agglutination
  factor)
magnesemia
magnesium
  chloride, m.
magnetic
  field, m.
  quantum number, m.
  resonance angiography, m. (MRA)
  resonance imaging, m. (MRI)
  resonance spectroscopy, m. (MRS)
Magnetrode
  cervical unit, M.
  magnetic loop induction, M.
magnetron
Magnevist (gadonepentate dimeglumine)
Mahurkar dual-lumen catheter
MAHA (microangiopathic hemolytic
  anemia)
MAI (Mycobacterium avium-
  intracellulare)
  bacteremia, M.

ADDITIONAL TERMS

MAID (mesna, Adriamycin, interleukin-3, dacarbazine)
MAID (Mesnex, Adriamycin, Ifex, dacarbazine)
mainstem bronchus
maintenance
    chemotherapy, m.
    dialysis, m.
    drug, m.
    level, m.
    therapy, m.
Mainz pouch
Maissoneuve amputation
Majocchi
    disease, M.
    granuloma, M.
major
    gene, m.
    histocompatibility complex, m. (MHC)
MAK-6 (monoclonal anticytokeratin) cocktail, M.
Makeham hypothesis
malabsorption
malacoma
malacoplakia
malacosarcosis
malaise
malaria therapy (for Lyme disease)
malate
    dehydrogenase, m.
Malgaigne amputation
Malherbe calcifying epithelioma
malignancy
malignant
    ascites, m.
    disease, m.
    effusion, m.
    exudate, m.
    fibrous histiocytoma, m. (MFH)
    foci, m.
    growth, m.
    hepatoma, m.
    histiocytic reticulosis, m.
    histiocytosis, m. (MH)
    insulinoma, m.
    lymphoma, m.
    melanoma, m.
    mesenchymal tumor, m.
    mesenchymoma, m.
    mixed mullerian tumor, m. (MMMT)
    mixed tumor, m.
    mole, m.
    neoplasm, m.
    pleural mesothelioma, m.
    polyp, m.
    process, m.
    trophoblastic teratoma, m.
    tumor, m.
    ulcer, m.
malignin
Malin syndrome
mallein
malnutrition
Maloney esophageal dilator
malpighian
    bodies, m.
    layer, m.
mamma (pl. mammae)
mammae (pl. of mamma)
mammal
mammalian
mammaplasty
mammary
    -derived growth inhibitor, m. (MDGI)
    dysplasia, m.
    gland, m.
    tumor agent, m.
    tumor virus, m. (MTV)
mammectomy
mammillary
    dimpling, m.
    duct, m.
mammo (mammogram)
mammogram
    film screen technique m.
    negative mode m.
    screening m.
    xeroradiographic m.
mammogram density pattern
    N1 (mainly fat; lowest risk)
    P1/P2 (ductal prominence; intermediate risk)
    Dy (extensive or diffuse densities or dysplasia; highest risk)
mammography
    Lintro-scan m.
Mammo-lock needle
Mammomat
mammoplasia
mammoplasty
Mammorex
m-AMSA or mAMSA (amsacrine)
Manchester

ADDITIONAL TERMS

classification, M.
dosage system, M.
interstitial single-plane implant, M.
ovoid, M.
Mancini plates
Mandelamine
mandible split
mandibular
  ostectomy, m.
  resection, m.
mandibulectomy
mandibulotomy
Mandol
mandrake
  root, m.
mandrin
manganese
Manhattan Project
mannitol
mannomustine
mannose
  -6-phosphate isomerase, m.
mannosidase
mannosidosis
Mann-Whitney U test
Mantel Haenzel stratified analysis
mantle
  blocks, m.
  field, m.
  irradiation, m.
  zone, m.
Mantoux test
manual differential
Manvene
Mann-Whitney U-test
MAO (monoamine oxidase)
  inhibitor, M. (MAOI)
MAOI (monoamine oxidase inhibitor)
map
  conjugation m.
  cytologic m.
  gene m.
  linkage m.
  restriction m.
MAP (megaloblastic anemia of
  pregnancy)
MAP (melphalan, Adriamycin,
  prednisone)
MAP (mitomycin-C, Adriamycin,
  Platinol)
map unit
mapping
  gene m.

marantic
marasmic
marasmus
march
  hemoglobin, m.
  tumor, m.
March disease
Marchand cell
Marchiafava-Micheli disease
Marek disease
Marfan syndrome
marfanoid
margaroid tumor
margin
  tumor m.
marginal granulocyte pool (MGP)
margination
margines (pl. of margo)
margo (pl. margines)
MARIA (macroaggregates of
  radioiodinated albumin)
marijuana
Marinol (dronabinol)
Marjolin ulcer
marker
  biologic m.
  CA-125 tumor m.
  cell-surface m.
  clonal m.
  cytogenetic m.
  genetic m.
  Ig m.
  immunologic m.
  tumor m.
Markov
  process, M.
  radiation, M.
Marlex
Marogen
Maroteaux-Lamy syndrome
Marplan
marrow
  aspiration, m.
  biopsy, m.
  cell, m.
  depression, m.
  donor, m.
  graft, m.
  harvesting, m.
  platelets, m.
  recipient, m.
  stem cells, m.
  storage, m.

ADDITIONAL TERMS

marrow—*Continued*
　stromal cells, m.
　transplant, m.
　transplantation, m.
marshmallow swallow test
marsupialization
Martinez technique
Martinotti cell
maschaladenitis
maschaloncus
masculation
masculinization
masculinize
masculinovoblastoma
maser (microwave amplification by
　stimulated emission of radiation)
Mason technique
Mason Pfizer monkey virus (MPMV)
mass
　-action law, m.
　effect, m.
　energy, m.
　lesion, m.
　number, m.
　spectrograph, m.
　spectrography, m.
　spectrometer, m.
　spectrometry, m.
massive
　involvement, m.
　radiation, m.
　tumor, m.
Masson
　hemangioendothelioma, M.
　stain, M.
　trichrome, M.
mast cell
　leukemia, m.
　tumor, m.
mastadenitis
mastadenoma
mastadenovirus
mastectomy
　Auchincloss-Madden m.
　extended radical m.
　Halsted m.
　Meyer m.
　modified m.
　modified radical m.
　nipple-areola m.
　palliative m.
　partial m.

Patey m.
　radical m.
　salvage m.
　Scanlon m.
　segmental m.
　simple m.
　subcutaneous m.
　superradical m.
　total m.
masthelcosis
mastitis
mastocarcinoma
mastochondroma
mastochondrosis
mastocyte
mastocytoma
mastocytosis
　diffuse m.
　diffuse cutaneous m.
　systemic m.
mastodynia
mastogram
mastography
mastoid
mastoidectomy
mastoiditis
mastoidotomy
mastoidotympanectomy
mastoncus
mastopathia
　cystica, m.
mastopathy
mastoscirrhus
mastosis
mastostomy
Masugi nephritis
masurium (Ma)
MAT (multiple agent therapy)
matagens
matched
　donor, m.
　lymphocyte transfusion, m.
　unrelated donor, m. (MUD)
maternal
　antibody, m.
　immunity, m.
　serum alpha-fetoprotein, m.
　(MSAFP)
maternohemotherapy
matrices (pl. of matrix)
matrix (pl. matrices)
Matuhasi-Ogata phenomenon

ADDITIONAL TERMS

Matulane (procarbazine)
maturation
Maunsell-Weir operation
Maurer
  dots, M.
  clefts, M.
Maxepa
maxillectomy
maxilloethmoidectomy
maxillofacial
  prosthesis, m.
maxillotomy
Maximow
  method, M.
  stain, M.
maximum
  dose, m. (Dmax)
  energy, m. (Emax)
  permissible concentration, m.
    (MPC)
  permissible dose, m. (MPD)
  permissible dose equivalent, m.
    (MPDE)
  target absorbed dose, m.
  tolerated dose, m. (MTD)
  velocity, m. (Vmax)
maxitron unit
maxwellian distribution
May apple
May-Grünwald stain
May-Grünwald-Giemsa stain
May-Hegglin anomaly
maytansine
MAZE (m-AMSA, azacitidine, etoposide)
mazoplasia
Mazzini test
Mb (brain metastases)
m-BACOD (moderate-dose
  methotrexate, bleomycin, Adriamycin,
  cyclophosphamide, Oncovin,
  dexamathasone)
M-BACOD (high-dose methotrexate,
  bleomycin, Adriamycin,
  cyclophosphamide, Oncovin,
  dexamethasone)
M-BACOS (methotrexate, bleomycin,
  Adriamycin, cyclophosphamide,
  Oncovin, Solu-Medrol)
M-BAM (cyclophosphamide, total body
  irradiation, monoclonal antibodies)
MBC (methotrexate, bleomycin,
  cisplatin)

MBD (methotrexate, bleomycin, DDP)
MBP (myelin basic protein)
MBq (megabecquerel)
MC (mitoxantrone, cytarabine)
MC29 myelocytomatosis virus
MCA (3-methylcholanthrene)
  -induced sarcoma, M.
MCBP (melphalan, cyclophosphamide,
  BCNU, prednisone)
MCC (mutated in colon cancer) gene
3M cesium 137 brachytherapy
McCort sign
McCoy
  antigen, M.
  media, M.
McCune-Albright syndrome
McDonough sarcoma virus
MCF (macrophage chemotactic factor)
  -7 tumor cells, M.
Mcg isotypic determinant
McGaw volumetric pump
McGhan
  breast implant, M.
  chin implant, M.
  facial implant, M.
McGill pain questionnaire
MCH (mean corpuscular hemoglobin)
MCHC (mean corpuscular hemoglobin
  concentration)
mCi (millicurie)
  mCi-d (millicurie-day)
  mCi-hr (millicurie-hour)
MCi (megacurie)
McKrae strain of herpes simplex virus
McLeod
  blood group system, M.
  phenotype, M.
McNaught keel
McNeer classification
McNemer test
MCP (melphalan, cyclophosphamide,
  prednisone)
M-CSF (macrophage colony-stimulating
  factor)
M-CSF (monocyte colony-stimulating
  factor)
MCTC (metrizamide CT cisternogram)
MCTD (mixed connective tissue disease)
MCV (mean corpuscular volume)
MCV (methotrexate, cisplatin,
  vinblastine)
McWhirter mastectomy

ADDITIONAL TERMS

Md (mendelevium)
MDA (minimum detectable activity)
MDF (multiple daily fractionation)
MDGI (mammary-derived growth
  inhibitor)
MDLO (metoclopramide,
  dexamethasone, larazepam,
  ondansetron)
MDLT-4 cell line
MDP (muramyl dipeptide)
MDR (multiple drug resistance)
  1 gene, M.
  2 gene, M.
  protein, M.
MDS (myelodysplastic syndrome)
M/E (myeloid/erythroid) ratio
MEA (multiple endocrine adenopathy)
mean
  corpuscular diameter, m.
  corpuscular hemoglobin, m. (MCH)
  corpuscular hemoglobin
    concentration, m. (MCHC)
  corpuscular volume, m. (MCV)
  dose, m.
  gonad dose, m.
  lethal dose, m.
  marrow dose, m. (MMD)
  organ dose, m.
meatoscope
meatoscopy
mebanazine
mebendazole
MEC (minimum effective concentration)
MeCCNU (methyl-CCNU or semustine)
MeCCNU (methyl-1-[2-chloroethyl]-3-
  cyclhexyl-1-nitrosurea)
mechanocyte
mechlorethamine (Mustargen)
  hydrochloride, m. (HN$_2$ or
    Mustargen or nitrogen mustard)
meclofenoxate
Meclomen
mecobalamine
MECY (methotrexate,
  cyclophosphamide)
MED (minimal effective dose)
MED (minimal erythema dose)
Medawar mechanism
media (pl. of medium)
median
  -effect equation, m.
  lethal dose, m. (MLD)
  survival time, m.

mediastinal
  adenopathy, m.
  dissection, m.
  germ cell tumor, m.
  irradiation, m.
  lymph node, m.
  lymphadenopathy, m.
  lymphangioma, m.
  lymphoma, m.
  mass, m. (MM)
  neoplasm, m.
  neuroblastoma, m.
  node biopsy, m.
  seminoma, m.
  teratocarcinoma, m.
  tumor, m.
mediastinitis
mediastinogram
mediastinography
mediastinoscope
mediastinoscopy
mediastinum
mediator cell
Medical Internal Radiation Dose (MIRD)
medical oncology
medication holiday
Medinger-Craver irradiation
MediPort
Medisperse
meditate
meditation
Mediterranean
  anemia, M.
  lymphoma, M.
  variant (B-), M.
medium (pl. media)
MEDLARS (Medical Literature and
  Retrieval System)
MEDLINE (computerized bibliography;
  see MEDLARS)
Medotopes
Medrate
medrogestone
Medrol
medroxyprogesterone (Depo-Provera)
  acetate, m.
medulla
medullary
medullated
medullation
medullectomy
medullization
medulloadrenal

ADDITIONAL TERMS

medulloarthritis
medulloblast
medulloblastoma
medulloepithelioma
medullomyoblastoma
medullosuprarenoma
MeFA (methyl-CCNU, 5-fluorouracil,
  Adriamycin)
mefloquine
Mefoxin
megabecquerel (MBq)
Megace (MEG or megestrol)
megacurie (MCi)
megaelectron volt (MeV)
MeGAG (mitoguazone)
megakaryoblast
megakaryocyte
  granular m.
  juvenile m.
  spent m.
megakaryocytic
megakaryocytopoiesis
megakaryocytopoietic
megakaryocytosis
megaloblast
  Sabin, m. of
megaloblastic
  anemia, m.
  anemia of pregnancy, m. (MAP)
megaloblastoid
megalocyte
megalocytic
megalokaryocyte
  colony-stimulating activity, m.
    (Meg-CSA)
megalosplenia
megathrombocyte
megavolt (MeV)
  photons, M.
megavoltage
  external beam radiation, m.
  irradiation, m.
  radiation, m.
  x-ray dosimetry, m.
  x-rays, m.
Meg-CSA (megakaryocyte colony-
  stimulating activity)
megestrol acetate (MEG or Megace)
Megostat
Meigs syndrome
meilolabial flap
meiogenic
meiosis

meiotic
Meirowski phenomenon
MEK (methionine enkephalin)
Mektec 99
Melacine (melanoma cell lysate vaccine)
melanemesis
melanemia
melanin
melanism
melanoacanthoma
melanoameloblastoma
melanoblast
melanoblastoma
melanoblastosis
melanocarcinoma
melanocyte
  dendritic m.
melanocyte-stimulating hormone (MSH)
  -inhibiting factor, m. (MSH-IF)
  -releasing factor, m. (MSH-RF)
melanocytic
  schwannoma, m.
melanocytoma
melanocytosis
melanoderma
melanodermatitis
melanoepithelioma
melanogen
melanogenesis
melanoglossia
melanoleukoderma
melanoma
  acral-lentiginous m.
  amelanotic m.
  benign juvenile m.
  chorionic m.
  Cloudman m. S91
  cutaneous malignant m.
  desmoplastic m.
  familial atypical mole-malignant m.
  Harding Passey m.
  intraocular m.
  juvenile m.
  lentigo maligna m. (LMM)
  malignant m.
  mucosal m.
  multiple m.
  nodular m.
  subungual m.
  superficial spreading m.
  uveal m.
melanoma cell lysate vaccine (Melacine)
melanomatosis

ADDITIONAL TERMS

melanomatous
melanonychia
melanophage
melanoplakia
melanoptysis
melanosarcoma
melanoscirrhus
melanosis
    bulbi, m.
    circumscribed precancerous m. of
    Dubreuilh
    coli, m.
    iridis, m.
    iris, m. of
    lenticularis progressiva, m.
    oculi, m.
    oculocutaneous m.
    Riehl m.
    sclerae, m.
    tar m.
melanosome
melanotic
    ameloblastoma, m.
    freckle of Hutchinson, m.
    neuroectodermal tumor, m.
    progonoma, m.
    sarcoma, m.
    whitlow, m.
melanotroph
melanotropic
melarsoprol
melasma
melena
melenemesis
melengestrol acetate
melenic
melioidosis
MeliBu (busulfan)
melioidosis
meloncus
meloplasty
Meloxine
melphalan (Alkeran or L-PAM or MEL)
Melzack-Wall gate control theory
MEM (macrophage electrophoretic
  mobility)
membrane
    attack complex, m. (MAC)
    attack complex-inhibitor, m. (MAC-
    INH)
    filter, m.
    fluidity, m.
    transport, m.

membranoproliferative
    glomerulonephritis (MPGN)
membranous
Memorial Sloan-Kettering Cancer
  Center
    protocol, M.
memory cells
memotine hydrochloride
MEN (multiple endocrine neoplasia)
    types I, II, III, M.
menadiol sodium diphosphate
menadione
Mendel law
mendelevium (Md)
mendelian
    allelic genes, m.
    dominant trait, m.
    inheritance, m.
    law, m.
Menest (esterified estrogen)
Menetrier disease
Menghini liver biopsy needle
meningeal
meninges (pl. of meninx)
meningioma
    angioblastic m.
meningiomatosis
meningitides (pl. of meningitis)
meningitis (pl. meningitides)
    carcinomatosa, m.
    cryptococcal m.
    eosinophilic m.
    leukemic m.
    lymphocytic m.
    mycobacterial m.
    septicemic m.
    serosa circumscripta, m.
    serous m.
    tubercular m.
    viral m.
meningoblastoma
meningocele
meningococcemia
meningococci (pl. of meningococcus)
menincococcosis
meningococcus (pl. meningococci)
meningoencephalitis
meningoencephalocele
meningoencephalopathy
meningofibroblastoma
meningogenic
meningoma
meningomyelocele

ADDITIONAL TERMS

meningomyeloencephalitis
meningomyeloencephalopathy
meningomyeloradiculitis
meningoradicular
menigoradiculitis
meningorecurrence
meningosis
meningothelioma
meninx (pl. meninges)
meniscocyte
meniscocytosis
menogaril
menopausal
menopause
menotropins
mentoplasty
Mentzer index
Mephyton
MePRDL (methylprednisolone)
meprednisone
mEq (milliequivalent)
MER (methanol extraction residue of BCG)
M/E ratio (myeloid/erythroid ratio)
merbarone
6-mercaptopurine (mercaptopurine or MP or 6-MP or Purinethol)
mercapturic acid
Merindino procedure
Meritene
Merkel cell
        carcinoma, M.
Merkel-Ranvier cell
merocyst
meromysin
meronecrosis
mesalamine
mesenchyma
mesenchymal
    bone sarcoma, m.
    chondrosarcoma, m.
    sex cord stromal tumor, m.
mesenchyme
mesenchymoma
    benign m.
    malignant m.
mesenteric
    fibromatosis, m.
    lymph node, m.
    lymphadenopathy, m.
mesenteritis
    retractile m.
mesentery

MeSH (Medical Subject Heading at National Library of Medicine; seeMEDLARS)
mesna (Mesnex)
Mesnex (mesna)
Mesnum
mesoblast
mesoblastic
mesocolon
mesocytoma
mesoderm
mesodermal
mesodermic
mesogastric
mesogastrium
mesoglioma
mesohyloma
mesolymphocyte
meson
mesonephric
mesonephroid
mesonephroma
mesosalpinx
mesosecrin
mesosigmoid
mesosome
mesothelial
mesothelioma
mesothelium
mesothorium
mesotron
mesovarium
messenger RNA (mRNA)
meta-analysis
metabolic
    alkalosis, m.
    analogue, m.
    antagonist, m.
    emergency, m.
    lesion, m.
    pathology, m.
metabolism
metabolimeter
metabolimetry
metabolite
metachromatic
metachromatophil
metachromophil
metagenesis
metagglutinin
metaglobulin
metaiodobenzylguanidine (MIBG)
metal complexing agent

ADDITIONAL TERMS

metallic
    clip, m.
    staple, m.
    taste, m.
metalloporphyrin
metalloprotease
metalloproteinase
metamorphosis
metamyelocyte
metaphase
metaphyseal
metaphysis
metaplasia
    agnogenic myeloid m.
    Barrett m.
    ciliated m.
    coelomic m.
    myeloid m.
    osseous m.
    patchy m.
    pseudosarcomatous m.
    squamous m.
metaplasm
metaplastic
metaraminol
metastases (pl. of metastasis)
metastasis (pl. metastases)
    advanced m.
    axillary m.
    biochemical m.
    bone m.
    brain m.
    calcareous m.
    chest wall m.
    contact m.
    crossed m.
    diffuse m.
    direct m.
    distant m.
    focal m.
    generalized m.
    hematogenous m.
    implantation m.
    intracranial m.
    liver m.
    local m.
    lung m.
    lymphangitic m.
    miliary m.
    nodular m.
    omental m.
    osseous m.
    osteoblastic m.
    ovarian m.
    paradoxical m.
    peritoneal m.
    pulmonary m.
    retrograde m.
    skeletal m.
    transplantation m.
    visceral m.
    widespread m.
metastasize
metastatic
    abscess, m.
    adenocarcinoma, m.
    bone lesion, m.
    calcification, m.
    carcinoid syndrome, m.
    carcinoma, m.
    cascade, m.
    deposits, m.
    disease, m.
    explosion, m.
    foci, m.
    implant, m.
    inflammation, m.
    involvement, m.
    lesion, m.
    melanoma, m.
    node, m.
    nodule, m.
    pneumonia, m.
    seeding, m.
    spread, m.
    studding, m.
    survey, m.
    tumor, m.
metathrombin
metatypical
Metchnikoff cellular immunity theory
metencephalon
met-enkephalin
    -like tumor immunoreactivity, m.
methadone
methaqualone
methemalbumin
methemalbuminemia
metheme
methemoglobin
    reductase, m. (NADPH)
    reduction test, m.
methemoglobinemia
methemoglobinuria
methenamine silver staining
methimazole

ADDITIONAL TERMS

methionine
  -enkephalin, m. (MEK)
  sulfatase, m.
methisazone
method
  Chou and Talalay, m. of
methodology
Methosarb
methotrexate (amethopterin or Folex or
  Mexate or MTX or Rheumatrex)
  toxicity, m.
methoxsalen
  topical solution, m.
8-methoxypsoralen
methyl
  -CCNU, m. (MeCCNU or semustine)
  FJ4 trap hypothesis, m.
  -GAG, m. (methyl-glycoxal
    bisguanylhydrazone)
  -glycoxal bisguanylhydrazone, m.
    (Me-GAG or MGBG)
  green dye, m.
  phosphonate, m.
  violet, m.
methylation
methylazoxymethanol
3-methylcholanthrene (MCA)
  -induced sarcoma, m.
methylcobalamin
5-methylcytosine
methyldichlorarsin
methyldopa
methylene blue
N-methylhydrazine (procarbazine)
methylmercaptopurine (MMPR)
methylmethacrylate
methylnitrosurea
methylprednisolone (MePRDL)
  pulse therapy, m. (MPPT)
methyltestosterone
5-methyltetrahydrofolate
methylthiouracil (MTU)
methylxanthine
methysergide
metiamide
Meticorten
Meticortilone
metmyoglobin
metoclopramide hydrochloride (Reglan)
metoprine
Metreton
metrizamide
metrocarcinoma

metrocystosis
metrocyte
metroendometritis
metrofibroma
metrolymphangitis
metronidazole
metroplasty
mets (metastases)
meturedepa
metyrapone
  test, m.
metyrosine (Demser)
MeV (megaelectron voltage)
MeV (megavolt)
MeV (megaelectron volt)
  electron beam, M.
  linear accelerator, M. (4 MeV/
    6 MeV/12 MeV/18 MeV)
  photons, M.
Mexate-AQ (methotrexate)
Mexican hat erythrocyte
mexiletine
Meyer mastectomy
Meynert cell
Mezlin (mezlocillin)
mezlocillin sodium
MF (methotrexate, 5-fluorouracil)
MF (mitomycin, 5-fluorouracil)
MFH (malignant fibrous histiocytoma)
MFP (melphalan, 5-fluorouracil,
  Provera)
Mg agglutinin
MGBG (methyl-glyoxal
  bisguanylhydrazone)
MGF (macrophage growth factor)
MGGH (methylglyoxal bisguanyl-
  hydrazone)
mg/kg (milligrams per kilogram)
MGP (marginal granulocyte pool)
Mh (hepatic metastases)
  tumor cells, M.
MH (malignant histiocytosis)
MH2 virus
MHA (microhemagglutination assay)
  -TP, M. (microhemagglutination
    assay-Treponema pallidum)
MHC (major histocompatibility complex)
  restriction, M.
MHD (minimum hemolytic dose)
mht oncogene
MIBG (metaiodobenzylguanidine)
  scan, M.
  scintigraphy, M.

ADDITIONAL TERMS

MIC (minimum inhibitory concentration)
mice
Michaelis
    constant, M.
    stain, M.
Michaelis-Menten saturation kinetics
miconazole
MICRhoGAM
microabscess
    Munro m.
    Pautrier m.
microadenocarcinoma
microadenoma
microadenopathy
microaggregate
microanatomy
microangiopathic
    anemia, m.
    hemolytic anemia, m. (MAHA)
microangiopathy
microbe
microbial
microbicidal
microbiology
microblast
microcalcification
microcephalic
microcephaly
microcurie (mC)
    hour, m. (mC-hr)
microcyst
microcystic
microcytase
microcyte
microcythemia
microcytic
microcytosis
microcytotoxicity
microdetermination
microdissection
microdrepanocytic
microdrepanocytosis
microdroplet
microelectrophoresis
microencapsulation assay
microerythrocyte
microfluorometry
MicroGeneSep
microglia
microgliocyte
microglioma
microgliomatosis
microglobulin

microhemagglutination assay (MHA)
    -Treponema pallidum, m. (MHA-
    TP)
microhematocrit
microimmunofluorescent
microinjection
microinvasion
microinvasive
microlesion
microleukoblast
Microlite
microlithiasis
microlymphoidocyte
micrometastases (pl. of micrometastasis)
micrometastasis (pl. micrometastases)
micrometastatic
micrometer
micromicrocurie
micromolecule
micromolecular
micromyeloblast
micromyelolymphocyte
microneedle
micronodular
micronormoblast
microorganism
microphage
microphagocyte
microphysics
micropinocytosis
microprobe
microprocessor
    -driven pump system, m.
microprolactinoma
microrefractometer
microroentgen (mR)
microsampling
microscopic
    agglutination, m.
    appearance, m.
    examination, m.
    indices, m.
    residual disease, m.
    section, m.
microscopy
    electron m.
    fluorescence m.
    immunofluorescence m.
    polarized light m.
    transmission electron m.
microsection
microsequencing
microslide

ADDITIONAL TERMS

MicroSkin urostomy pouch
microspectrophotometer
microspectrophotometry
microspectroscope
microspectroscopy
microsphere
microspherocyte
microspherocytosis
Microsporidia
microsporidiosis
microstaging
microsthenic
Microsulfon
microsurgery
microsurgical
microtiter
microtome
MicroTrak
microtransfusion
microtron
microtubule
microunit (mU)
microvolt (mV)
microvascular
microviscosimeter
microviscosimetry
microwave (MW)
microxycyte
MID (minimum infective dose)
Middeldorpf tumor
middle T
    antigen, m.
    protein, m.
Middlebrook
    agar, M.
    broth, M.
Middlebrook-Dubos hemagglutination
  test
midline
midlung
midplane
    depth, m.
    dose, m.
Mielke template bleeding time
MIF (macrophage-inhibiting factor)
MIF (macrophage-inhibitory factor)
MIF (migration-inhibitory factor)
mifepristone (RU 486)
Mignon eosinophilic granuloma
migrant pattern
migrated tumor
migration-inhibitory factor (MIF)
MIH (procarbazine)

Mijnhardt Volugraph
Mikulicz
    cells, M.
    colostomy, M.
    syndrome, M.
Miles operation
miliary
    carcinosis, m.
    tubercles, m.
milieu
milk
    anemia, m.
    factor, m.
Millen technique
millicurie (mCi)
    -day, m. (mCi-d)
    -hour, m. (mCi-hr)
milligamma
millijoule (mJ)
Millikan rays
millimicrocurie
millimole (mM)
milliosmole (mOsm)
Millipore filter
millirad (mrad)
millirem (mrem)
milliroentgen (mR)
millisecond (msec)
millivolt (mV)
Mill-Rose bronchial cytology brush
miltefosine
Miltenberger antigen
MINE (mesna, ifosfamide, Novantrone,
  etoposide)
miner's
    anemia, m.
    lung, m.
mineralocortocoid
    activity, m.
    deficiency, m.
Ming classification
minichromosome
mini-COAP (cyclophosphamide,
  Oncovin, ara-C, prednisone)
minicolpostat
mini-mantle treatment
minimum
    acceptable distance, m.
    detectable activity, m. (MDA)
    effective concentration, m. (MEC)
    effective dose, m. (MED)
    erythema dose, m. (MED)
    hemolytic dose, m. (MHD)

ADDITIONAL TERMS

minimum—*Continued*
  infective dose, m. (MID)
  inhibitory concentration, m. (MIC)
  lethal concentration, m. (MLC)
  lethal dose, m. (MLD)
  reacting dose, m. (MRD)
  target absorbed dose, m.
Minin light
miniradiochromatography
minisatellite DNA
Minitec
Minkowsky-Chauffard syndrome
minometer
Minot-Murphy diet
Minot-von Willebrand syndrome
minus-minus phenotype
minus-strand RNA
mioplasmia
miostagmin reaction
MIRD (Medical Internal Radiation Dose)
mirror image breast biopsy
mismatch
misonidazole
misoprostol (Cytotec)
missense mutation
mistletoe extract
MIT (monoiodotyrosine)
Mithracin (plicamycin)
mithramycin (plicamycin)
mitindomide
MITO (mitomycin)
Mitobronitol
mitocarcin
mitochondria (pl. of mitochondrion)
mitochondrial
  antibody, m.
  messenger RNA, m.
  ribosomal RNA, m.
mitochondrion (pl. mitochondria)
mitoclomine
mitocromin
mitogen
  pokeweed m. (PWM)
  T-cell m.
mitogenesis
mitogenetic
  radiation, m.
mitogenic
  factor, m.
  signal pathway, m.
mitogenicity
mitogillin
mitoguazone (MeGAG or methyl-GAG)

mitokinetic
mitolactol (dibromodulcitol)
mitomalcin
mitomycin (MITO or mitomycin-C or
  MMC or Mutamycin)
mitomycin-C (MMC)
mitopodozide
mitoschisis
mitoses (pl. of mitosis)
mitosis (pl. mitoses)
mitosome
mitosper
mitotane (Lysodren)
Mitotenamine
mitotic
  index, m.
  inhibitors, m.
  spindle, m.
mitoxantrone hydrochloride (DHAD or
  Novantrone)
Mitsuda
  antigen, M.
  reaction, M.
mixed
  agglutination reaction, m.
  amputation, m.
  cellularity, m.
  cellularity Hodgkin disease, m.
  chimerism, m.
  connective tissue disease, m.
    (MCTD)
  germ cell tumor, m.
  leukocyte culture, m. (MLC)
  leukocyte reaction, m. (MLR)
  lymphocyte culture, m. (MLC)
  lymphocyte reaction, m. (MLR)
  mullerian tumor, m.
  tumor, m.
Miyasato disease
mJ (millijoule)
MK-217 (biphosphonate)
MK-906 (finasteride)
M/L (monocyte/lymphocyte) ratio
MLC (minimum lethal concentration)
MLC (mixed leukocyte culture)
MLC (mixed lymphocyte culture)
MLD (median lethal dose)
MLD (minimum lethal dose)
MLNS (mucocutaneous lymph node
  syndrome)
MLR (mixed leukocyte reaction)
MLR (mixed lymphocyte reaction)
MLV (Moloney leukemia virus)

ADDITIONAL TERMS

MLV (mouse leukemia virus)
MLV-A virus
mM (millimole)
MM (mediastinal mass)
MM (mercaptopurine, methotrexate)
MM (multiple myeloma)
MMC (mitomycin-C)
MMD (mean marrow dose)
MMIF (macrophage migration inhibiting factor)
MMLV (Moloney murine leukemia virus)
MMMT (malignant mixed mullerian tumor)
MMOPP (methotrexate, mechlorethamine, Oncovin, procarbazine, prednisone)
MMPR (methylmercaptopurine)
MMT (mouse mammary tumor)
MMTV (mouse mammary tumor virus)
MN blood group system
Mo (molybdenum)
Mo cell
MoAb (monoclonal antibody)
MOAD (methotrexate, Oncovin, L-asparaginase, dexamethasone)
MOB (Mustargen, Oncovin, bleomycin)
MOB-III (mitomycin-C, Oncovin, bleomycin, cisplatin)
Mobin-Uddin filter
MOCA (methotrexate, Oncovin, cyclophosphamide, Adriamycin)
modality
modified
    Kopans breast lesion localization needle, m.
    radical hysterectomy, m.
    radical mastectomy, m.
    radical mastoidectomy, m.
Modrastane
modulated
modulation
    antigenic m.
modulator
MOF (MeCCNU, Oncovin, 5-fluorouracil)
MOF (methotrexate, Oncovin, 5-fluorouracil)
MOF-STREP (MeCCNU, Oncovin, 5-fluorouracil, streptozocin)
Mohs
    chemotherapy, M.
    excision of basal cell carcinoma, M.

micrographic chemosurgery, M.
micrography, M.
    surgery, M.
    technique, M.
moiety
molality
molar
    pregnancy, m.
    villous trophoblast, m.
molarity
mole
    atypical m.
    cystic m.
    false m.
    hydatid m.
    hydatidiform m.
    invasive m.
    malignant m.
    metastasizing m.
    vesicular m.
molecular
    biology, m.
    cloning, m.
    genetics, m.
    hybridization, m.
    immunopathology, m.
    lesion, m.
    mimicry, m.
    pharmacology, m.
    physics, m.
    structure, m.
    therapeutics, m.
    virology, m.
    weight, m.
molecularly
molecule
molgramostim (Leucomax)
Mol-Iron
Moll Catalog number
Moll gland
Moloney
    leukemia virus, m. (MLV)
    murine leukemia virus, m. (MMLV)
    sarcoma virus, M. (MSV)
    test, M.
Molulsky dye reduction test
molybdenum (Mo)
    radiation therapy, m.
    -technetium generator, m.
MOMP (mechlorethamine, Oncovin, methotrexate, prednisone)
monad
Monakow

ADDITIONAL TERMS

Monakow—*Continued*
 syndrome, M.
 theory, M.
monatomic
Monel metal radium applicator
Monilia
monilial
moniliasis
moniliid
moniliosis
monkey
 B virus, m.
 green m. kidney
mono (mononucleosis)
monoacylglycerol
monoamine oxidase (MAO)
 inhibitor, m. (MAOI)
monoaziridinyl putrescine
monoblast
monoblastic
monoblastoma
monobloc resection
monobutyrin
monocationic
monocellular
monochromatic
monochromaticity
monochromatophil
Monoclate
monoclonal
 antibody, m. (MAb or MoAb)
 antibody and rabbit complement,
  m.
 anticytokeratin, m. (MAK-6)
 anticytokeratin cocktail, m.
 gammopathy, m.
 spike, m.
monocyte
 colony-stimulating factor, m.
  (M-CSF)
 /lymphocyte ratio, m. (M/L ratio)
 -macrophage series, m.
monocytic
 leukemia, m.
 marrow, m.
 series, m.
monocytoid
monocytopenia
monocytopoiesis
monocytosis
monodermoma
Mono-Diff test
monogen

monohistiocytic
monoiodotyrosine (MIT)
monokine
monolaurin
monomer
 fibrin m.
monomeric
monomorphic
monomorphous
mononuclear
 leukocytosis, m.
 phagocyte system, m. (MPS)
mononucleate
mononucleosis
 cytomegalovirus m.
 infectious m.
 post-transfusion m.
mononucleotide
monophasic
 anaplasia, m.
monophenol
 monooxygenase, m.
monophosphoglycerate mutase (MPGM)
monophyletic
 theory, m.
monophyletism
monopoiesis
monopolymerase
monosome
monosomy
monospecific
Monospot test
Mono-Sure test
monotherapy
Monsel solution
monstrocellular
 sarcoma, m.
Monte Carlo calculation
Montenegro test
Montreal platelet syndrome
moon
 face, m.
 facies, m.
Mooser cell
MOP (mechlorethamine, Oncovin,
 prednisone)
MOP (mechlorethamine, Oncovin,
 procarbazine)
MOP (melphalan, Oncovin,
 methylprednisolone)
MOP-BAP (mechlorethamine, Oncovin,
 procarbazine, bleomycin, Adriamycin,
 prednisone)

ADDITIONAL TERMS

MOPP (mechlorethamine, Oncovin,
 procarbazine, prednisone)
MOPP (methotrexate, Oncovin,
 procarbazine, prednisone)
MOPP-ABV (mechlorethamine,
 Oncovin, procarbazine, prednisone,
 Adriamycin, bleomycin, vinblastine)
MOPP-ABV Hybrid (mechlorethamine,
 Oncovin, procarbazine, prednisone,
 Adriamycin, bleomycin, vinblastine,
 hydrocortisone)
MOPP-ABVD (mechlorethamine,
 Oncovin, procarbazine, prednisone,
 Adriamycin, bleomycin, vinblastine,
 dacarbazine)
MOPP-LO BLEO (mechlorethamine,
 Oncovin, procarbazine, prednisone,
 bleomycin)
MOPr (mechlorethamine, Oncovin,
 procarbazine)
Moranyl (suramin)
morbidity
morbilliform
morcellation
morcellement
Morgagni
 column, M.
 crypt, M.
Morganella
 morgagnii, M.
moribund
moroxydine
morphea
morphine sulfate (MS)
morphinization
morpholino-type
morphologic
morphological
 sex, m.
morphology
morrhuate sodium
mortality
 rate, m.
 trial, m.
morular cell
Morvan syndrome
mos oncogene
mosaic
mosaicism
Moschcowitz disease
Mosler sign
mOsm (milliosmole)
Moss classification

Mossbauer
 effect, M.
 spectrometer, M.
Mosse syndrome
Mossuril virus
mossy cell
mostly purine agent
mother
 cell, m.
 cyst, m.
motif
motility
Motilium (domperidone)
Mott
 body, M.
 cell, M.
moulage
mountain anemia
mouse
 Balb/C m.
 beige m.
 CFW (cancer-free white) m.
 DBA/2 m.
 HLA-transgenic m.
 nude (nu/nu) m.
 NZB (New Zealand black) m.
 pigmenting hairless m.
 SCID (severe combined
  immunodifficiency)-hu m.
 severe combined immunodifficiency
  (SCID)-hu m.
 Swiss nu/nu m.
 TIM (transgenic immunodeficient)
  m.
 transgenic immunodeficient m.
  (TIM)
 transgenic Mov m.
mouse erythroleukemia
mouse germ line DNA
mouse leukemia virus
mouse mammary tumor agent
mouse mammary tumor factor
mouse monoclonal antibody
mouse myeloma cells
mouse-specific lymphocyte antigen
 (MSLA)
mouse unit (MU)
Mousseau-Barbin prosthetic tube
mouth cells
mouthrinse
mouthwash
moving
 boundary electrophoresis, m.

ADDITIONAL TERMS

moving—*Continued*
gantry, m.
strip therapy, m.
Moynihan syndrome
MP (melphalan, prednisone)
6-MP (mercaptopurine)
MPC (maximum permissible
concentration)
MPD (maximum permissible dose)
MPDE (maximum permissible dose
equivalent)
M-PFL (methotrexate, Platinol,
5-fluorouracil, leucovorin)
MPGM (monophosphoglycerate mutase)
MPGN (membranoproliferative
glomerulonephritis)
MPI iodine 123
DPTA kit, M.
MPL+PRED (melphalan, prednisone)
MPM (malignant papillary
mesothelioma)
MPMV (Mason Pfizer monkey virus)
MPO (myeloperoxidase)
MPPT (methylprednisolone pulse
therapy)
M2 protocol (vincristine, carmustine,
cyclophosphamide, melphalan,
prednisone)
MPS (mononuclear phagocyte system)
μR (microroentgen)
mR (milliroentgen)
MRA (magnetic resonance angiography)
mrad (millirad)
MRD (minimum reacting dose)
MRI (magnetic resonance imaging)
mRNA (messenger RNA)
interleukin 2, m.
transcription, m.
translation, m.
MRS (magnetic resonance spectroscopy)
Ms (skin metastases)
MS (morphine sulfate)
MS (multiple sclerosis)
MS-1 hepatitis
MS-2 hepatitis
MSAFP (maternal serum alpha-
fetoprotein)
MS-Contin (morphine sulfate)
MSH (melanocyte-stimulating hormone)
MSH-IF (melanocyte-stimulating
hormone-inhibiting factor)
MSH-RF (melanocyte-stimulating
hormone-releasing factor)

MSL-109
MSLA (mouse-specific lymphocyte
antigen)
MSOF (multisystem organ failure)
MSV (Moloney sarcoma virus)
MSV (murine sarcoma virus)
MTD (maximum tolerated dose)
MTP-PE (muramyl-tripeptide)
MTT (methyl tetrazolium)
MTU (methylthiouracil)
MTV (mammary tumor virus)
MTX (methotrexate)
MTX+MP (methotrexate,
mercaptopurine)
MTX+MP+CTX (methotrexate,
mercaptopurine, Cytoxan)
MTZ (mitoxantrone)
MU (mouse unit)
Mu (Mache unit)
mu
chain, m.
heavy chain disease (HCD), m.
-meson, m.
receptors,m.
mucicarmine
stain, m.
mucin
clot test, m.
-producing adenocarcinoma, m.
-type antigens, m.
mucinase
mucinosis
mucinous
adenocarcinoma, m.
carcinoma, m.
cystadenocarcinoma, m.
tumor, m.
mucocele
mucocolitis
mucocutaneous
herpes, m.
lymph node syndrome, m. (MLNS)
mucocyst
mucoenteritis
mucoepidermoid
mucoid
mucolipidosis, types I through IV
mucolytic
mucopolypeptide
mucopolysaccharide
mucopolysaccharidosis
mucoprotein
mucopurulent

ADDITIONAL TERMS

mucormycosis
mucosal
    barrier, m.
    candidiasis, m.
    neuroma syndrome, m.
mucositis
mucosocutaneous
mucous
    colitis, m.
    cyst, m.
    enteritis, m.
    membrane, m.
mucoviscidosis
mucus
MUD (matched unrelated donor)
MUGA (multiple gated acquisition)
    scan, M. (blood pool
    ventriculography)
Muir-Torre syndrome
mule-spinners' cancer
Müller
    blood dust, M.
    cells, M.
    dust bodies, M.
    maneuver, M.
müllerian
    duct, m.
    tumor, m.
müllerianoma
multiagent
    chemotherapy, m.
    drug therapy, m.
    regimen, m.
    therapy, m.
multicellular
multicellularity
multicentric
multicentricity
multicystic
multidisciplinary
multidrug
    regimen, m.
    -resistance (MDR) gene, m.
    -resistant, m.
    therapy, m.
multifactorial
multifocal
multiforme
    erythema m.
    glioblastoma m.
multilocular
multiloculated
Multi-Med triple-lumen catheter

multimer
multimerization
multimodality
multinodular
    goiter, m.
    thyroiditis, m.
multinucleate
multioncological
multiplanar
    mode, m.
    technique, m.
multiple
    -agent therapy, m. (MAT)
    daily fractionation, m.
    drug resistance, m. (MDR)
    drug therapy, m.
    endocrine adenomatosis, m.
    endocrine adenopathy, m. (MEA)
    endocrine neoplasia types I, II, III,
      m. (MEN I, II, III)
    endocrine neoplasia type 2b, m.
    enhancing lesions, m.
    hamartoma syndrome, m.
    lentigines syndrome, m.
    lipomatosis, m.
    myeloma, m. (MM)
    organ system failure, m.
    sclerosis, m. (MS)
multipotential
multivalent
multivariant analysis
Munro microabscess
muon
muramidase
muramyl
    dipeptide, m. (MDP)
    tripeptide, m. (MTP-PE)
Murchison-Pel-Ebstein fever
Murchison-Sanderson syndrome
murine
    adenovirus, m.
    erythroleukemia, m.
    fibrosarcoma, m.
    leukemia virus, m.
    plasmacytoma, m.
    sarcoma virus, m. (MSV)
    T-cell phenotype, m.
murivirus
Muromonab-CD3 (murine monoclonal
    antibody to CD3 antigen)
Murri disease
Mus
    musculus, M.

ADDITIONAL TERMS

mushroom cloud
music therapy
musicotherapy
Mustard operation
mustard
  nitrogen m.
  L-phenylalanine m.
  uracil m.
mustard gas
Mustargen (mechlorethamine)
mustine
mutable
mutagen
mutagenesis
mutagenic
mutagenicity
mutagenize
Mutamycin (mitomycin)
mutant
  cell, m.
  gene, m.
mutase
mutate
mutation
  cold-sensitive m.
  conditional m.
  conditional lethal m.
  constitutive m.
  forward m.
  frameshift m.
  genomic m.
  homoeotic m.
  induced m.
  intervening sequence m.
  lethal m.
  missense m.
  natural m.
  nonsense m.
  opal m.
  point m.
  reading frameshift m.
  somatic m.
  suppressor m.
  temperature-sensitive m.
  transcription m.
  umber m.
  visible m.
mutational
  analysis, m.
mutein
mutogenic
mutogenicity
mutS gene

mV (millivolt)
MV (mitoxantrone, VP-16)
MVAC (methotrexate, vinblastine,
  Adriamycin, cisplatin)
MVF (mitoxantrone, vincristine,
  5-fluorouracil)
MVP (mitomycin-C, vinblastine,
  Platinol)
MVPP (mechlorethamine, vinblastine,
  procarbazine, prednisone)
MVT (mitoxantrone, VP-16, thiotepa)
MVVPP (mechlorethamine, vincristine,
  vinblastine, procarbazine, prednisone)
MX (presence of distant metastasis
  cannot be assessed)
Myambutol
myasthenia
  gravis, m.
  laryngis, m.
myasthenic
myb oncogene
myc oncogene
Mycelex
mycetoma
  actinomycotic m.
  eumycotic m.
mycoagglutinin
mycobacteria
mycobacterial
  adjuvant, m.
mycobacteriosis
Mycobacterium
  abscessus, M.
  africanum, M.
  aquae, M.
  avium, M.
  avium-intracellulare, M. (MAI)
  balnei, M.
  brunense, M.
  buruli, M.
  chelonei, M.
  fortuitum, M.
  gastri, M.
  giae, M.
  gordonae, M.
  habana, M.
  haemophilum, M.
  intracellulare, M.
  kansasii, M.
  leprae, M.
  luciflavum, M.
  marianum, M.
  marinum, M.

ADDITIONAL TERMS

minetti, M.
paraffinicum, M.
platypoecilus, M.
ranae, M.
scrofulaceum, M.
simiae, M.
tuberculosis, M.
ulcerans, M.
mycobacteriosis
Mycobutin (ansamycin or rifabutin)
mycohemia
Mycoplasma
    hominis, M.
    incognitus, M.
    orale, M.
    pneumoniae, M.
mycoplasma
    pneumonia, m.
mycoplasmal
mycoplasmosis
Mycosel agar
mycoside
mycosis
    fungoides, m.
    fungoides d'emblée, m.
    Gilchrist m.
    Posada m.
    splenic m.
    superficial m.
    systemic m.
mycostasis
mycostat
mycotic
    stomatitis, m.
mycotoxin
Mycotoruloides
myelin
    basic protein, m. (MBP)
myelitic
myelitis
myeloblast
myeloblastemia
myeloblastoma
myeloblastomatosis
myeloblastosis
myelocele
myelocyte
myelocythemia
myelocytic
myelocytoma
myelocytomatosis
myelocytosis
myelodysplasia

myelodysplastic
    syndrome, m. (MDS)
myeloencephalitis
    eosinophilic m.
myelofibrosis
    -osteosclerosis syndrome, m.
myelogenic
myelogenous
myelogram
myelography
myeloid
    cell, m.
    /erythroid ratio, m. (M/E ratio)
    granulocytic leukemia, m.
    leukemia, m.
    metaplasia, m.
    series, m.
myeloidosis
myelokentric
myelolipoma
myelolymphocyte
myeloma
    endothelial m.
    giant cell m.
    indolent m.
    localized m.
    malignant m.
    multiple m.
    nonsecretory m.
    osteosclerotic m.
    plasma cell m.
    solitary m.
myeloma cell
myeloma kidney
myeloma protein
myelomatoid
myelomatosis
myelomonoblast
myelomonocytic
myelomyces
myelopathic
    anemia, m.
    polycythemia, m.
myelopathy
myeloperoxidase
myelophthisic
    anemia, m.
myelophthisis
myeloplast
myeloplax
myeloplaxoma
myelopoiesis
    ectopic m.

ADDITIONAL TERMS

myelopoiesis—*Continued*
  extramedullary m.
myeloproliferation
myeloproliferative
  disease, m.
  disorder, m.
myelosarcoma
myelosarcomatosis
myelosis
  aleukemic m.
  chronic nonleukemic m.
  erythremic m.
  funicular m.
  megakaryocytic m.
  nonleukemic m.
myelostimulatory
  state, m.
myelosuppressed
myelosuppression
myelosuppressive
myelotherapy
myelotoxic
myelotoxicity
myelotoxin
Myleran (busulfan)
myoblastic
myoblastoma
    granular cell m.
myoblastomyoma
myocardial
myocardiectomy
myocardium
myocutaneous flap
myocyte
myocytoma
myoepithelioma
myofibroma
myofibromatosis
myofibrosis
myogenin
myoglobin
myohemoglobin
myohysterectomy
myolipoma
myoma (pl. myomata)
  ball m.
  epithelioid m.
  levicellulare, m.
  myoblastic m.
  nonstriated m.
  previum, m.
  sarcomatodes, m.
  striocellulare, m.

telangiectodes, m.
uteri, m.
uterine m.
myomagenesis
myomata (pl. of myoma)
myomatectomy
myomatosis
myomatous
myomectomy
myomelanosis
myometrial
  invasion, m.
myometritis
myometrium
myomohysterectomy
myomotomy
myoneuroma
myosarcoma
myoschwannoma
myosin
myosteoma
myristic acid
myristyl
  -src receptor, m.
myristylated
Mytillus edulis
myxadenoma
myxedema
myxedematoid
myxedematous
myxoblastoma
myxochondrofibrosarcoma
myxochondroma
myxochondrosarcoma
myxocystoma
myxoenchondroma
myxoendothelioma
myxofibroma
myxofibrosarcoma
myxoglioma
myxoid
  cyst, m.
  cystoma, m.
  liposarcoma, m.
myxoinoma
myxolipoma
myxoma (pl. myxomata)
  atrial m.
  cartilaginous m.
  cystic m.
  enchondromatous m.
  erectile m.
  fibrosum, m.

ADDITIONAL TERMS

fibrous m.
infectious m.
intracanalicular m. of mamma
lipomatous m.
odontogenic m.
sarcomatosum, m.
vascular m.
myxomata (pl. of myxoma)
myxomatosis
myxomatous
myxomyoma
myxoneuroma
myxopapillary
  ependymoma, m.
myxopapilloma
myxosarcoma
myxosarcomatous
myxovirus

N

N (regional lymph node
  grading)
    N0 (no regional lymph
    node metastasis)
N1, N2, N2a, N2b, N3, N3a, N3b,
  N3c (increasing involvement of
  regional lymph nodes)
  NX (regional lymph nodes cannot
  be assessed)
N antigen
n rays
N segment
N-stages (Nl, N2, N3)
N-terminal constant region
NA (neutralizing antibody)
nabilone
Naboth cyst
nabothian cyst
NAC (N-acetyl-L-cysteine)
NAC (neoadjuvant chemotherapy)
NAC (nitrogen mustard, Adriamycin,
  CCNU)
NAD (nicotinamide-adenine
  dinucleotide)
NAD+ (oxidized form of NAD)
NADH (reduced form of NAD)
  dehydrogenase, N.
  diaphorase, N.
  methemoglobin reductase, N.
  oxidase, N.
nadir
NADP (nicotinamide-adenine
  dinucleotide phosphate)

NADP+ (oxidized form of NADP)
NADPH (reduced form of NADP)
  -ferrihemoprotein reductase, N.
  methemoglobin reductase, N.
  oxidase, N.
Naegeli
  leukemia, N.
  macroblast, N.
nafoxidine hydrochloride
NAG vibrios
Naganol (suramin)
Nagasaki atomic bomb explosion
naked tubercles
NALL (null-cell acute lymphoblastic
  leukemia)
NALL (null-cell acute lymphocytic
  leukemia)
naloxazone
naloxonazine
naltrexone
Namalwa cell line
NANB (non-A, non-B)
  hepatitis, N. (NANBH)
NANBH (non-A, non-B hepatitis)
nanocurie (nCi)
nanogram
nanoparticle
napalm
naphthoquinone
naphthylpararosaniline
Naphuride (suramin)
napkin-ring obstruction
Naprosyn
naproxen
Narcan
narcotic
  agent, n.
  analgesic, n.
narcotism
nasal
  flap, n.
  glial heterotopia, n.
  glioma, n.
nascent
nasogastric
  feeding, n.
  tube, n.
nasojejunal (NJ)
  feeding, n.
  tube, n.
nasolabial
  flap, n.
nasopharyngeal

ADDITIONAL TERMS

nasopharyngeal—*Continued*
  angiofibroma, n.
  cancer, n.
  carcinoma, n.
  National
    Cancer Institute, N. (NCI)
    Institute of Allergy and Infectious
      Diseases, N. (NIAID)
  native
    immunity, n.
    L-asparaginase, n.
  natremia
  Natulan
  natural
    antibody, n.
    cytotoxic (NC) cells, n.
    immunity, n.
    killer (NK) cells, n.
    selection theory, n.
naturopathy
nausea
nauseant
nauseated
nauseous
Nazlin
Nb (niobium)
NB150 antigen
N901-BR (blocked ricin)
NBT (nitroblue tetrazolium)
n-butyl-deoxynojirimycin (DNJ)
NC (natural cytotoxic) cells
NCAM (neural cell adhesion molecule)
N-carboxymethychitosan-N, O-sulfate
  (NCMCS)
NCF (neutrophil chemotactic factor)
nCi (nanocurie)
NCI (National Cancer Institute)
NCMCS (N-carboxymethychitosan-N,
  O-sulfate)
NCS 254681 (5-iminodaunorubicin)
Nd (neodymium)
Nd:YAG (neodymium:yttrium-
  aluminum-garnet)
    laser, N.
NDA (new drug application)
NDK
nDNA test
Ne (neon)
nebularine
nebulization
nebulized
  mist, n.
  pentamidine, n.

nebulizer
NebuPent
NEC (necrotizing enterocolitis)
necrectomy
necrobiosis
necrobiotic
  nodule, n.
  rays, n.
necrocytosis
necrocytotoxin
necrogenic
necrogenous
necrolysis
  toxic epidermal n.
necrolytic
necronectomy
necropneumonia
necrosed
necroses (pl. of necrosis)
necrosis (pl. necroses)
  acute tubular n.
  anemic n.
  arteriolar n.
  aseptic n.
  avascular n.
  bacillary n.
  Balser fatty n.
  bone n.
  bridging n.
  caseous n.
  central n.
  cheesy n.
  coagulation n.
  colliquative n.
  cystic medial n.
  dry n.
  embolic n.
  epiphyseal ischemic n.
  Erdheim cystic medial n.
  exanthematous n.
  fat n.
  fibrinous n.
  focal n.
  gangrenous n.
  gangrenous pulp n.
  gummatous n.
  hepatic n.
  hyaline n.
  ischemic n.
  liquefaction n.
  liquefactive n.
  massive hepatic n.
  medial n.

Navelbine

ADDITIONAL TERMS

mercurial n.
moist n.
mummification n.
Paget quiet n.
peripheral n.
phosphorus n.
piecemeal n.
pressure n.
progrediens, n.
progressive emphysematous n.
putrefactive n.
radiation n.
radium n.
renal papillae, n. of
renal papillary n.
septic n.
simple n.
skin n.
soft-tissue n.
subacute hepatic n.
subcutaneous fat n.
submassive hepatic n.
syphilitic n.
thrombotic n.
total n.
ustilaginea, n.
warfarin-induced skin n.
Zenker n.
necrotic
necrotizing
   angiitis, n.
   enterocolitis, n. (NEC)
necrotoxin
NED (no evidence of disease)
needle
   biopsy, n.
   gun, n.
   localization, n.
   tracks, n.
needlestick
Negatan
negativity
negatol
negatron
Negri antibody
Negus stent
neighborhood symptom
neighborwise
Neill-Mooser
   body, N.
   reaction, N.
Neisser-Wechsberg leukocidin
Neisseria

flavescens, N.
gonorrhoeae, N.
lactamica, N.
meningitidis, N.
mucosa, N.
sicca, N.
subflava, N.
neisserial
Nelaton tumor
Nelson syndrome
NEM (N-ethylmaleimide)
   -sensitive factor, N.
neo gene
neoadjuvant chemotherapy (NAC)
neoantigen
neoantimosan
neoblastic
neocarzinostatin
neodymium (Nd)
   -yttrium-aluminum-garnet
   (Nd:YAG) laser, n.
neoformation
neogenesis
neoglottis
neomycin-resistance gene
neon (Ne)
   helium-n. laser (He-Ne laser)
   particle protocol, n.
neoplasia
   multiple endocrine n. (MEN)
neoplasm
   adrenal m.
   benign n.
   epithelial n.
   histoid n.
   malignant n.
   mixed n.
   organoid n.
   unicentric n.
neoplastic
   cell, n.
   disease, n.
   fibrosis, n.
   fracture, n.
   lesion, n.
   pericarditis, n.
   polyp, n.
   transformation, n.
neoplastigenic
neopterin
   plasma n. level
Neosar (cyclophosphamide)
neostibosan

ADDITIONAL TERMS

neostomy
Neovox Electrolarynx
nephelometric
  immunoassay, n.
  inhibition assay, n.
nephelometry
nephradenoma
NephrAmine
nephrectomize
nephrectomy
nephrelcosis
nephric
nephritic
nephritis
nephroblastoma
  cystic differentiated n.
  polycystic n.
nephroblastomatosis
nephrocalcinosis
nephrocystosis
nephrogram
nephrolithiasis
nephrolysis
nephrolytic
nephroma
  embryonal n.
  malignant mesenchymal n.
  mesoblastic n.
  multicystic n.
  multilocular cystic n.
nephromalacia
nephromegaly
nephroncus
nephronophthisis
  familial juvenile n.
nephropathy
  Balkan n.
  diabetic n.
  hypercalcemic n.
  hypokalemic n.
  IgA n.
  membranous n.
nephrophthisis
nephropoietin
nephropyelography
nephrosclerosis
nephrosis
nephrosonephritis
nephrostomy
nephrotic
  syndrome, n.
nephrotomogram
nephrotomography

nephrotoxic
nephrotoxicity
nephroureterectomy
nephroureterocystectomy
neptunium (Np)
Nequinate
nerve growth factor (NGF)
nesidiectomy
nesidioblast
nesidioblastoma
nesidioblastosis
nest
  cancer n's
N-ethylmaleimide (NEM)
Netromycin
network
  idiotype-anti-idiotype n.
network theory
Neufeld reaction
NEU-GENES
Neumann cells
Neupogen
neural
  cell adhesion molecule, n. (NCAM)
  crest, n.
  nevus, n.
neuraminidase
neuraxis
  irradiation, n.
neurilemma
neurilemmitis
neurilemoma
  acoustic n.
neurinoma
  acoustic n.
neurinomatosis
neuroastrocytoma
neuroblast
neuroblastoma
neurocytoma
neuroectodermal
neurodegenerative
neuroepithelioma
neurofibroma
  plexiform n.
neurofibromatosis
  multiple n.
  von Recklinghausen n.
neurofibrosarcoma
neurogenic
  bladder, n.
  sarcoma, n.
  tumor, n.

ADDITIONAL TERMS

neurogenous
neurogliocyte
neurogliocytoma
neuroglioma
    ganglionare, n.
neurogliomatosis
neurogliosis
neurohypophysectomy
neurohypophysial
neurohypophysis
neuroid
    nevus, n.
neuroimmunologic
neuroimmunology
neuroleptic
Neuroleukin
neurolymphomatosis
    gallinarum, n.
neuroma
    acoustic n.
    amputation n.
    amyelinic n.
    appendiceal n.
    cutis, n.
    false n.
    fascicular n.
    ganglionar n.
    ganglionated n.
    ganglionic n.
    malignant n.
    medullated n.
    mucosal n.
    multiple n.
    myelinic n.
    nevoid n.
    plexiform n.
    telangiectodes, n.
    traumatic n.
    trigeminal n.
    true n.
    Verneuil n.
neuromatosis
neuromatous
neuromuscular
neuromyasthenia
neuromyopathy
neuron
    -specific enolase, n. (NSE)
neuronectin
neuronevus
neuronopathy
neuronophage
neuronophagia

neuro-oncology
neuro-ophthalmology
neuropathic
neuropathy
neuropeptide
    Y, n.
neuropharmacology
neurophysin
neuropil
neuroradiologic
neuroradiology
neuroroentgenology
neurosarcoma
neurospongioma
neurotropic virus
neurotropin
neurovirulent
Neusser granules
neutral
    endopeptidase, n.
    protamine Hagedorn, n. (NPH)
    red dye, n.
neutralizing antibody (NA)
neutramycin
neutrino
neutrocyte
neutrocytopenia
neutrocytosis
neutron
    epithermal n.
    fast n.
    slow n.
    thermal n.
neutron absorption process
neutron beam therapy
neutron bombardment
neutron brachytherapy
neutron capture analysis
neutron dose
neutron irradiation
neutron radiation
neutron radiography
neutron shield
neutropenia
    autoimmune n.
    chronic benign n. of childhood
    chronic hypoplastic n.
    congenital n.
    cyclic n.
    familial benign chronic n.
    hypersplenic n.
    idiopathic n.
    immune n.

ADDITIONAL TERMS

neutropenia—*Continued*
  Kostmann n.
  malignant n.
  neonatal n.
  periodic n.
  peripheral n.
  primary splenic n.
  splenic n.
neutrophil
  band n.
  filamented n.
  giant n.
  juvenile n.
  nonfilamented n.
  polymorphonuclear n.
  rod n.
  segmented n.
  stab n.
  stabnuclear n.
neutrophil chemotactic factor (NCF)
neutrophil lobe count
neutrophilia
neutrophilic
  leukemia, n.
  leukocytosis, n.
  lymphocytosis, n.
nevi (pl. of nevus)
Neville tracheobronchial prosthesis
nevirapine (BIRG-587)
nevoblast
nevocarcinoma
nevocyte
nevoid
  basal cell carcinoma syndrome, n.
  basiloma syndrome, n.
  cyst, n.
nevolipoma
nevoxanthoendothelioma
nevus (pl. nevi)
  achromatic n.
  amelanotic n.
  anemicus, n.
  angiectodes, n.
  angiomatodes, n.
  araneus, n.
  basal cell n.
  bathing trunk n.
  Becker n.
  blue n.
  blue rubber bleb n.
  cellular blue n.
  chromatophore n. of Naegeli
  comedonicus, n.

compound n.
congenital pigmented n.
connective tissue n.
cutaneous n.
depigmentosus, n.
dermal n.
dysplastic n.
elasticus, n.
elasticus of Lewandowsky, n.
epidermal n.
epithelial n.
fatty n.
flammeus, n.
fuscoceruleus acromiodeltoideus, n.
fuscoceruleus ophthalmomaxillaris, n.
giant congenital pigmented n.
giant hairy n.
giant pigmented n.
hairy n.
halo n.
hepatic n.
intradermal n.
Ito, n. of
Jadassohn-Tieche n.
junction n.
junctional n.
linear n.
lipomatosus, n.
lipomatosus cutaneous superficialis, l.
maternus, n.
melanocytic n.
neural n.
neuroid n.
nevocellular n.
nevocytic n.
nevus cell n.
nuchal n.
Ota, n. of
pigmented n.
pigmented hairy epidermal n.
pigmentosus, n.
pilosus, n.
port-wine n.
sebaceous n.
sebaceus, n.
spider n.
spilus, n.
spilus tardus, n.
spindle and epithelioid cell n.
Spitz n.

ADDITIONAL TERMS

spongiosus albus mucosae, n.
stellar n.
strawberry n.
Sutton n.
unius lateris, n.
Unna n.
vascular n.
vascularis, n.
vasculosus, n.
venosus, n.
verrucous, n.
white sponge n.
new growth
New International Staging System (NISS)
New Zealand black mouse (NZBM)
newtonian physics
Neysman bias
Nezelof syndrome
NFl gene
N-formyl-1-methionyl-1-leucyl-1-phenylaline (FMLP)

NGF (nerve growth factor)
NHL (non-Hodgkin lymphoma)
Niagestin
NIAID (National Institute of Allergy and Infectious Diseases)
nialamide
Nichols radioimmunoassay
nick translation
nicoduozide
Nicolas-Favre disease
nicotinamide-adenine
    dinucleotide, n. (NAD)
    dinucleotide phosphate, n. (NADP)
nicotine
nicotinism
Nicozide
NIDD (noninsulin-dependent diabetes)
NIDDM (noninsulin-dependent diabetes mellitus)
nidus
Niemann-Pick
    cells, N.
    disease, N.
night sweats
nigricans
Nigrin
nigrities
NIH 3T3 cells
Nikiforoff method
Nikolsky sign

Nile blue dye
Nimeh method
nimodipine
nimustine
niobium (Nb)
Nipent (pentostatin)
Nippe test
nipple
    crater n.
    everted n.
    retracted n.
nipple-areolar complex
nipple-areolar mastectomy
nipple-areolar reconstruction
nipple discharge
nipple inversion
nipple marker
nipple retraction
nipple shadow
niridazole
NISS (New International Staging System)
Nissl
    bodies, N.
    granules, N.
    stain, N.
niton (Nt)
nitroaromatics
nitroblue tetrazolium (NBT)
4-nitro-estrone-3-methyl-ether (NSC 321803)
nitrogen mustard (HN2 or mechlorethamine or Mustargen)
nitroprusside
nitropyrene
nitrosamine
nitrosurea
Nizoral
NJ (nasojejunal)
    feeding, N.
    tube, N.
NK (natural killer)
    cell, N.
N-linked glycosylation sites
NM (mechlorethamine)
N-methylformamide
N-methylhydrazine (procarbazine)
NMR (nuclear magnetic resonance)
    spectroscopy, N.
NMRI (nuclear magnetic resonance imaging)
NMSC (nonmelanoma skin cancer)
n-myc oncogene

ADDITIONAL TERMS

N-myristyl transferase
No (nobelium)
nobelium (No)
Nocardia
    asteroides, N.
    brasiliensis, N.
    caviae, N.
    farcinica, N.
    lutea, N.
    madurae, N.
    otitidis-caviarum, N.
    rubra, N.
nocardial
Nocardiopsis
nocardiosis
nociceptor
nocodazole
Noctec
nodal
    involvement, n.
    metastases, n.
    spread, n.
node
    axillary n.
    cervical n.
    Cloquet n.
    Delphian n.
    Ewald n.
    hemal n's
    hemolymph n's
    inguinal n.
    Irish n.
    lymph n.
    prelaryngeal n.
    pretracheal n.
    Ranvier, n's of
    Rosenmüller n.
    Rotter n's
    sentinel n.
    signal n.
    solitary n.
    sump n's
    Troisier n.
    Virchow n.
node-negative
node-positive
nodular
    density, n.
    goiter, n.
    histiocytic lymphoma, n.
    melanoma, n.
    mixed lymphoma, n.

    poorly differentiated lymphocytic,
        n. (NPDL)
    thyroid, n.
    tumor, n.
nodule
    Busacca n's
    cold n.
    Gamna n's
    Gandy-Gamna n's
    Koeppe n's
    lymphatic n's
    siderotic n's
    Sister Mary Joseph n.
    tabac n's
    thyroid n.
    warm n.
noduli (pl. of nodulus)
nodulus (pl. noduli)
no evidence of disease (NED)
nogalamycin
Noguchi test
noli me tangere (rodent ulcer)
Nolvadex (tamoxifen)
noma
    pudendae, n.
    vulvae, n.
nominal
    antigen, n.
    single dose, n. (NSD)
    standard dose, n. (NSD)
nonagglutinating
    vibrios, n.
nonalpha chain
non-A, non-B hepatitis (NANB)
    hepatitis, n. (NANBH)
nonbacterial
non-B
    cell leukemia, n.
    hepatitis, n.
non-Bowen squamous cell carcinoma
non-Burkitt lymphoma
noncaseating granuloma
nonchromaffin paraganglioma
nonclathrin coat
noncleaved
nondisjunction
nonepithelial
nonfilamented neutrophils
non-Hodgkin lymphoma (NHL)
noninfiltrating
noninsulin-dependent
    diabetes, n. (NIDD)

ADDITIONAL TERMS

diabetes mellitus, n. (NIDDM)
noninvasive
    disease, n.
    neoplasm, n.
    tumor, n.
nonionizing radiation
nonlymphocytic
nonmalignant
nonmelanoma skin cancer (NMSC)
nonmetastatic
nonnarcotic
    analgesia, n.
nonnecrotic
nonneoplastic
nonnucleated
nonnucleoside RT inhibitor
non-oat cell carcinoma
nononcogenic
nonopaque
nonoxynol 4, 9, 15, 30
nonpalpable
nonproliferating
nonproliferative
nonradiable
nonradioactive
nonradioisotopic
nonreactive
nonreactivity
nonsecreting
nonsecretor
nonself
nonseminomatous
    germ cell tumor, n. (NSGCT)
    testicular cancer, n.
nonsense mutation
non-small cell
    bronchogenic cancer, n. (NSCBC)
    lung cancer, n. (NSCLC)
nonspecific
nonspherocytic
nonsteroidal
    anti-inflammatory agent, n.
    (NSAIA)
    anti-inflammatory drug, n. (NSAID)
nonstructural gene
nonsuppressible insulinlike activity
    (NSILA)
nonsuppurative
non–T-cell leukemia
nontoxic
nontumorigenic
norethisterone enanthate

Norland-Cameron photon densitometry
normoblast
    acidophilic n.
    basophilic n.
    early n.
    eosinophilic n.
    intermediate n.
    late n.
    orthochromatic n.
    oxyphilic n.
    polychromatic n.
normoblastic
normoblastosis
normochromia
normochromic
    anemia, n.
normocyte
normocytic
    anemia, n.
    normochromic anemia, n.
Normocytin
normocytosis
normoerythrocyte
normoglycemia
normoglycemic
normokalemia
normokalemic
normo-orthocytosis
Normosang
normoskeocytosis
normovolemia
normovolemic
Norport pump
Norpramine
Norris corpuscle
North American blastomycosis
Northern
    analysis, N.
    blot test, N.
    blotting, N.
Norton-Simon hypothesis
Norum-Gjone disease
Norwalk
    agent, N.
    virus, N.
nosocomial
nosomycosis
nosotoxic
nosotoxicosis
Nothnagel syndrome
notochord
notochordoma

ADDITIONAL TERMS

no-touch technique
not-self
Nottingham introducer
Novantrone (mitoxantrone)
Novapren
novobiocin
Nowell hypothesis
Np (neptunium)
NP (nucleoside phosphorylase)
NPC (nasopharyngeal carcinoma)
NPDL (nodular poorly differentiated
  lymphocytic)
NPH (neutral protamine Hagedorn)
  insulin, N.
NPY (neuropeptide Y)
n-ras
  oncogene, n.
  proto-oncogene, n.
NRBC (nucleated red blood cell)
nRNA (nuclear RNA)
NSAIA (nonsteroidal anti-inflammatory
  agent)
NSAID (nonsteroidal anti-inflammatory
  drug)
NSC 321803 (4-nitro-estrone-3-methyl
  ether)
NSCLC (non-small-cell lung cancer)
NSD (nominal single dose)
NSD (nominal standard dose)
NSE (neuron-specific enolase)
NSGCT (nonseminomatous germ cell
  tumor)
NSILA (nonsuppressible insulinlike
  activity)
Nt (niton)
5′NT (5′nucleotid)
nuclear
  antigens, n.
  bomb, n.
  chemistry, n.
  decay, n.
  disintegration, n.
  energy, n.
  envelope, n.
  enzyme, n.
  factor, n.
  fallout, n.
  fission, n.
  fusion, n.
  imaging, n.
  isomer, n.
  medicine, n.
  particles, n.

physics, n.
polarity, n.
probe, n.
radiation, n.
reaction, n.
reactor, n.
resonance, n.
RNA, n. (nRNA)
scanning, n.
scintigraphy, n.
spin, n.
spin quantum number, n.
nuclear magnetic resonance (NMR)
  imaging, n. (NMRI)
  scan, n.
  spectra, n.
  spectrometer, n.
  spectroscopy, n.
  spin-warp method, n.
nuclease
nucleated
  erythrocyte, n.
  red blood cell, n. (NRBC)
nucleation
nuclei (pl. of nucleus)
nucleic acid
nuclein
  bases, n.
nucleization
nucleize
nucleocapsid
nucleocytoplasmic
nucleohistone
nucleoid
nucleoli (pl. of nucleolus)
nucleolus (pl. nucleoli)
nucleon
  number, n.
nucleonics
nucleophagocytosis
nucleophile
Nucleopore filter
nucleoprotein
nucleoside
  analogue, n.
  diphosphate kinase, n.
  inhibitor, n.
  monophosphate kinase, n.
  phosphorylase, n. (NP)
nucleosome
nucleosynthesis
5′-nucleotidase
5′nucleotide (5′NT)

ADDITIONAL TERMS

nucleotide
cyclic n's
pyridine n.
nucleotide cyclase
nucleotide polymerase
nucleotide sequence analysis
nucleotidyltransferase
nucleotoxin
Nuclesa Cervitron II afterloader
Nucletron Selectron afterloader
nucleus (pl. nuclei)
nuclide
radioactive n.
Nuclide-4 emulsion
nude (nu/nu) mouse
null
allele, n.
cell, n.
-cell acute lymphoblastic leukemia,
n. (NALL)
-cell acute lymphocytic leukemia,
n. (NALL)
phenotype, n.
-type non-Hodgkin lymphoma, n.
nummular
Numorphan
nu/nu (nude) mouse
nutrition
nutritional
anemia, n.
status, n.
support, n.
NX (regional lymph nodes cannot be
assessed)
Nyberg factor
nymphoncus
nystatin
pastilles, n.
NZBM (New Zealand black mouse)

O₂ (oxygen)
O agglutinin
O antigen
O-core polysaccharide
O-specific polysaccharide
OAF (osteoclast-activating factor)
Oak Ridge National Laboratory
Oakley-Fullthorpe technique
o-aminoazotoluene
OAP (Oncovin, ara-C, prednisone)
OAP-BLEO (Oncovin, ara-C,
prednisone, bleomycin)

oat cell
carcinoma, o.
oat-shaped cells
Obecalp (placebo spelled backwards)
obligate aerobes
obliterate
obliteration
observed survival rate
obstipated
obstipation
obstructing
carcinoma, o.
lesion, o.
mass, o.
obstructive
carcinoma, o.
lesion, o.
mass, o.
obstruent
obtundation
obtunded
occipitothalamic irradiation
occlusion
occlusive
lesion, o.
occult
bleeding, o.
blood, o.
cancer, o.
lesion, o.
malignancy, o.
mass, o.
neoplasm, o.
primary malignancy, o. (OPM)
occupational
exposure, o.
radiation, o.
risk, o.
octad
octet theory
octreotide acetate (Sandostatin)
ocular
herpes, o.
rhabdomyosarcoma, o.
O-DAP (Oncovin, dianhydrogalactitol,
Adriamycin, Platinol)
odontoameloblastoma
odontoblast
odontoblastoma
odontogenic
cyst, o.
fibroma, o.
fibromyxoma, o.

ADDITIONAL TERMS

odontoma
    adamantinum, o.
    ameloblastic o.
    composite o.
    coronal o.
    coronary o.
    dilated o.
    embryoplastic o.
    fibrous o.
    follicular o.
    mixed o.
    radicular o.
odynophagia
OER (oxygen enhancement ratio)
OF (osmotic fragility)
ofloxacin
Ogilvie syndrome
OGS (orbital granulocytic sarcoma)
ohne Hauch (O antigen)
OI (opportunistic infection)
oil red O stain
OK 432 (picibanil)
Okazaki fragment
OKT4 cells
OKT8 cells
OK 10 virus
Oldfield syndrome
oleogranuloma
oleoma
Oleotope
olfactory
    esthesioneuroma, o.
    groove meningioma, o.
    neuroblastoma, o.
    neuroepithelioma, o.
oligemia
oligo analogue
oligoastrocytoma
oligochromemia
oligoclonal bands
oligocythemia
oligocythemic
oligocytosis
oligodendroblastoma
oligodendrocyte
oligodendroglia
oligodendroglioma
oligodynamic
oligoleukocythemia
oligomer
oligonucleotide
    probe, o.
oligopeptide

oligopnea
oligoptyalism
oligoribonucleotide
    synthesis, o.
oligosaccharide
oligosialia
Oliver-Rosalki method
Ollier disease
olsalazine
Olshevsky tube
Olympus
    bronchoscope, O.
    esophagoscope, O.
    gastroscope, O.
    sigmoidoscope, O.
OMAD (Oncovin, methotrexate,
    Adriamycin, dactinomycin)
omega
    -3 fatty acid, o.
    particle, o.
omentectomy
omeprazole
Omphalotus illudens
Ommaya reservoir
Omnipaque
omoblastoma
omohyoid muscle
omphalelcosis
omphaloma
omphaloncus
OMS (oral morphine sulfate in solution)
    Concentrate
ONCOCIN system
oncocyte
oncocytic
oncocytoma
oncodevelopmental
    proteins, o.
oncodnavirus
oncoembryonic
    antigens, o.
oncofetal
    antigen, o.
    proteins, o.
oncogene (listed under "gene")
    activation, o.
    location, o.
    peptide growth factor, o.
oncogenesis
ongogenetic
oncogenic
    virus, o.
oncogenically

ADDITIONAL TERMS

oncogenicity
oncogenous
oncologic
oncologist
oncology
   radiation o.
oncology mix
oncolysate
oncolysis
oncolytic
oncoma
oncometer
onconeural
   antigens, o.
oncoprotein
OncoRAD OV103
oncornavirus
OncoScint CR103 monoclonal antibody
OncoScint OV103 monoclonal antibody
oncosis
oncotaxonomy
oncotherapy
oncothlipsis
oncotic
oncotomy
Oncotrac
oncotropic
Oncovin (vincristine)
Oncovirinae
oncovirus
ondansetron (Zofran)
One-Alpha
one-dimensional
   double electroimmunodiffusion, o.
   isoelectric focusing, o. (1D-IEF)
   isoelectric focusing gel
   electrophoresis, o.
   single electroimmunodiffusion, o.
one gene
   -one enzyme hypothesis, o.
   -one polypeptide hypothesis, o.
onlay graft
ontogony
onychoma
oogenesis
oophorectomize
oophorectomy
oophorocystectomy
oophorocytosis
oophorohysterectomy
oophoroma
   folliculare, o.
oophorosalpingectomy

oothecohysterectomy
O&P (ova and parasites)
opacification
opacify
OPAL (Oncovin, prednisone,
   L-asparaginase)
opaque
open
   amputation, o.
   biopsy, o.
   label protocol, o.
   pleural biopsy, o.
   reading frame, o. (ORF)
operable
   cancer, o.
   disease, o.
operator
   gene, o.
   locus, o.
operon
Ophelia syndrome
ophthalmopathy
ophthalmoplegia
opiate
opioid
   peptides, o.
   receptors, o.
Opitz disease
opium
OPM (occult primary malignancy)
OPP (Oncovin, procarbazine,
   prednisone)
OPPA (Oncovin, procarbazine,
   prednisone, Adriamycin)
opportunist
   infection, o.
   organism, o.
opportunistic
   infection, o. (OI)
   organism, o.
opposed
   fields, o.
   portals, o.
opsinogen
opsinogenous
opsoclonus
opsonic
opsonification
opsonin
   immune o.
opsonization
opsonize
opsonizing antibodies

ADDITIONAL TERMS

opsonocytophagic
opsonometry
Opti-fluor
Optimmune
oral
    alpha interferon, o.
    bleeding, o.
    cancer, o.
    candidiasis, o.
    contraceptives, o.
    copulation, o.
    eroticism, o.
    intercourse, o.
    iron, o.
    lesion, o.
    sex, o.
    submucous fibrosis, o. (OSF)
    thrush, o.
    transmucosal fentanyl citrate, o.
        (OTFC)
orality
Oramorph SR
OraQuick test
OraSure test
Ora-Testryl (fluoxymesterone)
orbital
    contents, o.
    exenteration, o.
    floor, o.
    granulocytic sarcoma, o. (OGS)
    pseudotumor, o.
    rhabdomyosarcoma, o.
    rim, o.
orbitotomy
orbivirus
orchidectomy
orchidoepididymectomy
orchidoncus
orchiectomy
orchiencephaloma
orchilytic
orchioblastoma
orchiocele
orchiomyeloma
orchioncus
orchioscheocele
orchioscirrhus
orchitis
orchitolytic
orexigenic
ORF (open reading frame)
organ
    -absorbed dose, o.

dysfunction, o.
perfusion system, o.
-specific, o.
-specific antigen, o.
system failure, o.
-tolerance dose, o. (OTD)
transplant, o.
organic
    brain syndrome, o.
    psychoses, o.
organism
organoid
organoma
organomegaly
organoplatinum
organotropism
Oriental sore
original antigenic sin
Orimune
ormaplatin
Ornidyl
ornithine decarboxylase
ornotherapy
orogenital
orolingual
Oromorph
oropharyngeal
oropharynx
orosomucoid
orphan drug
Ortho HCV 2.0 ELISA test system
orthochromatic
orthochromia
Orthoclone OKT3
orthocytosis
ortho-dihydroxybenzene
orthomolecular
Ortho-mune
orthovoltage
orthovoltate
    unit, o.
Orudis
Os (osmium)
OS (overall survival)
oscheocele
oscheoma
oscheoncus
OSF (oral submucous fibrosis)
Osler triad
Osler-Vaquez disease
Osler-Weber-Rendu syndrome
Osm (osmole)
Osmitrol

ADDITIONAL TERMS

osmium (Os)
osmolality
osmolarity
osmole (Osm)
osmolute
osmometer
osmometry
osmosis
osmotherapy
osmotic
    fragility test, o.
osseous
ossification
ossifying
    fibroid, o.
    fibroma, o.
    leiomyoma, o.
ostectomy
osteoarthritis
osteoarthropathy
osteoblast
osteoblastic
osteoblastoma
osteocachectic
osteocachexia
osteocarcinoma
osteocele
osteocephaloma
osteochondrofibroma
osteochondroma
    fibrosing o.
osteochondromatosis
    synovial o.
osteochondromyxoma
osteochondropathy
ostochondrophyte
osteochondrosarcoma
osteochondrosis
osteoclasia
osteoclasis
osteoclast
    -activating factor, o. (OAF)
osteoclastic
osteoclastoma
osteocopic
osteocyte
osteocystoma
osteodensitometer
osteodentinoma
osteodynia
osteodystrophia
osteodystrophy
osteoencephaloma

osteoenchondroma
osteofibrochondrosarcoma
osteofibroma
osteofibromatosis
osteogen
osteogenesis
osteogenetic
osteogenic
    sarcoma, o.
osteogram
osteohydatidosis
osteoid
    osteoma, o.
    tumor, o.
osteolipochondroma
osteolipoma
osteolysis
osteolytic
osteoma
    cancellous o.
    cavalryman's o.
    compact o.
    cutis, o.
    dental o.
    durum, o.
    eburneum, o.
    fibrous o.
    giant osteoid o.
    medullare, o.
    multiplex intermusculare, o.
    osteoid o.
    parosteal o.
    sarcomatosum, o.
    spongiosum, o.
    tropical ulcer o.
osteomalacia
osteomalacic
osteomatoid
osteomatosis
osteomiosis
osteomyelitic
osteomyelitis
    conchiolin o.
    Garre o.
    malignant o.
    salmonella o.
    sclerosing nonsuppurative o.
    typhoid o.
    variolosa, o.
osteomyelodysplasia
osteomyelodysplastic
osteomyelography
osteomyoinvasion

ADDITIONAL TERMS

osteomyoinvasive
osteomyxochondroma
osteon
osteoncus
osteonecrosis
osteonectin
osteonosus
osteo-odontoma
osteopenia
osteopenic
osteoperiosteal
osteoperiostitis
osteopetrosis
osteophage
osteophyma
osteophyte
osteoplast
osteoplastic
   necrotomy, o.
osteopoikilosis
osteopontin
osteoporosis
osteoporotic
osteoradionecrosis
osteosarcoma
   classic o.
   fibroblastic o.
   parosteal o.
   periosteal o.
   telangiectatic o.
osteosarcomatous
Osteoscan
osteosclerosis
osteosclerotic
   anemia, o.
osteospongioma
osteosteatoma
osteotabes
osteotabetic
osteotelangiectasia
osteotomy
ostomate
ostomy
   adhesive, o.
   appliance, o.
   bag, o.
   care, o.
   club, o.
OTD (organ tolerance dose)
Oto nevus
Ouchterlony
   double diffusion technique, O.
   immunodiffusion, O.

Oudin
   immunodiffusion, O.
   resonator, O.
oulectomy
ova and parasites (O&P)
Ovaban
ovalbumin
ovalocytosis
ovarian
   ablation, o.
   cancer, o.
   carcinoma, o.
   carcinoma antigen, o. (CA-125)
   cyst, o.
   cystectomy, o.
   dysfunction, o.
   fibroid, o.
   malignancy, o.
   mass, o.
   seminoma, o.
   teratoma, o.
   tumor, o.
ovariectomy
ovariocele
ovariohysterectomy
ovariosalpingectomy
ovariosteresis
ovariotomy
ovariprival
ovary
   polycystic o.
overall survival (OS)
overexpression
   gene o.
ovoid
ovotransferrin
Owren disease
ox
   cell hemolysin test, o.
   red blood cells, o.
oxafuradene
oxagrelate
oxalate plasma
oxamisole hydrochloride
oxamniquine (Vansil)
oxamyristic acid
Oxandrin (oxandrolone)
oxandrolone (Oxandrin)
oxidant
oximeter
oximetry
oxisuran
oxoformycin B

ADDITIONAL TERMS

oxophenarsine
5-oxoprolinase
5-oxoproline
5-oxoprolinuria
oxothiazolidine carboxylate
  (Procysteine)
Oxycel
oxygen (O_2)
    affinity, o.
    binding, o.
    cisternography, o.
    enhancement ratio, o. (OER)
    -hemoglobin dissociation curve, o.
    transport, o.
oxygenase
oxygenate
oxygenation
oxyhemoglobin
oxyhemogram
oxyhyperglycemia
oxymetholone (Adroyd or Anadrol-50 or
  HMD)
oxymorphone hydrochloride
oxyphenisatin
oxyphil
    adenoma, o.
    cell, o.
    cell tumor, o.
oxyphilic
    erythroblasts, o.
    granular cell adenoma, o.
Oz
    allotype, O.
    antigen, O.
    isotypic determinant, O.
ozone
ozonophore

P P24
    antibody, P.
    antigen, P.
    antigen capture assay, P.
^{32}P (radioactive phosphorus)
P32 (colloidal chromic phosphate)
    intraperitoneal treatment, P.
P 231 (radioactive phosphorus)
P antigen
P blood group system
P-cell growth factor
p (pathologic) classification of tumor
P factor

P53 gene
P-glycoprotein (P-170)
P-170 glycoprotein
P 32 isotope
P-30 protein
Pa (protactinium)
PA (pernicious anemia)
PABA (para-aminobenzoic acid)
Pabanol
PAB-Esc-C (Platinol, Adriamycin,
  bleomycin, escalating doses of
  cyclophosphamide)
PAC (Platinol, Adriamycin,
  cyclophosphamide)
PAC-4D 5-day infusion
PACE (Platinol, Adriamycin,
  cyclophosphamide, etoposide)
pachydermatocele
pachyhematous
pachytene
Pacific yew tree
packed
    cell volume, p. (PCV)
    field, p.
    marrow syndrome, p.
    red cells, p. (PRC)
packing fraction
pack-year
    history, p.
    smoking history, p.
PAF (platelet activating factor)
    acether, P.
PAF (platelet aggregating factor)
PAGE (polyacrylamide gel
  electrophoresis)
Pageblot system
Paget
    carcinoma, P.
    cells, P.
    disease, P.
    disease of nipple, P.
    extramammary P. disease
    quiet necrosis of bone, P.
    test, P.
pagetoid
    cell, p.
    reticulosis, p.
PAH (p-aminohippuric acid or para-
  aminohippuric acid)
PAH (polycyclic aromatic hydrocarbons)
PAHA (p-aminohippuric acid or para-
  aminohippuric acid)
PAI-1 (plasminogen activator inhibitor)

ADDITIONAL TERMS

PAIDS (pediatric AIDS)
PAIgG (platelet-associated IgG)
pain
    control, p.
    management, p.
painful bruising syndrome
paired
    lateral ports, p.
    rotational arcs, p.
PALA (N-phosphonoacetyl-L-aspartate)
palatal
palate
palatectomy
palatoglossal
palatomaxillary
palatopharyngeal
palatoplasty
Palex ostomy appliances
palindrome
palindromia
palindromic
palisade
palisading
Pall filter
palladium (Pd)
    103, p. (Pd 103)
palliate
palliation
palliative
    surgery, p.
    treatment, p.
pallid
pallidectomy
pallor
palmar
    erythema, p.
    fibromatosis, p.
Palmitoylcarnitine
palpable
palpation
2-PAM (pralidoxime)
L-PAM (melphalan or L-phenylanaline
    mustard)
pamaquine
pamidronate disodium (Aredia)
p-aminobenzoic acid (PABA)
p-aminohippurate
    sodium, p.
p-aminohippuric acid (PAH or PAHA)
panagglutinable
panagglutination
panagglutinin
Panax ginseng

pan-B-cell antigen
pancake coil
Pancoast
    syndrome, P.
    tumor, P.
pancolectomy
pancreas
pancreatectomy
pancreatelcosis
pancreatic
    cancer, p.
    endocrine neoplasia, p.
    hamartoma, p.
    insufficiency, p.
    islet cell tumor, p.
    oncofetal antigen, p. (POA)
    polypeptide, p. (PP)
    pseudocyst, p.
pancreaticoduodenal
pancreaticoduodenostomy
pancreaticohepatic syndrome
pancreaticosplenic
pancreatoduodenectomy
pancreatitis
pancreatoblastoma
pancreatogenous
pancreatogram
pancreatography
pancreatolienal
pancreatolytic
pancreatoncus
pancreatopathy
pancreatotropic
pancreectomy
pancreolysis
pancreolytic
pancreopathy
pancreoprivic
pancreotherapy
pancreozymin
Pancretide
pancytopenia
    -dysmelia syndrome, p.
    Fanconi p.
Pander islands
panendoscope
panendoscopy
Paneth cells
panhematin
panhematopenia
    primary splenic p.
panhematopoietic
panhemocytophthisis

ADDITIONAL TERMS

Panheprin
panhypogammaglobulinemia
panhypopituitarism
panhysterectomy
panhysterocolpectomy
panhystero-oophorectomy
panhysterosalpingectomy
panhysterosalpingo-oophorectomy
panimmunity
Panje
    implant, P.
    voice button, P.
    voice valve, P.
panleukopenia
panlymphopenia
panmyeloid
panmyelopathy
    constitutional infantile p.
panmyelophthisis
panmyelosis
Panorex radiograph
panproctocolectomy
pan-T antigen
Panton-Vallentine leukocidin
pantothenic acid
Panwarfin
Pap (Papanicolaou)
    smear, P.
    stain, P.
    test, P.
PAP (peroxidase-antiperoxidase)
    immunoperoxidase, P.
    technique, P.
PAP (prostatic acid phosphatase)
papain
    cleavage, p.
Papanicolaou (Pap)
    smear, P.
    stain, P.
    test, P.
papaverine
paperadioimmunosorbent test (PRIST)
papilla (pl. papillae)
papillae (pl. of papilla)
papillary
    adenocarcinoma, p.
    adenocystoma, p.
    adenoma, p.
    carcinoma, p.
    cystadenocarcinoma, p.
    cystadenoma lymphomatosum, p.
    cystic adenoma, p.
    necrosis, p.

    serocystadenocarcinoma, p.
    serous cystadenocarcinoma,
      p.
    thyroid carcinoma, p.
    tumor, p.
papillectomy
papilledema
papilliform
papillitis
papilloadenocystoma
papillocarcinoma
papilloma
papillomatosis
papillomatous
papillomavirus
papillopathy
papillotomy
Papnet system
papovavirus
Pappenheim stain
Pappenheimer bodies
papular
papule
papulosis
papulosquamous
para-aminobenzoic acid (PABA)
para-aminohippuric acid (PAH
    or PAHA)
parablast
paracanthoma
paracentesis
Paracoccidioides
    brasiliensis, P.
paracoccidioidomycosis
paracolitis
paracolpitis
paracrine
    growth factor, p.
paradoxical
    metastasis, p.
paraffin
    block, p.
    cancer, p.
    section, p.
paraffinoma
parafollicular
paraganglia (pl. of paraganglion)
paraganglioma
paraganglion (pl. paraganglia)
paraganglionic
parageusia
Paragon immunofixation
  electrophoresis

ADDITIONAL TERMS

paragranuloma
parahemophilia
parahormone
paralingual
parallel
  grid, p.
  -opposed fields, p.
  -opposed technique, p.
  plate dialyzer, p.
  track, p.
parameningeal rhabdomyosarcoma
paramomycin sulfate
paramyloidosis
paramyxovirus
Parana virus
paraneoplastic
  acrokeratosis, p.
  cerebellar degeneration, p.
  changes, p.
  lesion, p.
  leukemoid reaction, p.
  pemphigus syndrome, p.
  syndrome, p.
paranephroma
paraparesis
parapharyngeal
paraplasm
Paraplatin (carboplatin)
paraplegia
paraplegic
parapneumonia
paraproctitis
paraprostatitis
paraprotein
  spike, p.
paraproteinemia
paraquat
pararectal
pararosaniline pamoate
parasagittal
parasialadenoma
parasite
parasitemia
parasitic
  fibroma, p.
  infestation, p.
  thrombus, p.
parasitism
paraspinal mass
parasternal
parastruma
paratesticular
parathion

parathormone
parathyroid
  adenoma, p.
  extract, p.
  hormone, p. (PTH)
  insufficiency, p.
parathyroidal
parathyroidectomize
parathyroidectomy
parathyroidoma
parathyropathy
parathyroprival
parathyroprivia
parathyroprivic
parathyrotropic
paratope
paratracheal
  nodes, p.
parenchyma
parenchymal
parent cell
parenteral
  alimentation, p.
  chemotherapy, p.
  feeding, p.
  iron, p.
  nutrition, p.
  total p. nutrition
paresis
paresthesia
paresthetic
paretic
paries (pl. parietes)
parietes (pl. of paries)
parieto-occipital
Parinaud syndrome
Paris classification
parity
parocrine
Parodi-Irgens sarcoma virus
paromomycin
paromphalocele
parophthalmoncus
parosteal
  desmoid, p.
  osteosarcoma, p. (POS)
parotid
  gland, p.
  lymph node, p.
  tumor, p.
parotidectomy
parotidoscirrhus
parotitis

ADDITIONAL TERMS

parous
parovarian
 cyst, p.
parovariotomy
paroxysmal
 cold hemoglobinuria, p. (PCH)
 nocturnal hemoglobinuria, p.
  (PNH)
Parrot ulcer
Parry disease
partial
 antigen, p.
 exchange transfusion, p.
 gastrectomy, p.
 mastectomy, p.
 penectomy, p.
 resection, p.
 thromboplastin time, p. (PTT)
particle
 alpha p.
 beta p.
 C p.
 Dane p.
 elementary p.
 high-velocity p's
 nuclear p's
 Zimmerman elementary p's
particle accelerator
particle beam
particle beam radiotherapy
particle bombardment
particle counter
particle irradiation
particle radiation
particulate
 irradiation, p.
 radiation, p.
parvicellular
parvovirus
PAS (para-aminosalicylic acid)
PAS (periodic acid-Schiff)
 orange G, P.
 reagent, P.
 stain, P.
 test, P.
PAS (peripheral access system)
 port, P.
Passavant
 bar, P.
 ridge, P.
passenger leukocytes
passive
 cutaneous anaphylaxis, p.

hemagglutination, p.
immunization, p.
immunity, p.
immunotherapy, p.
smoking, p.
Pasteur theory
pasteurization
pastille
 radiometer, p.
Patch mutation
patchwork radiation therapy
patchy infiltrate
PATCO (prednisone, ara-C, thioguanine,
 cyclophosphamide, Oncovin)
Patey mastectomy
pathema
pathogen
pathogenesis
pathogenic
pathologic
 fracture, p.
 mitosis, p.
 process, p.
pathophysiologic
pathophysiology
pathway
 alternative complement p.
 amphibolic p.
 biosynthetic p.
 classical complement p.
 de novo p.
 Embden-Meyerhof p.
 Embden-Meyerhof-Parnas p.
 final common p.
 lipoxygenase p.
 pentose phosphate p.
 properdin p.
patient-controlled analgesia (PCA)
 administered epidurally, p. (PCAE)
Patil stereotactic system
Patterson-Kelly syndrome
patulous
Paul-Bunnell test
Paul-Bunnell-Davidsohn test
Pautrier microabscess
PAVe (procarbazine, Alkeran, Velban)
pavementing
PBI (protein-bound iodine)
PBLs (peripheral blood lymphocytes)
PBMC (peripheral blood mononuclear
 cells)
PBPC (peripheral blood progenitor
 cells)

ADDITIONAL TERMS

PB-1 polypeptide
PBV (Platinol, bleomycin, vinblastine)
PC-55
PCA (patient-controlled analgesia)
    pump, P.
PCA-1 antigen
PCAE (patient-controlled analgesia
    administered epidurally)
P. carinii (Pneumocystis carinii)
PCB (polychlorinated biphenyl)
PCB (procarbazine)
PCC (pheochromocytoma)
PCE (perchlorethylene)
PCE (Platinol, cyclophosphamide,
    Eldesine)
PCH (paroxysmal cold hemoglobinuria)
pCi (picocurie)
Pck-1 gene
PCL (plasma cell leukemia)
PCNU
PCO (polycystic ovary)
pCO_2 (carbon dioxide pressure)
pCO_2 (carbon dioxide tension)
PCP (Pneumocystis carinii pneumonia)
PCR (polymerase chain reaction)
PCT (plasmacytoma)
PCV (packed cell volume)
PCV (procarbazine, CCNU, vincristine)
Pd (palladium)
    ^{103}Pd seed implantation, P.
PD (peritoneal dialysis)
PDBu (phorbol 12,13-dibutyrate)
PDD (percentage depth dose)
PDGA (pteroyldiglutamic acid)
PDGF (platelet-derived growth factor)
PDLL (poorly differentiated lymphocytic
    lymphoma)
PDQ (Physician's Data Query)
    Cancer Treatment Database, P.
    information system, P.
PDT (photodynamic therapy)
PE (phycoerythrin)
    dye, P.
peak-and-trough levels
Pean operation
pearl tumor
pearly tumor
Pearson chi-square analysis
peau d'orange
PEB (Platinol, etoposide, bleomycin)
PEC (Platinol, etoposide,
    cyclophosphamide)
PECHO (prostatic echogram)

Pecquet cistern
pectoralis major myocutaneous pedicle
    flap
pediatric
    AIDS, p. (PAIDS)
    lymphoma, p.
Pediatric BLITZ (B4 blocked ricin)
Pediatric Oncology Group (POG)
pedicle flap
peduncle
peduncular
pedunculated
pefloxacin
PEG (polyethylene glycol)
    -ADA, P. (polyethylene glycol-
    adenosine deaminase)
    -adenosine deaminase, P. (PEG-
    ADA)
    -IL2, P. (polyethylene glycol-
    modified interleukin-2)
    -interleukin-2, p. (PEG-IL-2)
    -L-ASP, P. (polyethylene glycol-
    conjugated L-asparaginase)
    -L-asparaginase, P. (polyethylene
    glycol-conjugated L-asparaginase)
pegademase bovine (Adagen or Imudon
    or PEG-ADA)
pegaspargase
PEL (permissible exposure limits)
Pel-Ebstein fever
pelade
Pelger nuclear anomaly
Pelger-Huet
    cells, P.
    nuclear anomaly, P.
pelgeroid
peliomycin
peliosis
    hepatis, p.
    liver, p. of
Pelizaeus-Merzbacher disease
pelvic
    endometriosis, p.
    exenteration, p.
    floor, p.
    irradiation, p.
    lymph node, p.
    lymphadenectomy, p.
    malignancy, p.
    mass, p.
    metastasis, p.
    sidewall, p.
    studding, p.

ADDITIONAL TERMS

washings, p.
pelvioileoneocystostomy
pelvioprostatic capsule
pelviradiography
pelviroentgenography
pelvioscopy
pelvirectal
pelviureteroradiography
pelvoscopy
pemphigoid
pemphigus
    paraneoplastic p. syndrome
PEN (pharmacy equivalent names)
Penbritin
penectomy
penetrability
penetrable
penetrate
penetrometer
penetrometry
Penfield method
penile
    carcinoma, p.
    implant, p.
    prosthesis, p.
    resection, p.
penis
penitis
Penn seroflocculation reaction
pentad
pentagastrin
Pentam 300 (pentamidine)
pentamethylmelamine (PMM)
pentamidine
    aerosolization, p.
    isethionate, p.
    nebulizer, p.
    spray, p.
pentamustine
Pentaspan
Pentastarch
pentazocine
pentetate
    calcium trisodium, p.
    indium disodium In 111, p.
pentobarbital
pentosan polysulfate (PPS)
pentose phosphate
    pathway, p.
    shunt, p.
pentostatin (DCF or 2′-deoxycoformycin or Nipent)
pentoxifylline (Trental)

peotomy
PEP (Procytox, epipodophyllotoxin-derivative, prednisolone)
PEPA (protective environment and prophylactic antibiotics)
Pepper
    syndrome, P.
    -type neuroblastoma, P.
pepsin
pepstatin
Peptamen
peptic
peptidase
peptide
    -binding groove, p.
    growth factors, p.
    hormone, p.
    -producing islet tumor, p.
    synthetase, p.
    T, p.
peptidoglycan
Peptococcus
    anaerobius, P.
    asaccharolyticus, P.
    constellatus, P.
    magnus, P.
peptone plasma
Peptostreptococcus
    anaerobius, P.
    lanceolatus, P.
    micros, P.
    parvulus, P.
    productus, P.
percentage depth dose (PDD)
perchlorethylene (PCE)
Percocet
Percodan
Percoll technique
PercuCut biopsy needle
PercuGuide
percutaneous
    needle biopsy, p. (PNB)
    transhepatic biopsy, p. (PTHB)
Perez sign
perfluorochemical (PFC)
perforin
perfusate
perfusing
perfusion
Pergamid
periadenitis
    mucosa necrotica recurrens, p.
perianal

ADDITIONAL TERMS

perianal—*Continued*
 herpes, p.
 Paget disease, p.
periangioma
periaortic
 irradiation, p.
 lymph nodes, p.
periareolar
pericardectomy
pericardiectomy
pericarditis
 radiation p.
pericardium
pericholangitis
perichondritis
perichondroma
pericolitis
 membranous p.
pericolonic
pericolpitis
pericyte
pericytoma
Peridex
periendothelioma
periepithelioma
periesophageal
perihepatitis
perihilar
perilesional
perimetry testing
perineal
 dissection, p.
 needle biopsy, p.
 prostatectomy, p.
perineocolporectomyomectomy
perineoscrotal
perineoplasty
perineovaginal
perineovaginorectal
perineovulvar
perineum
perineural
periodic acid-Schiff (PAS)
 stain, p.
 test, p.
perioral
periosteal
 osteosarcoma, p.
periosteoma
periosteomedullitis
periosteomyelitis
periosteophyte
periosteoplastic

amputation, p.
periostitis
periostoma
periostomedullitis
periostosis
peripancreatic
peripheral
 access system, p. (PAS)
 blood, p.
 blood lymphocytes, p. (PBLs)
 blood mononuclear cells, p.
 (PBMC)
 blood progenitor cells, p. (PBPC)
 blood stem cells, p.
 circulation, p.
 cyanosis, p.
 line, p.
 nerve block anesthesia, p.
 nerve lesion, p.
 nervous system, p.
 neurectomy, p.
 neuroectodermal tumor, p.
 palisading, p.
 perfusion, p.
 smear, p.
 stem cell harvesting, p. (PSCH)
 stem cells, p.
 tumor, p.
peripherally inserted
 catheter, p. (PIC)
 central line catheter, p. (PICC)
periphery
peripolesis
periportal
 carcinoma, p.
 cirrhosis, p.
periproctic
periproctitis
periprostatic
periprostatitis
perirectal
peristalsis
peristaltic
perithelial
perithelioma
peritoneal
 dialysis, p.
 mesothelioma, p.
 washings, p.
peritoneography
peritoneoplasty
peritoneoscopy
peritoneovenous shunt

ADDITIONAL TERMS

peritoneum
peritonitic
peritonitis
periventricular
perivesical
periwinkle plant
perleche
Perlman tumor
permanent
    colostomy, p.
    loop ileostomy, p.
    remission, p.
    section, p.
permeability
permeable
permeability
permeate
permeation
permissible
    dose, p.
    exposure limits, p. (PEL)
permitted exposure dose/rodent
  potency dose (PERP)
permutation
permuted
pernicious
    anemia, p. (PA)
peroral
per os
peroxidase
    -antiperoxidase, p. (PAP)
    hemolysis, p.
    reaction, p.
    stain, p.
peroxide
    mouthwash, p.
    swishes, p.
Peroxyl
PERP (permitted exposure dose/rodent
  potency dose)
perphenazine
per primam intentionam
per rectum
per secundam intentionam
persistent generalized lymphadenopathy
  (PGL)
person with AIDS (PWA)
Pertscan 99m
Peruvian balsam
pessary cell
pesticide
    exposure, p.
    residue, p.

PET (positron emission tomography)
petechia (pl. petechiae)
petechiae (pl. of petechiae)
petechial
Petit constant
Petri dish
Petriellidium
    boydii, P.
petrolatoma
petrosal
    ganglion, p.
petrosphenoidal
petrous
Peutz-Jeghers syndrome
PEV (poussée evolutirie)
    classification, P.
Peyer patches
PF (protection factor)
PF4 (platelet factor 4)
    RIA, P.
PFA (phosphonoformic acid)
PFC (perfluorochemical)
PF+E (Platinol, 5-fluorouracil plus
  etoposide, methotrexate, leucovorin)
PFGE (pulsed field gradient gel
  electrophoresis)
Pfieffer
    bacillus, P.
    disease, P.
    phenomenon, P.
Pfiffner and Myers method
PFL (Platinol, 5-fluorouracil,
  leucovorin)
PFM (Platinol, 5-fluorouracil, moderate-
  dose methotrexate)
PFS (progression-free survival)
PFT (phenylalanine mustard,
  5-fluorouracil, tamoxifen)
PFT (pulmonary function test)
pg (picogram)
PG (prostaglandin)
PGE (percutaneous gastroenterostomy)
PGL (persistent generalized
  lymphadenopathy)
pH (hydrogen ion concentration)
Ph (Philadelphia) chromosome
PHA (phytohemagglutinin)
PHA (phytohemagglutinin antigen)
phacomatosis
phagadena
phagadenic
    ulcer, p.
phage

ADDITIONAL TERMS

phage—*Continued*
  typing, p.
phagelysis
phagocytable
phagocyte
  alveolar p's
  mononuclear p.
phagocytic
phagocytin
phagocytize
phagocytoblast
phagocytolysis
phagocytolytic
phagocytosis
  induced p.
  spontaneous p.
  surface p.
phagocytotic
phagokaryosis
phagosome
phagotype
phakoma
phakomatosis
phalangeal
phalangectomy
phalanges (pl. of phalanx)
phalangophalangeal
  amputation, p.
phalanx (pl. phalanges)
phallectomy
phallic
phalliform
phallitis
phalloid
phalloidin
phalloncus
phalloplasty
phallus
phantogeusia
phantom
  corpuscle, p.
  limb, p.
  pain, p.
  tumor, p.
pharmacochemistry
pharmacodynamics
pharmacoendocrinology
pharmacogenetic
pharmacokinetics
pharmacologic
pharmacoradiography
pharmacoroentgenography
pharmacotherapy

pharmacy
  body p.
  human p.
pharmacy equivalent name (PEN)
pharmokinetic
pharyngeal
  herpes, p.
  pouch syndrome, p.
pharyngectasia
pharyngectomy
pharyngitis
pharyngodynia
pharyngoesophageal
  prosthesis, p.
  reconstruction, p.
pharyngolaryngeal
  prosthesis, p.
  reconstruction, p.
pharyngopathy
pharyngoplasty
pharyngoscleroma
pharyngoscope
pharyngoscopy
pharyngostenosis
pharyngostoma
pharyngostomy
pharyngotome
pharyngotomy
pharyngoxerosis
pharynx
Phase I, II, III studies
phased array
phasein
phasen
phase-specific
phene
phenethicillin
  sodium, p.
phenolsulfonphthalein (PSP)
phenotype
  Bombay p.
  McLeod p.
  myeloid p.
  null p.
phenotypic
phenprocoumon
phentolamine
  hydrochloride, p.
  mesylate, p.
phenylalanine
  hydroxylase, p.
  hydroxylase gene, p.
  4-mono-oxygenase, p.

ADDITIONAL TERMS

mustard, p. (L-PAM)
phenylbutazone
phenylhydrazine
    anemia, p.
phenylketonuria (PKU)
phenylpyruvic acid
pheochromoblast
pheochromoblastoma
pheochromocytoma (PCC)
pheresis
Phi bodies
phi-meson
Philadelphia (Ph) chromosome
Phillips
    contact therapy unit, P.
    radiation treatment gun, P.
phimosis
phimotic
PHK (platelet phosphohexokinase)
phlebitic
phlebitis
phlebotomize
phlebotomy
phlegm
phlogocyte
phlogocytosis
phlorhizin test
phloxine
    -tartrazine stain, p.
Phocas disease
Phoma
phorbol
    12,13-dibutyrate, p. (PDBu)
    ester, p.
    myristate acetate, p. (PMA)
phoroblast
phorocyte
phorocytosis
phosgene
    oxime, p.
PhosLo
phosphatase
    acid p.
    alkaline p. (ALP)
phosphate
    polyestradiol p.
phosphatemia
phosphatidylcholine
phosphatidylethanolamine
phosphatidylinositol
    -specific phospholipase C, p.
phosphatidylserine
phosphatemia

N-phosphoacetyl-L-aspartate (PALA)
phosphocreatine
phosphocol P32
phosphodiesterase
phosphoenolpyruvate carboxykinase
    (GTP)
6-phosphofructokinase
phosphoglucokinase
phosphogluconate dehydrogenase
phosphoglycerate
    kinase, p.
    mutase, p.
phosphogluceromutase
phosphoglyceride
phosphokinase
phospholipase
phospholipid
phosphomonoesterase
phosphonate
phosphonecrosis
phosphonoformate
phosphonoformic acid (PFA)
phosphoprotein
phosphopyruvate
    carboxykinase, p.
    carboxlyase, p.
phosphoramidate
phosphoramide mustard
phosphoribosylpyrophosphate
    aminotransferase, p.
    synthetase, p.
phosphoribosyltransferase
PhosphorImager
phosphorothoate analogue
phosphorus (P)
    labeled p.
    radioactive p.
phosphorylase
    kinase, p.
    phosphatase, p.
    purine nucleoside p.
phosphorylated
phosphorylation
phosphorylcholine
Phosphotope oral solution
phosphotransferase
phosphotungstic acid
phossy jaw
photoablation
photoactinic
photoactive
photoallergy
photocarcinogenesis

ADDITIONAL TERMS

photochemical
photochemistry
photochemotherapeutic
photochemotherapy
photochromagen
photochromogenicity
photocoagulation
photoculdoscope
photodegradation
photodermatitis
photodisintegration
photodynamic
photoelectric
photoelectron
photofluorography
photofluoroscope
Photofrin II
photoisomerization
photoluminescence
photoluminescent
photometer
photomethemoglobin
photometry
photomicrograph
photomicroscope
photomicroscopy
photon
    beam densitometry, p.
    bombardment, p.
    contamination, p.
    -deficient lesion, p.
    energy, p.
    fluence, p.
    symmetry, p.
photoneutron
photonosus
photonscan
photonuclear
photo-oxidation
photopheresis
photoprotection
photoradiation
photoradiometer
photoreaction
photoreactivation
photoreception
photoreceptive
photoscan
photoscanner
photosensitivity
photosensitization
photosensitizer
phototherapy

photothermy
phototoxic
phototoxicity
phototoxis
photovaporization
phrenectomy
PHRT (procarbazine, hydroxyurea, radiotherapy)
phthisis
phycoerythrin (PE)
    dye, p.
phycomycosis
phyllode
phyllolith
phylloquinone
phylogenetic
phylogenic
phyma (pl. phymata)
phymata (pl. of phyma)
phymatoid
phymatology
phymatorhusin
phymatorrhysin
phymatosis
physalides (pl. of physalis)
physaliphore
physalis (pl. physalides)
physical
    chemistry, p.
    half-life, p.
Physician's Data Query (PDQ)
physicochemical
physiochemical
physiologic
    anemia, p.
    hypogammaglobulinemia, p.
    jaundice, p.
    leukocytosis, p.
    salt solution, p. (PSS)
    staging, p.
physocele
physostigmine
phytagglutinin
phytanic acid
phytase
phytoagglutinin
phytoanaphylactogen
phytohemagglutinin (PHA)
    antigen, p. (PHA)
phytomitogen
phytonadione
phytoprecipitin
phytosensitinogen

ADDITIONAL TERMS

pi
  lines, p.
  -meson, p.
PIA (Platinol, ifosfamide, Adriamycin)
piastrinemia
PIC (peripherally inserted catheter)
PICC (peripherally inserted central line
  catheter)
Pichinde virus
picibanil (OK-432)
Pick
  adenoma, P.
  bodies, P.
  cells, P.
  disease, P.
  inclusion body, P.
  tubular adenoma, P.
pickwickian syndrome
picocurie (pCi)
picodnavirus
picogram (pg)
picolinic acid
picomole
picopicogram (ppg)
picornavirus
picrogeusia
PID (plasma-iron disappearance)
PIDT (plasma-iron disappearance time)
piecrusting
pie-shaped dose
PIF (prolactin-inhibiting factor)
PIFT (platelet immunofluorescence test)
piggyback
  intravenous p. (IVP)
piggybacking
pigment
pigmentation
  hematogenous p.
  macroscopic p.
  radiation p.
pigmented
  ameloblastoma, p.
  basal cell carcinoma, p.
  lesion, p.
  mole, p.
  nevus, p.
  xerodermoid, p.
pigmenting hairless mouse
pigmentogenesis
pika
pilocytic
  astrocytoma, p.
pilomatricoma

pilomatrixoma
pilonidal cyst
pilot dose
Pimaricin
pimeloma
pi-meson
PIMS (programmable implantable
  medication system)
Pindborg tumor
pine cone extract
pineal
  body, p.
  teratoma, p.
pinealectomy
pinealoblastoma
pinealocyte
pinealocytoma
pinealoma
pinealopathy
pineoblastoma
pineocytoma
pineocytosis
Pinkus fibroepithelioma
pinocyte
pinocytosis
pion
  beam, p.
  dosimetry, p.
  therapy, p.
Pipell endometrial suction catheter
piperazenedione
piperoxan hydrochloride
pipe-smoker's
  carcinoma, p.
  lip, p.
PIPIDA (p-isopropylacetanilide-
  iminodiacetic acid)
  scan, P.
pipobroman (Vercyte)
piposulfan
pirarubicin
Pirigoff amputation
piritrexim isoethionate (BW 301U)
piroplasmosis
piroxantrone hydrochloride (PXT)
PIT (plasma iron turnover)
pitch
  -workers' cancer, p.
  wart, p.
Pitfield fluid
PITR (plasma iron turnover rate)
pits
Pitt talking tracheostomy tube

ADDITIONAL TERMS

Pittsburgh pneumonia agent
pituitarism
pituitary
    ablation, p.
    adamantinoma, p.
    adenoma, p.
    ameloblastoma, p.
    basophilism, p.
    gland, p.
    stalk, p.
    tumor, p.
pivhydrazine
pixel
PK (pyruvate kinase)
P-K (Prausnitz-Küstner)
    antibody, P.
    reaction, P.
    transfer test, P.
PKC inhibition
PLA-1 (platelet antigen)
placebo
    -controlled study, p.
    -effect, p.
placenta
placental
    alkaline phosphatase, p. (PLAP)
    blood flow, p.
    lactogen, p.
    transfusion, p.
placentoma
Planck
    constant, P.
    quantum theory, P.
planocellular
planocyte
plant
    alkaloids, p.
    extracts, p.
PLAP (placental alkaline phosphatase)
plaque
    atheromatous p.
    eye p.
plaque-forming cell assay
plaque irradiation
plaqueing
Plasbumin
plasma
    acid phosphatase, p.
    activation, p.
    aldosterone, p.
    amino acids, p.
    catecholamines, p.
    cell, p.

    cell antigen, p.
    cell dyscrasia, p.
    cell granuloma, p.
    cell leukemia, p.
    cell myeloma, p.
    clotting time, p.
    dyscrasia, p.
    exchange, p.
    expander, p.
    ferritin, p.
    immune factor, p.
    iron clearance half-time, p.
    iron disappearance, p. (PID)
    iron disappearance time, p. (PIDT)
    iron turnover, p. (PIT)
    iron turnover rate, p. (PITR)
    kallikrein, p.
    neopterin level, p.
    protein, p.
    protein fraction, p. (PPF)
    prothrombin conversion factor, p.
      (PPCF)
    renin, p.
    skimming, p.
    -thrombin clot method, p.
    thromboplastin, p.
    thromboplastin antecedent, p.
      (PTA)
    thromboplastin component, p.
      (PTC)
    thromboplastin factor, p. (PTF)
    transfusion, p.
    volume extender, p.
plasmablast
plasmacrit
plasmacyte
plasmacytic
plasmacytoid
plasmacytoma (PCT)
    chest wall p.
    extramedullary p.
    multiple p. of bone
plasmacytosis
plasmagene
plasmahaut
plasmal
plasmalogen
Plasmalyte 148
Plasmanate
plasmapheresis
Plasma-Plex
Plasmatein
plasmatherapy

ADDITIONAL TERMS

plasmatofibrous
   astrocytes, p.
plasmatosis
plasmid
   library, p.
   vector system, p.
plasmin
   prothrombin conversion factor, p.
plasminogen
   activator, p.
   activator inhibitor, p. (PAI-1)
plasmocyte
plasmocytoma
Plasmodium
   falciparum, P.
   malariae, P.
   ovale, P.
   vivax, P.
plasmodium
   exoerythrocytic p.
plasmoma
plasmonucleic acid
plasmotropism
plastein
Plasti-Pore
Platamine
platelike atelectasis
platelet
   -activating factor, p. (PAF)
   adhesion, p.
   adhesiveness, p.
   agglutinin, p.
   -aggregating factor, p. (PAF)
   aggregation, p.
   antigen, p.
   -associated IgG, p. (PAIgG)
   clumping, p.
   clustering, p.
   coagulation factor, p.
   concentrate, p.
   count, p.
   -derived growth factor, p. (PDGF)
   fibrinogen, p.
   -free plasma, p.
   heparitinase, p.
   immunofluorescence test, p. (PIFT)
   inhibition, p.
   isoantibodies, p.
   membrane-bound IgG, p.
   migration inhibition, p.
   nadir, p.
   peroxidase, p.
   phosphohexokinase, p. (PHK)

   -poor, p.
   radioactive antiglobulin test, p.
     (PRAT)
   -rich, p.
   -specific antigen, p.
   suspension immunofluorescence
     test, p. (PSIFT)
   transfusion, p.
Platelet Factor 4
plateletpheresis
plating
Platinol (cisplatin)
platinum
   diamminodichloride, p.
platycyte
PLD (potentially lethal damage)
PLDR (potentially lethal damage repair)
Pleatman Sac
pleiotropic
   drug resistance, p.
   gene, p.
pleiotropin
pleiotropism
pleocytosis
   mononuclear p.
pleokaryocyte
pleomorphic
   adenoma, p.
   epithelial cells, p.
   lipoma, p.
   salivary adenoma, p.
pleomorphism
   nuclear p.
plesiotherapy
pleura (pl. pleurae)
pleurae (pl. of pleura)
pleural
   biopsy, p.
   bleb, p.
   effusion, p.
   fluid, p.
   loculation, p.
   mass, p.
   metastasis, p.
   plaque, p.
   plaquing, p.
   thickening, p.
pleurectomy
Pleur-Evac
pleurocentesis
pleuroclysis
pleurodesis
pleurography

ADDITIONAL TERMS

pleuroperitoneal shunt
pleuropneumonectomy
pleuropneumonia
   -like organisms, p. (PPLO)
pleurorrhea
pleuroscopy
plexiform
   neurofibroma, p.
   tumorlet, p.
PLH (pulmonary lymphoid hyperplasia)
plicamycin (Mithracin)
plicate
plication
Plimmer bodies
PLL (prolymphocytic leukemia)
ploidy
plombage
PLT (primed lymphocyte typing)
Plummer-Vinson
   radium applicator, P.
   syndrome, P.
pluriglandular
   adenomatosis, p.
pluripotent
   stem cells, p.
pluripotential
pluripotentiality
pluriresistant
plus-stranded
   RNA genome virus, p.
plutonium (Pu)
pM (pathologic assessment of distant
   metastasis)
Pm (promethium)
PM (prednimustine)
PMA (phorbol myristate acetate)
PMB (Platinol, methotrexate,
   bleomycin)
PMB (polymorphonuclear basophil
   leukocyte)
PME (polymorphonuclear eosinophil
   leukocyte)
PMF (L-phenylalanine mustard,
   methotrexate, 5-fluorouracil)
PMFAC (prednisone, methotrexate, and
   FAC protocol [5-fluorouracil,
   Adriamycin, cyclophosphamide])
PML (progressive multifocal
   leukoencephalopathy)
PMM (pentamethylmelamine)
PMN (polymorphonuclear neutrophil
   leukocyte)
PMR (polymorphic reticulosis)

P-MVAC (Platinol, methotrexate,
   vinblastine, Adriamycin, carboplatin)
pN (pathologic assessment of regional
   lymph nodes, written as pN1bi, pN1bii,
   pN1biii, pN1biv; subsets of pathologic
   classification)
PNB (percutaneous needle biopsy)
PNET (primitive neuroectodermal
   tumor)
PNET-MB (primitive neuroectodermal
   tumor-medulloblastoma)
pneumatic
pneumatization
pneumatocele
   cranii, p.
   extracranial p.
   intracranial p.
pneumatosis
pneumatotherapy
pneumectomy
pneumocele
pneumocentesis
pneumococcal
pneumococci (pl. of pneumococcus)
pneumococcus (pl. pneumococci)
pneumocolon
pneumoconiosis
pneumocystic
Pneumocystis
   carinii, P.
   carinii pneumonia, P. (PCP)
pneumocystis
   pneumonia, p.
   pneumonitis, p.
pneumocystosis
pneumoempyema
pneumoencephalogram
pneumoencephalography (PEG)
pneumoencephalomyelogram
pneumoencephalomyelography
pneumofasciogram
pneumogalactocele
pneumogastrography
pneumogram
pneumography
pneumogynogram
pneumolithiasis
pneumomalacia
pneumomediastinogram
pneumomediastinography
pneumomediastinum
pneumomelanosis
pneumomelanotic

ADDITIONAL TERMS

pneumomycosis
pneumonectomize
pneumonectomy
pneumonia
 abortive p.
 acute p.
 alba, p.
 alcoholic p.
 amebic p.
 anthrax p.
 apex p.
 apical p.
 apostematosa, p.
 Aspergillus p.
 aspiration p.
 atypical p.
 bacterial p.
 bilious p.
 bronchial p.
 Buhl desquamative p.
 Candida p.
 caseous p.
 catarrhal p.
 central p.
 cerebral p.
 cheesy p.
 chronic p.
 chronic eosinophilic p.
 cold agglutinin p.
 congenital aspiration p.
 contusion p.
 core p.
 Corrigan p.
 croupous p.
 deglutition p.
 desquamative p.
 desquamative interstitial p.
 dissecans, p.
 double p.
 Eaton agent p.
 embolic p.
 eosinophilic p.
 ephemeral p.
 ether p.
 fibrinous p.
 fibrous p.
 Friedländer p.
 Friedländer bacillus p.
 gangrenous p.
 giant cell p.
 Hecht p.
 hypostatic p.
 indurative p.

influenza virus p.
influenzal p.
inhalation p.
interlobularis purulenta, p.
interstitial p.
interstitial plasma cell p.
intrauterine p.
Kaufman p.
Legionella pneumophila p.
lipid p.
lipoid p.
lobar p.
lobular p.
Löffler p.
Louisiana p.
lymphoid interstitial p.
malleosa, p.
massive p.
metastatic p.
migratory p.
miliary p.
mycoplasmal p.
Nocardia p
obstructive p.
oil-aspiration p.
parasitic p.
parenchymatous p.
Pittsburgh p.
plague p.
plasma cell p.
pleuritic p.
pleurogenetic p.
pleurogenic p.
pneumococcal p.
pneumocystis p.
Pneumocystis carinii p.
primary atypical p.
purulent p.
rheumatic p.
Riesman p.
round p.
secondary p.
septic p.
staphylococcal p.
streptococcal p.
suppurative p.
terminal p.
toxemic p.
traumatic p.
tuberculous p.
tularemic p.
typhoid p.
unresolved p.

ADDITIONAL TERMS

pneumonia—*Continued*
vagus p.
varicella p.
viral p.
walking p.
wandering p.
white p.
woolsorter's p.
pneumonic
pneumonitis
acute interstitial p.
aspiration p.
chemical p.
cholesterol p.
desquamative interstitial p.
granulomatous p.
hypersensitivity p.
interstitial p.
lymphocytic interstitial p. (LIP)
malarial p.
pneumocystis p.
radiation p.
uremic p.
pneumonocele
pneumonocentesis
pneumonocirrhosis
pneumonoconiosis
pneumonocyte
pneumonograph
pneumonogram
pneumonolipoidosis
pneumonolysis
pneumonomelanosis
pneumonomycosis
pneumonopathy
pneumonopexy
pneumonopathy
pneumonoresection
pneumonosis
pneumopathy
Pneumopent
pneumoperitoneum
pneumopexy
pneumopleuroparietopexy
pneumopreperitoneum
pneumopyopericardium
pneumopyothorax
pneumoradiography
pneumoroentgenogram
pneumoroentgenography
pneumosepticemia
pneumoserothorax
pneumosilicosis

pneumotherapy
pneumothorax
complete p.
partial p.
spontaneous p.
tension p.
pneumotomography
pneumotoxin
Pneumovax
pneumoventriculography
PNH (paroxysmal nocturnal
hemoglobinuria)
PNP (purine-nucleoside
phosphorylase)
PNS Unna boot
Pnu-Imune 23
Po (polonium)
pO_2 (partial oxygen pressure)
pO_2 (partial oxygen tension)
POA (pancreatic oncofetal antigen)
POC (procarbazine, Oncovin, CCNU)
POCA (prednisone, Oncovin, cytarabine,
Adriamycin)
POCC (procarbazine, Oncovin,
cyclophosphamide, CCNU)
podophyllin
podophyllotoxin
Podophyllum
peltatum, P.
podophyllum resin
podofilox
POEMS (polyneuropathy,
organomegaly, endocrinopathy,
monoclonal protein, skin change)
syndrome
POG (Pediatric Oncology Group)
Pohl test
poietin
poikiloblast
poikilocarynosis
poikilocyte
poikilocythemia
poikilocytosis
poikiloderma
poikilodermatomyositis
poikiloploid
poikiloploidy
poikilosmosis
poikilothrombocyte
point mutation
Poirier gland
poison ivy extract
Poisson distribution

ADDITIONAL TERMS

pokeroot
pokeweed mitogen (PWM)
pol (polymerase) gene
polar
    anemia, p.
    planar molecules, p.
polarity
polkissen (juxtaglomerular cells)
pollutant
pollute
pollution
polonium (Po)
Poloxamer 188
poly (polymorphonuclear leukocyte)
poly A (polyadenylate)
    tail, p.
poly A:U (polyadenylate:polyuridylate)
Poly ENA test system
Poly I:C
    (polyriboinosinic:polyribocytidylic acid)
Polya operation
polyacrylamide gel electrophoresis
    (PAGE)
polyadenitis
polyadenoma
polyadenomatosis
polyadenomatous
polyadenopathy
polyadenous
polyadenylate (poly A)
    :polyuridylate, p. (poly A:U)
polyadenylation
polyagglutinability
polyagglutination
polyamine
    synthesis, p.
polyangiitis
polyarteritis
    nodosa, p.
polyarthritis
polychemotherapy
polychorinated biphenyl (PCB)
polychromasia
polychromatic
polychromatophil
polychromatophilic
polychromatosis
polyclonal
    activator, p.
    antibody, p.
    hypergammaglobulinemia, p.
    hyperglobulinemia, p.
polycyclic

aromatic hydrocarbons, p. (PAH)
    hydrocarbons, p.
polycycloidal
    tomography, p.
polycystic
    breast, p.
    disease, p.
    kidney, p.
    liver, p.
    nephroblastoma, p.
    ovary, p. (PCO)
    renal disease, p.
polycystoma
polycyte
polycythemia
    absolute p.
    appropriate p.
    benign p.
    compensatory p.
    hypertonica, p.
    inappropriate p.
    myelopathic p.
    primary p.
    relative p.
    rubra, p.
    rubra vera, p.
    secondary p.
    splenomegalic p.
    spurious p.
    stress p.
    vera, p. (PV)
polydeoxyribonucleotide synthase (ATP)
polydrug
    abuse, p.
    overdose, p.
    therapy, p.
polyembryoma
polyemia
    polycythaemica, p.
polyendocrine
    adenomatosis, p.
    autoimmune disease, p.
    deficiency syndrome, p.
    neoplasia, p.
polyendocrinoma
polyendocrinopathy
polyestradiol (Estradurin)
    phosphate, p.
polyethylene glycol (PEG)
    -conjugated L-asparaginase, p.
    (PEG-L-ASP)
    -modified interleukin-2, p.
    (PEG-IL-2)

ADDITIONAL TERMS

polyferose
polygen
polygene
polygenic
polyglandular
polyglutamylation
polyhedral
polyhemia
polyimmunoglobulin
polyinfection
polykaryocyte
polylymphocytic
polylysine
polymer
    addition p.
    condensation p.
polymerase
    chain reaction, p. (PCR)
polymeric
polymerid
polymerism
polymerization
    fibrin p.
polymerizing
polymethyl
    methacrylate, p.
polymicrobial
polymicrobic
polymicrolipomatosis
polymorphic
    reticulosis, p. (PMR)
polymorphism
polymorphocellular
polymorphocyte
polymorphonuclear
    basophil leukocyte, p. (PMB)
    eosinophil leukocyte, p. (PME)
    neutrophil leukocyte, p. (PMN)
polymyalgia
    arterica, p.
    rheumatica, p.
polymyositis
polyneuritis
polyneuroradiculitis
polyneuropathy
polynuclear
    aromatic hydrocarbons, p. (PAH)
polynucleotide
    adenyltransferase, p.
    ligase, p.
    phosphatase, p.
    phosphorylase, p.
polyoma

    virus, p. (PV)
polyomavirus (PV)
polyp
    adenomatous p.
    antral p.
    ascending colon p.
    cardiac p.
    cecal p.
    cervical p.
    choanal p's
    colonic p.
    descending colon p.
    duodenal p.
    endocervical p's
    endometrial p's
    fibrinous p.
    gastric p.
    gelatinous p.
    gum p.
    hepatic flexure p.
    Hopmann p.
    hydatid p.
    juvenile p's
    laryngeal p.
    larynx, p's of
    lymphoid p's
    nasal p's
    pedunculated p.
    retention p's
    sentinel p.
    sessile p.
    sigmoid p.
    splenic flexure p.
    transverse colon p.
    uterine p.
    vocal cord p.
polypathia
polypectomy
polypeptidase
polypeptide
    cytokeratin p.
    gastric inhibitory p. (GIP)
    intestinal p.
    pancreatic p.
    vasoactive intestinal p. (VIP)
polypeptide hormones
polypeptidemia
polypharmaceutical
polypharmacy
polyphasic anaplasia
polyphyletic
    theory, p.
polypi (pl. of polypus)

ADDITIONAL TERMS

polyploid
polyploidy
polypoid
   adenocarcinoma, p.
   adenoma, p.
   cystic structure, p.
   lesion, p.
   mass, p.
polypoidosis
polyposis
   coli, p.
   familial p.
   familial intestinal p.
   gastrica, p.
   intestinalis, p.
   multiple familial p.
polyprotein
polypus (pl. polypi)
polyriboinosinic
   :polyribocytidylic acid, p. (Poly I:C)
polyribonucleotide
   nucleotidyltransferase, p.
polyribosome
polysaccharide
polysaccharidosis
polyvinyl
   alcohol, p.
   chloride, p.
POMP (prednisone, Oncovin,
  methotrexate, Purinethol)
Pomp-Siemens cabinet
pons (pl. pontes)
pontes (pl. of pons)
pool
   gene p.
   lymphocyte p.
   stem cell progenitor p.
poorly
   defined, p.
   differentiated, p.
   marginated, p.
popcorn pattern
popin
poppers (amyl nitrite)
porencephalic cyst
porfiromycin
Porites coral
Porod-Kratky wormlike chain theory
poroma
   eccrine p.
porphobilinogen
   deaminase, p.
   synthase, p.

porphyria
   acquired p.
   acute intermittent p.
   congenital erythropoietic p.
   congenital photosensitive p.
   cutanea tarda hereditaria, p.
   erythropoietic p.
   erythropoietica, p.
   hepatic p.
   hepatica, p.
   mixed p.
   South African genetic p.
   variegata, p.
   variegate p.
   X, p.
porphyrin
porphyrinemia
porphyrinogen
porphyrinuria
port
   size, p.
   wine stain, p.
Port-A-Cath
Porter-Silber chromogen
Portex tracheostomy tube
Portland hemoglobin
Portmann classification
Portner-Koolpe biliary biopsy set
porton asparaginase (Erwinia
  L-asparaginase)
POS (parosteal osteosarcoma)
Posada mycosis
Posada-Wernicke disease
positional cloning
positive
   electron, p.
   -ion accelerator, p.
positrocephalogram
positron
   coincidence, p.
   decay, p.
   emission tomography, p. (PET)
   scintillation camera, p.
positronium
postadrenalectomy
   pituitary adenoma, p.
postcricoid pharyngeal cancer
postgastrectomy
postherpetic
postirradiation
   malignancy, p.
   syndrome, p.
postlaryngectomy

ADDITIONAL TERMS

postlaser
postmastectomy
postmediastinal
postmenopausal
postnatal
postperfusion syndrome
postphlebitic
postpneumonectomy irradiation
postprandial
postpump syndrome
postradiation
    dysplasia, p. (PRD)
    fibromatosis, p.
    fibrosarcoma, p.
postsplenectomy
postsplenic
postsurgical
    TNM classification, p. (pTNM)
posttransfusion
    AIDS, p.
    hepatitis, p. (PTH)
    mononucleosis, p.
    purpura, p.
    syndrome, p.
posttransplant
posttransplantation
potassium (K)
potassemia
potato tumor
potential
potentialization
potentially
    lethal damage, p. (PLD)
    lethal damage repair, p. (PDLR)
potentiation
potentiator
Pott puffy tumor
poudrage
poussée évolutirie (PEV)
    classification, P.
poxvirus
power-breeder reactor
PP (pancreatic polypeptide)
PPCF (plasma prothrombin conversion factor)
PPD (purified protein derivative)
PPF (plasma protein fraction)
ppg (picopicogram)
PPLO (pleuropneumonia-like organisms)
Pr (praseodymium)
PR (progesterone receptor)

    antigen, P.
PR-225 (redox-acyclovir)
PR-239 (redox-penicillin G)
Prague strain of Rous sarcoma virus
pralidoxime (2-PAM)
praseodymium (Pr)
PRAT (platelet reactive antiglobulin test)
Prausnitz-Küstner (P-K)
    antibody, P.
    reaction, P.
pRb (retinoblastoma protein)
PRC (packed red cells)
PRD (postradiation dysplasia)
PRDL (prednisolone)
preauricular
    irradiation, p.
    lymph nodes, p.
pre-B cell
    acute lymphocytic leukemia, p.
precancer
precancerosis
precancerous
    dermatitis, p.
    lesion, p.
precarcinomatous
Precef
precipitable
precipitate
precipitin
    curve, p.
    reaction, p.
    ring, p.
precipitinogen
precipitinoid
precipitophore
precipitum
precursor
PRED (prednisone)
Pred-G
Pred-G-SOP
predictive value
predilection
predisposing
predisposition
    genetic p.
prednimustine
prednisolone
prednisone
preelacin
pregnancy serum
pregnanetriol

ADDITIONAL TERMS

pregnant mare's serum
preinvasive
    carcinoma, p.
    lesion, p.
Preisz-Nocard bacillus
prekallikrein
prelaryngeal node
preleukemia
preleukemic
premalignancy
premalignant
premammary
    abscess, p.
Premarin (conjugated estrogens)
premenopausal
pre-messenger RNA (pre-mRNA)
premitotic
premonocyte
premorbid
pre-mRNA (pre-messenger RNA)
premunition
premyeloblast
premyolocyte
preneoplastic
Pre-Pen
preradiation
prerandomization
pressure
    alopecia, p.
    sore, p.
pre-T cell
    acute lymphocytic leukemia, p.
pretracheal
    fascia, p.
    lymph node, p.
    space, p.
pretreatment
    procedure, p.
    staging, p.
pretumorous
prezone
PRF (prolactin-releasing factor)
PRH-E (Platinol, etanidazole)
priA gene
priapism
priB gene
priC gene
Price-Jones curve
prickle-cell
    carcinoma, p.
Priest assay
primaquine

    -sensitive anemia, p.
primary
    anemia, p.
    brain tumor, p.
    bubo, p.
    carcinoma, p.
    chemotherapy, p.
    colostomy, p.
    immune response, p.
    immunodeficiency, p.
    intra-axial brain tumor, p.
    lesion, p.
    radiation, p.
    splenic panhematopenia, p.
    tumor, p.
primase
primate
    studies, p.
Primaxin
PRIME (procarbazine, isophosphamide,
    methotrexate)
primed
    cells, p.
    lymphocyte typing, p. (PLT)
primer
primethamine
priming dose
primitive
    cells, p.
    erythroblasts, p.
    neurodectal tumor, p. (PNET)
    neurodectal tumor-
        medulloblastoma, p. (PNET-MB)
    polar spongioblastoma, p.
    white cells, p.
primordial cyst
primosome
Principen
Pringle
    maneuver, P.
    type, P.
PRIST (paperadioimmunosorbent test)
private antigens
pro time (prothrombin time)
proaccelerin
proactivator
    C3 p. (C3PA)
proagglutinoid
proantithrombin
proband
probe
    diagnostic system, p.

ADDITIONAL TERMS

probenecid
Probit analysis
Probitron readings for radium inserts
procarbazine hydrochloride (Matulane
  or N-methylhydrazine or MIH or PCB)
procarboxypeptidase
procarcinogen
prochlorperazine
procoagulant
procollagen
procollagenase
proconvertin (Factor VII)
Procrit
proctalgia
proctectomy
proctitis
    factitial p.
    obliterans, p.
    radiation p.
    traumatic p.
procto (proctoscopy)
proctocolectomy
proctocolitis
proctocolonoscopy
proctocolpoplasty
proctodynia
proctopexy
proctopolypus
proctoscope
proctoscopic
proctoscopy
proctosigmoid
proctosigmoidectomy
proctosigmoiditis
proctosigmoidoscope
proctosigmoidoscopic
proctosigmoidoscopy
proctostomy
proctotomy
Procysteine (oxothiazolidine
  carboxylate)
Procytox (cyclophosphamide)
Pro-Depo (hydroxyprogesterone)
prodromal
prodrome
product
    analogue, p.
    -limit estimate, p.
proerythroblast
proerythrocyte
profibrinolysin
Profilinine Heat-Treated
progenitor

cells, p.
Progens (conjugated estrogens)
progestational
progesteroid
progesterone
    receptor, p. (PR)
progestin
progestogen
progestomimetic
prognostic
prognostication
progonoma
    melanotic p.
programmable implantable medication
    system (PIMS)
programmed cell death
progranulocyte
progranulocytic
    leukemia, p.
progression
    disease, p. of
    -free survival, p. (PFS)
progressive
    disease, p.
    multifocal leukoencephalopathy, p.
        (PML)
    systemic sclerosis, p. (PSS)
Progynon
prohormone
Project Inform
prokaryocyte
prokaryocytic
prokaryote
Prokine
prolactin
    adenoma, p.
    -producing tumor, p.
    -releasing factor, p. (PRF)
prolactinoma
Prolastin
Proleukin (aldesleukin)
proleukocyte
proliferating
proliferation
    cell p.
    macrophage p.
    melanocyte p.
    tumor p.
proliferative
proline
Proloprim (trimethoprim)
prolymphocyte
prolymphocytic

ADDITIONAL TERMS

leukemia, p.
ProMACE (prednisone, methotrexate,
Adriamycin, cyclophosphamide,
etoposide)
ProMACE-CytaBOM (prednisone,
Adriamycin, cyclophosphamide,
etoposide, cytarabine, bleomycin,
Oncovin, methotrexate)
ProMACE-MOPP (procarbazine,
methotrexate, Adriamycin,
cyclophosphamide, etoposide,
Mustargen, Oncovin, procarbazine,
prednisone)
promegakaryocyte
promegaloblast
promethium (Pm)
promiscuity
promiscuous
promitosis
promitotic
promonocyte
promoter/enhancer sequence
promyelocyte
promyelocytic
leukemia, p.
pronormoblast
pro-opiocortin
pro-opiomelanocortin
propeptide
properdin (factor P)
prophage
prophase
prophylactic
prophylax
prophylaxis
propidium iodine
propiolactone
Propionibacterium
acnes, P.
proplasmacyte
proplasmin
Proplast implant
Proplex
propolis
proportional
counter, p.
ionization chamber, p.
propylthiouracil (PTU)
prorubricyte
Prosorba Column
prostacyclin
prostaglandin (PG)
prostata

prostalgia
prostate
cancer, p.
chips, p.
gland, p.
hypertrophy, p.
lobe, p.
nodule, p.
-specific antigen, p. (PSA)
transurethral resection of p.
(TURP)
prostatectomy
bag, p.
prostathelcosis
prostatic
acid phosphatase, p. (PAP)
benign p. hypertrophy (BPH)
biopsy, p.
cancer, p.
capsule, p.
echogram, p. (PECHO)
hypertrophy, p.
lobe, p.
nodule, p.
tumor, p.
prostaticovesical
prostaticovesiculectomy
prostatism
prostatitis
prostatocystomy
prostatodynia
prostatography
prostatomegaly
prostatomyomectomy
prostatovesiculectomy
prostheses (pl. of prosthesis)
prosthesis (pl. prostheses)
prosthetic
prosthodontics
prostratin
protactinium (Pa)
protamine sulfate
protease
inhibitor, p.
protection factor (PF)
protector
LATS (long-acting thyroid
stimulator) p.
proteid
proteidic
proteidogenous
protein
A, p.

ADDITIONAL TERMS

protein—*Continued*
  allosteric p.
  amyloid A p.
  amyloid light chain p.
  bacterial cellular p.
  Bence Jones p.
  C, p.
  C4 binding p.
  carrier p.
  cationic p's
  coagulated p.
  complete p.
  constitutive p's
  C-reactive p. (CRP)
  derived p.
  encephalitogenic p.
  fibrillar p.
  folate-binding p.
  globular p.
  Hektoen, Kretschmer, and Welker
    p.
  immune p's
  iron-sulfur p.
  M p.
  myelin basic p. (MBP)
  myeloma p.
  origin-binding (UL9) p.
  plasma p's
  racemized p.
  RAP 1 p.
  S, p.
  S p.
  serum p's
  serum amyloid p's
  staphylococcal p. A
  STOP p.
  synthetic p.
  Tus p.
  UL9 (origin-binding) p.
  Y p.
  Z p.
  zinc-finger p.
protein-A column
protein-A-peroxidase conjugate
  immunoperoxidase
protein binding
protein-bound
protein-bound iodine (PBI)
protein buffer
protein electrophoresis
protein folding
protein-glutamine
protein kinase

protein quotient
protein sequencing
protein spike
protein synthesis
proteinaceous
proteinase
proteinemia
  Bence-Jones p.
proteinosis
proteinuria
Protenate
proteoglycan
proteolipid
  gene, p.
proteolysis
proteolytic
  enzyme, p.
Proteus
  mirabilis, P.
  morganii, P.
  vulgaris, P.
prothrombin (factor II)
  -consumption test, p.
  -converting principle, p.
  -proconvertin test, p.
  time, p. (PT)
prothrombinase
prothrombinemia
prothrombinogen
prothrombinogenic
prothrombinopenia
prothymocyte
protide
protirelin
protium
protocol
  AA (ara-C, Adriamycin)
  AAA (adenosine-adenosine-
    adenosine)
  ABC (Adriamycin, BCNU,
    cyclophosphamide)
  ABCD (Adriamycin, bleomycin,
    CCNU, dacarbazine)
  ABCM (Adriamycin, bleomycin,
    cyclophosphamide, mitomycin-C)
  ABCX (Adriamycin, bleomycin,
    cisplatin, radiation therapy)
  ABD (Adriamycin, bleomycin,
    DTIC)
  ABDIC (Adriamycin, bleomycin,
    dacarbazine, CCNU, prednisone)
  ABDV (Adriamycin, bleomycin,
    DTIC, vinblastine)

ADDITIONAL TERMS

ABP (Adriamycin, bleomycin, prednisone)

ABV (actinomycin-D, bleomycin, vincristine)

ABVD (Adriamycin, bleomycin, vinblastine, dacarbazine)

ABVE (Adriamycin, bleomycin, vincristine, etoposide)

AC (Adriamycin, carmustine)

AC (Adriamycin, CCNU)

AC (Adriamycin, cisplatin)

ACe (Adriamycin, cyclophosphamide)

ACE (Adriamycin, cyclophosphamide, etoposide)

ACE-II (Adriamycin, cyclophosphamide, etoposide in high-dose infusion)

ACFUCY (actinomycin D, 5-FU, cyclophosphamide)

ACID (Adriamycin, cyclophosphamide, imidazole, dactinomycin)

ACM (Adriamycin, cyclophosphamide, methotrexate)

ACOAP (Adriamycin, cyclophosphamide, Oncovin, cytosine arabinoside, prednisone)

ACOP (Adriamycin, cyclophosphamide, Oncovin, prednisone)

ACOPP (Adriamycin, cyclophosphamide, Oncovin, prednisone, procarbazine)

ACT-FU-Cy (actinomycin-D, 5-FU, cyclophosphamide)

A+D or 7+3 (ara-C, daunorubicin)

ADBC (Adriamycin, DTIC, bleomycin, CCNU)

ADE (ara-C, daunorubicin, etoposide)

ADIC (Adriamycin, DTIC)

AdOAP (Adriamycin, Oncovin, ara-C, prednisone)

AdOP (Adriamycin, Oncovin, prednisone)

Adria+BCNU (Adriamycin, BCNU)

Adria-L-PAM (Adriamycin, melphalan)

AFM (Adriamycin, 5-fluorouracil, methotrexate)

AID (Adriamycin, ifosfamide, dacarbazine, mesna)

AIM (L-asparaginase, ifosfamide, methotrexate)

ALOMAD (Adriamycin, Leukeran, Oncovin, methotrexate, actinomycin D, dacarbazine)

Alpha-Beta (alpha tocopherol and beta carotene)

ALT-RCC (autolymphocyte-based treatment for renal cell carcinoma)

anti-MY9 BMT (bone marrow transplant) p.

anti-T12 allogeneic BMT (bone marrow transplant) p.

AOPA (ara-C, Oncovin, prednisone, asparaginase)

AOPE (Adriamycin, Oncovin, prednisone, etoposide)

APC (AMSA, prednisone, chlorambucil)

APE (Adriamycin, Platinol, etoposide)

APO (Adriamycin, prednisone, Oncovin)

ara-C+ADR (cytarabine, Adriamycin)

ara-C+DNR+PRED+HP (cytarabine, daunorubicin, prednisolone, mercaptopurine)

ara-C+6TG (cytarabine, thioguanine)

A-SHAP (Adriamycin, Solu-Medrol, high-dose ara-C, Platinol)

AV (Adriamycin, vincristine)

AVM (Adriamycin, vinblastine, methotrexate)

AVM (Adriamycin, vincristine, mitomycin-C)

AVP (actinomycin D, vincristine, Platinol)

AVP (Adriamycin, vincristine, procarbazine)

BACO (bleomycin, Adriamycin, CCNU, Oncovin)

BACOD (bleomycin, Adriamycin, cyclophosphamide, Oncovin, dexamethasone)

BACON (bleomycin, Adriamycin, CCNU, Oncovin, nitrogen mustard)

BACOP (bleomycin, Adriamycin,

ADDITIONAL TERMS

protocol—*Continued*
    cyclophosphamide, Oncovin,
    prednisone)
BACT (BCNU, ara-C,
    cyclophosphamide,
    6-thioguanine)
BACT (bleomycin, Adriamycin,
    cyclophosphamide, tamoxifen)
BAM/BLITZ (B4 blocked ricin)
BAMON (bleomycin, Adriamycin,
    methotrexate, Oncovin, nitrogen
    mustard)
BAP (bleomycin, Adriamycin,
    prednisone)
BAVIP (bleomycin, Adriamycin,
    vinblastine, imidazole
    carboxamide, prednisone)
BBVP-M (BCNU, bleomycin,
    VePesid, prednisone,
    methotrexate)
BCAVe (bleomycin, CCNU,
    Adriamycin, Velban)
BCD (bleomycin,
    cyclophosphamide, dactinomycin)
BCOP (BCNU, cyclophosphamide,
    Oncovin, prednisone)
BCP (BCNU, cyclophosphamide,
    prednisone)
BCVP (BCNU, cyclophosphamide,
    vincristine, prednisone)
BCVPP (BCNU, cyclophosphamide,
    vinblastine, procarbazine,
    prednisone)
B-DOPA (bleomycin, dacarbazine,
    Oncovin, prednisone, Adriamycin)
BEAC (BCNU, etoposide, ara-C,
    cyclophosphamide)
BEMP (bleomycin, Eldisine,
    mitomycin, Platinol)
BEP (bleomuycin, etoposide,
    Platinol)
BHD (BCNU, hydroxyurea,
    dacarbazine)
BHDV (BCNU, hydroxyurea,
    dacarbazine, vincristine)
BLEO-MOPP (bleomycin, nitrogen
    mustard, Oncovin, procarbazine,
    prednisone)
B-MOPP (bleomycin,
    mechlorethamine, Oncovin,
    procarbazine, prednisone)
BMP (BCNU, methotrexate,
    procarbazine)
BLITZ (monoclonal antibodies)

BOAP (bleomycin, Oncovin,
    Adriamycin, prednisone)
BOLD (bleomycin, Oncovin,
    lomustine, dacarbazine)
BONP (bleomycin, Oncovin,
    Natulan, prednisolone)
BOP (BCNU, Oncovin, prednisone)
BOP (bleomycin, Oncovin, Platinol)
BOPAM (bleomycin, Oncovin,
    prednisone, Adriamycin,
    mechlorethamine, methotrexate)
BOPP (BCNU, Oncovin,
    procarbazine, prednisone)
BT (BCNU, triazinate)
BVAP (BCNU, vincristine,
    Adriamycin, prednisone)
BVCPP (BCNU, vinblastine,
    cyclophosphamide, procarbazine,
    prednisone)
BVD (BCNU, vincristine,
    dacarbazine)
BVDS (bleomycin, Velban,
    doxorubicin, streptozocin)
BVPP (BCNU, vincristine,
    procarbazine, prednisone)
CABOP (cyclophosphamide,
    Adriamycin, bleomycin, Oncovin,
    prednisone)
CABS (CCNU, Adriamycin,
    bleomycin, streptozotocin)
CAC (cisplatin, ara-C, caffeine)
CAD (cyclophosphamide,
    Adriamycin, dacarbazine)
CAD (cytosine arabinoside,
    daunorubicin)
CADIC (cyclophosphamide,
    Adriamycin, DTIC)
CAE (cyclophosphamide,
    Adriamycin, etoposide)
CAF (cyclophosphamide,
    Adriamycin, 5-fluorouracil)
CAFFI (cyclophosphamide,
    Adriamycin, 5-fluorouracil by
    continuous infusion)
CAFP (cyclophosphamide,
    Adriamycin, 5-fluorouracil,
    prednisone)
CAFTH (cyclophosphamide,
    adriamycin, 5-fluorouracil,
    tamoxifen, Halotestin)
CAFVP (cyclophosphamide,
    Adriamycin, 5-fluorouracil,
    vincristine, prednisone)
CALF (cyclophosphamide,

ADDITIONAL TERMS

Adriamycin, leucovorin calcium,
5-fluorouracil)
CALF-E (cyclophosphamide,
Adriamycin, leucovorin calcium,
5-fluorouracil, ethinyl estradiol)
CAM (cyclophosphamide,
Adriamycin, methotrexate)
CAMB (cyclophosphamide,
Adriamycin, methotrexate,
bleomycin)
CAMELEON (cytosine arabinoside,
high-dose methotrexate,
leucovorin, Oncovin)
CAMEO (cyclophosphamide,
Adriamycin, methotrexate,
etoposide, Oncovin)
CAMF (cyclophosphamide,
Adriamycin, methotrexate,
5-fluorouracil)
CAMF (cyclophosphamide,
Adriamycin, methotrexate, folic
acid)
CAMLO (cytosine arabinoside,
methotrexate, leucovorin,
Oncovin)
CAMP (cyclophosphamide,
Adriamycin, methotrexate,
procarbazine)
CAO (cyclophosphamide,
Adriamycin, Oncovin)
CAP (cyclophosphamide,
Adriamycin, Platinol)
CAP (cyclophosphamide,
Adriamycin, prednisone)
CAP-I (cyclophosphamide,
Adriamycin, Platinol)
CAP-II (cyclophosphamide,
Adriamycin, high-dose Platinol)
CAP-BOP (cyclophosphamide,
Adriamycin, procarbazine,
bleomycin, Oncovin, prednisone)
CAPPr (cyclophosphamide,
Adriamycin, Platinol, prednisone)
CAT (cytosine arabinoside,
Adriamycin, 6-thioguanine)
CAT (cytosine arabinoside,
thioguanine)
CAV (cyclophosphamide,
Adriamycin, Velban)
CAV (cyclophosphamide,
Adriamycin, vincristine)
CAVe (CCNU, Adriamycin, Velban)
CAVP (cyclophosphamide,
Adriamycin, VM-26, prednisone)

CAVP-I (cyclophosphamide,
Adriamycin, vincristine,
prednisone)
CAVP-16 (cyclophosphamide,
Adriamycin, VP-16)
CAVPM (cyclophosphamide,
Adriamycin, VP-16, prednisone,
methotrexate)
CBPPA (cyclophosphamide,
bleomycin, procarbazine,
prednisone, Adriamycin)
CBV (cyclophosphamide, BCNU,
VP-16-213)
CBVD (CCNU, bleomycin,
vinblastine, dexamethasone)
CCAVV (CCNU, cyclophosphamide,
Adriamycin, vincristine, VP-16)
CCFE (cyclophosphamide,
cisplatin, 5-fluorouracil,
estramustine)
CCM (cyclophosphamide, CCNU,
methotrexate)
CCMA (CCNU, cyclophosphamide,
methotrexate, Adriamycin)
CCNU-OP (CCNU, Oncovin,
prednisone)
CCOB (CCNU, cyclophosphamide,
Oncovin, bleomycin)
CCV (CCNU, cyclophosphamide,
vincristine)
CCV-AV (CCNU,
cyclophosphamide, vincristine
plus Adriamycin, vincristine)
CCVB (CCNU, cyclophosphamide,
vincristine, bleomycin)
CCVPP (CCNU, cyclophosphamide,
Velban, procarbazine, prednisone)
CCVV (cyclophosphamide, CCNU,
VP-16, vincristine)
CCVVP (cyclophosphamide, CCNU,
VP-16, vincristine, Platinol)
CD (cytarabine, daunorubicin)
CDC (carboplatin, doxorubicin,
cyclophosphamide)
CDE (cyclophosphamide,
doxorubicin, etoposide)
CEB (carboplatin, etoposide,
bleomycin)
CECA (cisplatin, etoposide,
cyclophosphamide, Adriamycin)
CEF (cyclophosphamide,
epirubicin, 5-fluorouracil)
CEM (cytosine arabinoside,
etoposide, methotrexate)

ADDITIONAL TERMS

protocol—*Continued*

CEP (CCNU, etoposide, prednimustine)

CEP (cyclophosphamide, etoposide, Platinol)

CF (cisplatin, 5-fluorouracil)

CFL (cisplatin, 5-fluorouracil, leucovorin calcium)

CFM (cyclophosphamide, 5-fluorouracil, mitoxantrone)

CFP (cyclophosphamide, 5-fluorouracil, prednisone)

CFPT (cyclophosphamide, 5-fluorouracil, prednisone, tamoxifen)

CHAD (cyclophosphamide, hexamethylmelamine, Adriamycin, DDP)

CHAP (cyclophosphamide, Hexalen, Adriamycin, Platinol)

CHD (cyclophosphamide, hexamethylmelamine, DDP)

CHD-R (cyclophosphamide, hexamethylmelamine, DDP, radiotherapy)

CHEX-UP (cyclophosphamide, hexamethylmelamine, 5-fluorouracil, Platinol)

CHF (cyclophosphamide, hexamethylmelamine, 5-fluorouracil)

CHL+PRED (chlorambucil, prednisone)

Chl-VPP (chlorambucil, vinblastine, procarbazine, prednisone)

CHO (cyclophosphamide, hydroxydaunomycin, Oncovin)

CHOB (cyclophosphamide, hydroxydaunomycin, Oncovin, bleomycin)

CHOD (cyclophosphamide, hydroxydaunomycin, Oncovin, dexamethasone)

CHOP (cyclophosphamide, Halotestin, Oncovin, prednisone)

CHOP (cyclophosphamide, hydroxydaunomycin, Oncovin, prednisone)

CHOP-BLEO (cyclophosphamide, hydroxydaunomycin, Oncovin, prednisone, bleomycin)

CHOPE (cyclophosphamide, Halotestin, Oncovin, prednisone, etoposide)

CHOR (cyclophosphamide, hydroxydaunomycin, Oncovin, radiotherapy)

CHVP (cyclophosphamide, hydroxydaunomycin, VM-26, prednisone)

CIA (CCNU, isophosphamide, Adriamycin)

CISCAii/BViv (cisplatin, cyclophosphamide, Adriamycin, vinblastine, bleomycin)

CMC (cyclophosphamide, methotrexate, CCNU)

CMC-VAP (cyclophosphamide, methotrexate, CCNU, vincristine, Adriamycin, procarbazine)

CMF (cyclophosphamide, methotrexate, 5-fluorouracil)

CMF-AV (cyclophosphamide, methotrexate, 5-fluorouracil, Adriamycin, vincristine)

CMFAVP (cyclophosphamide, methotrexate, 5-fluorouracil, Adriamycin, vincristine, prednisone)

CMF-BLEO (cyclophosphamide, methotrexate, 5-fluorouracil, bleomycin)

CMF-FLU (cyclophosphamide, methotrexate, 5-fluorouracil, fluoxymesterone)

CMFH (cyclophosphamide, methotrexate, 5-fluorouracil, hydroxurea)

CMFP (cyclophosphamide, methotrexate, 5-fluorouracil, prednisone)

CMFpT (cyclophosphamide, methotrexate, 5-fluorouracil, low-dose prednisone, tamoxifen)

CMFPTH (cyclophosphamide, methotrexate, 5-fluorouracil, prednisone, tamoxifen, Halotestin)

CMFP-VA (cyclophosphamide, methotrexate, 5-fluorouracil, prednisone, vincristine, Adriamycin)

CMFT (cyclophosphamide, methotrexate, 5-fluorouracil, tamoxifen)

ADDITIONAL TERMS

CMF-TAM (cyclophosphamide, methotrexate, 5-fluorouracil, tamoxifen)

CM-5-FU (cyclophosphamide, methotrexate, 5-fluorouracil)

CMFV (cyclophosphamide, methotrexate, 5-fluorouracil, vincristine)

CMFVAT (cyclophosphamide, methotrexate, 5-fluorouracil, vincristine, Adriamycin, testosterone)

CMFVP, also called Cooper CMFVP, Cooper regimen, or SWOG CMFVP (cyclophosphamide, methotrexate, 5-fluorouracil, vincristine, prednisone)

CMH (cyclophosphamide, m-AMSA, hydroxyurea)

C-MOPP (cyclophosphamide, mechlorethamine, Oncovin, procarbazine, prednisone)

CMP (CCNU, methotrexate, procarbazine)

CMPF (cyclophosphamide, methotrexate, prednisone, 5-fluorouracil)

CMV (cisplatin, methotrexate, vinblastine)

CNF (cyclophosphamide, Novantrone, 5-fluorouracil)

CNOP (cyclophosphamide, Novantrone, Oncovin, prednisone)

COAP (cyclophosphamide, Oncovin, ara-C, prednisone)

COAP-BLEO (cyclophosphamide, Oncovin, ara-C, prednisone, bleomycin)

COB (cisplatin, Oncovin, bleomycin)

COBMAM (cyclophosphamide, Oncovin, bleomycin, methotrexate, Adriamycin, MeCCNU)

COF/COM (cyclophosphamide, Oncovin, 5-fluorouracil plus cyclophosphamide, Oncovin, methotrexate)

COM (cyclophosphamide, Oncovin, MeCCNU)

COM (cyclophosphamide, Oncovin, methotrexate)

COMA-A (cyclophosphamide, Oncovin, methotrexate, Adriamycin, ara-C)

COMB (cyclophosphamide, Oncovin, MeCCNU, bleomycin)

COMB (cyclophosphamide, Oncovin, methotrexate, bleomycin)

COMBAP (cyclophosphamide, Oncovin, methotrexate, bleomycin, Adriamycin, prednisone)

COMe (cyclophosphamide, Oncovin, methotrexate)

COMET-A (cyclophosphamide, Oncovin, methotrexate, leucovorin, etoposide, ara-C)

COMF (cyclophosphamide, Oncovin, methotrexate, 5-fluorouracil)

COMLA (cyclophosphamide, Oncovin, methotrexate, leucovorin, ara-C)

COMP (cyclophosphamide, Oncovin, methotrexate, prednisone)

Cooper CMFVP (cyclophosphamide, methotrexate, 5-fluorouracil, vincristine, prednisone)

COP (cyclophosphamide, Oncovin, prednisolone)

COP (cyclophosphamide, Oncovin, prednisone)

COPA (cyclophosphamide, Oncovin, prednisone, Adriamycin)

COPAC (CCNU, Oncovin, prednisone, Adriamycin, cyclophosphamide)

COP-B (cyclophosphamide, Oncovin, prednisone, bleomycin)

COP-BAM (cyclophosphamide, Oncovin, prednisone, bleomycin, Adriamycin, Matulane)

COP-BLEO (cyclophosphamide, Oncovin, prednisone, bleomycin)

COPE (cyclophosphamide, Oncovin, Platinol, etoposide)

COPP (CCNU, Oncovin, procarbazine, prednisone)

COPP (cyclophosphamide, Oncovin, procarbazine, prednisone)

ADDITIONAL TERMS

protocol—*Continued*

CP (Cytoxan, Platinol)

CPB (cyclophosphamide, Platinol, BCNU)

CPC (cyclophosphamide, Platinol, carboplatin)

CPOB (cyclophosphamide, prednisone, Oncovin, bleomycin)

CROP (cyclophosphamide, rubidazone, Oncovin, prednisone)

CROPAM (cyclophosphamide, rubidazone, Oncovin, prednisone, L-asparaginase, methotrexate)

CTCb (cyclophosphamide, thiotepa, carboplatin)

CTX-Plat (cyclophosphamide, Platinol)

CV (cisplatin, VP-16)

CVA (cyclophosphamide, vincristine, Adriamycin)

CVA-BMP (cyclophosphamide, vincristine, Adriamycin, BCNU, methotrexate, procarbazine)

CVAD (cyclophosphamide, vincristine, Adriamycin, dexamethasone)

CVB (CCNU, vinblastine, bleomycin)

CVD (cisplatin, vinblastine, dacarbazine)

CVEB (cisplatin, Velban, etoposide, bleomycin)

CVI (carboplatin, VePesid, ifosfamide, Mesnex uroprotection)

CVM (cyclophosphamide, vincristine, methotrexate)

CVP (cyclophosphamide, vincristine, prednisone)

CVP-BLEO (cyclophosphamide, vincristine, prednisone, bleomycin)

CVPP (CCNU, vinblastine, prednisone, procarbazine)

CVPP (cyclophosphamide, vinblastine, procarbazine, prednisone)

CVPP-CCNU (cyclophosphamide, vinblastine, procarbazine, prednisone, CCNU)

CyADIC (cyclophosphamide, Adriamycin, DTIC)

CyHOP (cyclophosphamide, Halotestin, Oncovin, prednisone)

CyVADACT (cyclophosphamide, vincristine, Adriamycin, dactinomycin)

CyVADIC (cyclophosphamide, vincristine, Adriamycin, DTIC)

CyVMAD (cyclophosphamide, vincristine, methotrexate, Adriamycin, DTIC)

Dana Farber series p.

DAP I (dianhydrogalactitol, Adriamycin, Platinol)

DAP II (dianhydrogalactitol, Adriamycin, high-dose Platinol)

DAP/TMP (dapsone, trimethoprim)

DAT (daunomycin, ara-C, 6-thioguanine)

DATVP (daunomycin, ara-C, thioguanine, vincristine, prednisone)

DAV (dibromodulcitol, Adriamycin, vincristine)

DAVH (dibromodulcitol, Adriamycin, vincristine, Halotestin)

DBV (dacarbazine, BCNU, vincristine)

DC (daunorubicin, cytarabine)

DCCMP (daunorubicin, cyclocytidine, 6-mercaptopurine, prednisone)

DCMP (daunorubicin, cytarabine, 6-mercaptopurine, prednisone)

DCT (daunorubicin, cytarabine, thioguanine)

DCV (dacarbazine, CCNU, vincristine)

DECAL (dexamethasone, etoposide, cisplatin, ara-C, L-asparaginase)

DFV (DDP, 5-fluorouracil, VePesid)

DHAP (dexamethasone, high-dose ara-C, Platinol)

DIMOPP (dose-intensified MOPP)

DOAP (daunorubicin, Oncovin, ara-C, prednisone)

DTIC-ACTD (DTIC, actinomycin D)

DVB (DDP, vindesine, bleomycin)

DVP (daunorubicin, vincristine, prednisone)

DVPL-ASP (daunorubicin, vincristine, prednisone, L-asparaginase)

ADDITIONAL TERMS

DZAPO (daunorubicin, azactidine, ara-C, prednisone, Oncovin)

EAP (etoposide, Adriamycin, Platinol)

EBAP (Eldisine, BCNU, Adriamycin, prednisone)

ECHO (etoposide, cyclophosphamide, hydroxydaunomycin, Oncovin)

EDAP (etoposide, dexamethasone, ara-C, Platinol)

Einhorn chemotherapy regimen

ELF (etoposide, leucovorin, 5-fluorouracil)

E-MVAC (escalated methotrexate, vinblastine, Adriamycin, cisplatin)

E-MVAC (escalated methotrexate, vinblastine, Adriamycin, cyclophosphamide)

EP (etoposide, Platinol)

EPOCH (etoposide, prednisone, Oncovin, cyclophosphamide, Halotestin)

ESHAP (etoposide, Solu-Medrol, ara-C, Platinol)

EVA (etoposide, vinblastine, Adriamycin)

expanded access p.

FAC (5-fluorouracil, Adriamycin, cyclophosphamide)

FAC-BCG (Ftorafur, Adriamycin, cyclophosphamide, bacille Calmette-Guérin)

FAC-LEV (5-fluorouracil, Adriamycin, cyclophosphamide, levamisole)

FAC-M (5-fluorouracil, Adriamycin, cyclophosphamide, methotrexate)

FACP (Ftorafur, Adriamycin, cyclophosphamide, Platinol)

FACS (5-fluorouracil, Adriamycin, cyclophosphamide, streptozocin)

FACVP (5-fluorouracil, Adriamycin, cyclophosphamide, VP-16)

FAM (5-fluorouracil, Adriamycin, mitomycin-C)

FAM-C (5-fluorouracil, Adriamycin, methyl-CCNU)

FAM-CF (5-fluorouracil, Adriamycin, mitomycin, citrovorum factor)

FAME (5-fluorouracil, Adriamycin, MeCCNU)

FAMMe (5-fluorouracil, Adriamycin, mitomycin-C, MeCCNU)

FAM-S (5-fluorouracil, Adriamycin, mitomycin-C, streptozocin)

FAMTX (5-fluorouracil, Adriamycin, high-dose methotrexate)

FAP (5-fluorouracil, Adriamycin, Platinol)

FCAP (5-fluorouracil, cyclophosphamide, Adriamycin, Platinol)

FCE (5-fluorouracil, cisplatin, etoposide)

F-CL (5-fluorouracil, leucovorin calcium)

FCP (5-fluorouracil, cyclophosphamide, prednisone)

FEC (5-fluorouracil, epirubicin, cyclophosphamide)

FED (5-fluorouracil, etoposide, DDP)

FIMe (5-fluorouracil, ICRF-159, MeCCNU)

FL (flutamide, leuprolide acetate)

FL (flutamide, Lupron Depot)

FLAC (5-fluorouracil, leucovorin calcium, Adriamycin, cyclophosphamide)

FLAP (5-fluorouracil, leucovorin calcium, Adriamycin, Platinol)

FLe (5-fluorouracil, levamisole)

Fluosol/BCNU (fluosol-DA20, BCNU)

FMS (5-fluorouracil, mitomycin-C, streptozocin)

FMV (5-fluorouracil, methyl CCNU, vincristine)

FNM (5-fluorouracil, Novantrone, methotrexate)

FOAM (5-fluorouracil, Oncovin, Adriamycin, mitomycin-C)

FOM (5-fluorouracil, Oncovin, mitomycin-C)

FOMi (5-fluorouracil, Oncovin, mitomycin-C)

FRACON (framycetin, colistin, nystatin)

FUM (5-FU, methotrexate)

ADDITIONAL TERMS

protocol—*Continued*
FURAM (Ftorafur, Adriamycin,
mitomycin-C)
FUVAC (5-FU, vinblastine,
Adriamycin, cyclophosphamide)
HAD (hexamethylmelamine,
Adriamycin, DDP)
HAM (hexamethylmelamine,
Adriamycin, melphalan)
HAM (hexamethylmelamine,
Adriamycin, methotrexate)
HAMP (hexamethylmelamine,
Adriamycin, methotrexate,
Platinol)
HCAO (hexamethylmelamine,
cyclophosphamide, Adriamycin,
Platinol)
H-CAP (hexamethylmelamine,
cyclophosphamide, Adriamycin,
Platinol)
HDPEB (high-dose PEB or
Platinol, etoposide, bleomycin)
HD-VAC (high-dose methotrexate
plus vinblastine, Adriamycin
cisplatin)
Hexa-CAF (Hexalen,
cyclophosphamide, Adrucil,
Folex)
HiC-COM (ara-C, citrovorum
factor, allopurinol, Elliot B
solution, cyclophosphamide,
Oncovin, methotrexate)
HIDAC (high-dose ara-C)
high-risk ATAC (L-asparaginase,
ara-C, VP-16, anti-J2 26
monoclonal antibody, anti-CALLA
hybridoma antibody)
HMTX (high-dose methotrexate)
HOAP-BLEO (hydroxydaunomycin,
Oncovin, ara-C, prednisone,
bleomycin)
HOP (hydroxydaunomycin,
Oncovin, prednisone)
ICE (ifosfamide, carboplatin,
etoposide)
IMF (Ifex, Mesnex, Folex,
5-fluorouracil)
IMVP-16 (ifosfamide,
methotrexate, VP-16)
KGC (Keflin, gentamicin,
carbenicillin)
LAM (L-asparaginase,
methotrexate)

LAPOCA (L-asparaginase,
prednisone, Oncovin, cytarabine,
Adriamycin)
LMF (Leukeran, methotrexate,
5-fluorouracil)
L-VAM (Lupron, Velban,
Adriamycin, Mutamycin)
LVVP (Leukeran, vinblastine,
vincristine, prednisone)
M2 (vincristine, carmustine,
cyclophosphamide, melphalan,
prednisone)
MABOP (Mustargen, Adriamycin,
bleomycin, Oncovin, prednisone)
MAC (methotrexate, actinomycin
D, cyclophosphamide)
MAC (methotrexate, Adriamycin,
cyclophosphamide)
MAC (mitomycin-C, Adriamycin,
cyclophosphamide)
MACC (methotrexate, Adriamycin,
cyclophosphamide, CCNU)
MACHO (methotrexate,
asparaginase, cyclophosphamide,
hydroxydaunomycin, Oncovin)
MACOP-B (methotrexate,
Adriamycin, cyclophosphamide,
Oncovin, prednisone,
bleomycin)
MAD (MeCCNU, Adriamycin)
MADDOC (mechlorethamine,
Adriamycin, dacarbazine, DDP,
Oncovin, cyclophosphamide)
MAID (mesna, Adriamycin,
interleukin-3, dacarbazine)
MAID (Mesnex, Adriamycin, Ifex,
dacarbazine)
MAP (melphalan, Adriamycin,
prednisone)
MAP (mitomycin-C, Adriamycin,
Platinol)
MAT (multiple agent therapy)
MAZE (m-AMSA, azacitidine,
etoposide)
m-BACOD (moderate dose
methotrexate, bleomycin,
Adriamycin, cyclophosphamide,
Oncovin, dexamethasone)
M-BACOD (high-dose
methotrexate, bleomycin,
Adriamycin, cyclophosphamide,
Oncovin, dexamethasone)
M-BACOS (methotrexate,

ADDITIONAL TERMS

bleomycin, Adriamycin,
cyclophosphamide, Oncovin,
Solu-Medrol)

M-BAM (cyiclophosphamide, total
body irradiation, monoclonal
antibodies)

MBC (methotrexate, bleomycin,
cisplatin)

MBD (methotrexate, bleomycin,
DDP)

MC (mitoxantrone, cytarabine)

MCBP (melphalan,
cyclophosphamide, BCNU,
prednisone)

MCP (melphalan,
cyclophosphamide, prednisone)

MCV (methotrexate, cisplatin,
vinblastine)

MDLO (metoclopramide,
dexamethasone, lorazepam,
ondansetron)

MECY (methotrexate,
cyclophosphamide)

MeFA (methyl-CCNU,
5-fluorouracil, Adriamycin)

Memorial Sloan-Kettering
protocol

MF (methotrexate, 5-fluorouracil)

MF (mitomycin, 5-fluorouracil)

MFP (melphalan, 5-fluorouracil,
Provera)

MINE (mesna, ifosfamide,
Novantrone, etoposide)

mini-COAP (cyclophosphamide,
Oncovin, ara-C, prednisone)

MM (mercaptopurine,
methotrexate)

MMOPP (methotrexate,
mechlorethamine, Oncovin,
procarbazine, prednisone)

MMPT (methylprednisolone pulse
therapy)

MOAD (methotrexate, Oncovin,
L-asparaginase, dexamethasone)

MOB (Mustargen, Oncovin,
bleomycin)

MOB-III (mitomycin-C, Oncovin,
bleomycin, cisplatin)

MOCA (methotrexate, Oncovin,
cyclophosphamide, Adriamycin)

MOF (MeCCNU, Oncovin,
5-fluorouracil)

MOF (methotrexate, Oncovin,

5-fluorouracil)

MOF-STREP (MeCCNU, Oncovin,
5-fluorouracil, streptozocin)

MOMP (mechlorethamine,
Oncovin, methotrexate,
prednisone)

MOP (mechlorethamine, Oncovin,
prednisone)

MOP (mechlorethamine, Oncovin,
procarbazine)

MOP (melphalan, Oncovin,
methylprednisolone)

MOP-BAP (mechlorethamine,
Oncovin, procarbazine,
bleomycin, Adriamycin,
prednisone)

MOPP (mechlorethamine, Oncovin,
procarbazine, prednisone)

MOPP (methotrexate, Oncovin,
procarbazine, prednisone)

MOPP-ABV (mechlorethamine,
Oncovin, procarbazine,
prednisone, Adriamycin,
bleomycin, vinblastine)

MOPP-ABV Hybrid
(mechlorethamine, Oncovin,
procarbazine, prednisone,
Adriamycin, bleomycin,
vinblastine, hydrocortisone)

MOPP-ABVD (mechlorethamine,
Oncovin, procarbazine,
prednisone, Adriamycin,
bleomycin, vinblastine,
dacarbazine)

MOPP-LO BLEO
(mechlorethamine, Oncovin,
procarbazine, prednisone,
bleomycin)

MOPr (mechlorethamine, Oncovin,
procarbazine)

MP (melphalan, prednisone)

M-PFL (methotrexate, Platinol,
5-fluorouracil, leucovorin
calcium)

MPL + PRED (melphalan,
prednisone)

MTX + MP (methotrexate,
mercaptopurine)

MTX + MP + CTX (methotrexate,
mercaptopurine, Cytoxan)

MV (mitroxantrone, VP-16)

MVAC (methotrexate, vinblastine,
Adriamycin, cisplatin)

ADDITIONAL TERMS

protocol—*Continued*

MVF (mitoxantrone, vincristine, 5-fluorouracil)

MVP (mitomycin-C, vinblastine, Platinol)

MVPP (mechlorethamine, vinblastine, procarbazine, prednisone)

MVT (mitoxantrone, VP-16, thiotepa).

MVVPP (mechlorethamine, vincristine, vinblastine, procarbazine, prednisone)

NAC (nitrogen mustard, Adriamycin, CCNU)

neon particle p.

OAP (Oncovin, ara-C, prednisone)

OAP-BLEO (Oncovin, ara-C, prednisone, bleomycin)

O-DAP (Oncovin, dianhydrogalactitol, Adriamycin, Platinol)

OMAD (Oncovin, methotrexate, Adriamycin, dactinomycin)

OPAL (Oncovin, prednisone, L-asparaginase)

OPP (Oncovin, procarbazine, prednisone)

OPPA (Oncovin, procarbazine, prednisone, Adriamycin)

PAB-Esc-C (Platinol, Adriamycin, bleomycin, escalating doses of cyclophosphamide)

PAC (Platinol, Adriamycin, cyclophosphamide)

PAC-4D 5-day infusion (Platinol, Adriamycin, cyclophosphamide)

PACE (Platinol, Adriamycin, cyclophosphamide, etoposide)

PATCO (prednisone, ara-C, thioguanine, cyclophosphamide, Oncovin)

PAVe (procarbazine, Alkeran, Velban)

PBV (Platinol, bleomycin, vinblastine)

PCE (Platinol, cyclophosphamide, Eldesine)

PCV (procarbazine, CCNU, vincristine)

PEB (Platinol, etoposide, bleomycin)

PEC (Platinol, etoposide, cyclophosphamide)

Pediatric BLITZ (B4 blocked ricin)

PEP (Procytox, epipodophyllotoxin-derivative, prednisolone)

PF+E (Platinol, 5-fluorouracil plus etoposide, methotrexate, leucovorin)

PFL (Platinol, 5-fluorouracil, leucovorin calcium)

PFM (Platinol, 5-fluorouracil, moderate-dose methotrexate)

PFT (phenylalanine mustard, 5-fluorouracil, tamoxifen)

PHRT (procarbazine, hydroxyurea, radiotherapy)

PIA (Platinol, ifosfamide, Adriamycin)

PMB (Platinol, methotrexate, bleomycin)

PMF (L-phenylalanine mustard, methotrexate, 5-fluorouracil)

PMFAC (prednisone, methotrexate, and FAC protocol [5-fluorouracil, Adriamycin, cyclophosphamide])

P-MVAC (Platinol, methotrexate, vinblastine, Adriamycin, carboplatin)

POC (procarbazine, Oncovin, CCNU)

POCA (prednisone, Oncovin, cytarabine, Adriamycin)

POCC (procarbazine, Oncovin, cyclophosphamide, CCNU)

POMP (prednisone, Oncovin, methotrexate, Purinethol)

PRH-E (Platinol, etanidazole)

PRIME (procarbazine, isophosphamide, methotrexate)

ProMACE (prednisone, methotrexate, Adriamycin, cyclophosphamide, etoposide)

ProMACE-CytaBOM (prednisone, Adriamycin, cyclophosphamide, etoposide, cytarabine, bleomycin, Oncovin, methotrexate)

ProMACE-MOPP (procarbazine, methotrexate, Adriamycin, cyclophosphamide, etoposide, Mustargen, Oncovin, procarbazine, prednisone)

protocol 019

ADDITIONAL TERMS

pulse VAC (vincristine, actinomycin D, cyclophosphamide)
PUVA (psoralens, ultraviolet A)
PVA (prednisone, vincristine, asparaginase)
PVB (Platinol, vinblastine, bleomycin)
PVDA (prednisone, vincristine, daunorubicin, asparaginase)
PVP (Platinol, VP-16)
RIDD (recombinant interleukin-2, dacarbazine, DDP)
ROAP (rubidazone, Oncovin, ara-C, prednisone)
St. Jude Research Children's Hospital p.
SAM (streptozocin, Adriamycin, methyl-CCNU)
SCAB (streptozocin, CCNU, Adriamycin, bleomycin)
SIMAL-pilot (ara-C, hydrocortisone, mesna, prednisone, VP-16, leucovorin)
SIMAL—2nd induction/ maintenance (prednisone, L-asparaginase, daunomycin, VM-26, methotrexate, ara-C, VP-16, leucovorin)
SIMAL—BMT [bone marrow transplant] (ara-C, methotrexate, prednisone)
SK (Sloan-Kettering) p.
Sloan-Kettering (SK) p.
SMF (streptozocin, mitomycin-C, 5-fluorouracil)
STAMP p.
St. Jude Research Children's Hospital p.
super-CM regimen (cyclophosphamide, methotrexate, 5-fluorouracil)
SWOG CMFVP (cyclophosphamide, methotrexate, 5-fluorouracil, vincristine, prednisone)
T-2 p. (dactinomycin, Adriamycin, vincristine, cyclophosphamide, radiation)
T-10 p. (methotrexate, calcium leucovorin rescue, Adriamycin, cisplatin, bleomycin, cyclophosphamide, dactinomycin)

TAD (6-thioguanine, ara-C, daunomycin)
TC (6-thioguanine, cytarabine)
T-CAP (Baker Antifol, cyclophosphamide, Adriamycin, Platinol)
T-CAP III (triazinate, cyclophosphamide, Adriamycin, Platinol)
TEC (Thiotepa, etoposide, carboplatin)
TEMP (tamoxifen, etoposide, mitoxantrone, Platinol)
T-MOP (6-thioguanine, methotrexate, Oncovin, prednisone)
TOAP (thioguanine, Oncovin, cytosine arabinoside, prednisone)
TPDCV (thioguanine, procarbazine, DBC, CCNU, vincristine)
TRAP (thioguanine, rubidomycin, ara-C, prednisone)
VA (vincristine, Adriamycin)
VAAP (vincristine, asparaginase, Adriamycin, prednisone)
VAB 1 (vinblastine, actinomycin D, bleomycin)
VAB 2 (vinblastine, actinomycin D, bleomycin, cisplatin)
VAB 3 (vinblastine, actinomycin D, bleomycin, cisplatin, chlorambucil, cyclophosphamide)
VAB 4 (vinblastine, actinomycin D, bleomycin, cisplatin, cyclophosphamide)
VAB 5 (vinblastine, actinomycin D, bleomycin, cisplatin, cyclophosphamide)
VAB 6 (cyclophosphamide, dactinomycin, vinblastine, bleomycin, cisplatin)
VABCD (vinblastine, Adriamycin, bleomycin, CCNU, DTIC)
VAC (vincristine, actinomycin D, cyclophosphamide)
VAC (vincristine, Adriamycin, cyclophosphamide)
VAC pulse (vincristine, actinomycin D, cyclophosphamide) administered periodically
VAC standard (vincristine,

ADDITIONAL TERMS

protocol—*Continued*
Adriamycin, cyclophosphamide)
administered daily
VACA (vincristine, actinomycin D,
cyclophosphamide, Adriamycin)
VACAD (vincristine, Adriamycin,
cyclophosphamide, actinomycin
D, dacarbazine)
VACP (VePesid, Adriamycin,
cyclophosphamide, Platinol)
VAD (vincristine, Adriamycin,
dexamethasone)
VAD/V (vincristine, Adriamycin,
dexamethasone, verapamil)
VAFAC (vincristine, amethopterin,
5-fluorouracil, Adriamycin,
cyclophosphamide)
VAI (vincristine, actinomycin D,
ifosfamide)
VAM (VP-26–213, Adriamycin,
methotrexate)
VAMP (vincristine, Adriamycin,
methotrexate, prednisone)
VAMP (vincristine, amethopterin,
6-mercaptopurine, prednisone)
VAP (vincristine, Adriamycin,
procarbazine)
VAP (vincristine, asparaginase,
prednisone)
VAP-II (vinblastine, actinomycin D,
Platinol)
VAT (vinblastine, Adriamycin,
thiotepa)
VAT (vincristine, ara-A,
6-thioguanine)
VATD (vincristine, ara-C,
6-thioguanine, daunorubicin)
VATH (vinblastine, Adriamycin,
thiotepa, Halotestin)
VAV (VP-26–213, Adriamycin,
vincristine)
VBA (vincristine, BCNU,
Adriamycin)
VBAP (vincristine, BCNU,
Adriamycin, prednisone)
VBC (VePesid, BCNU,
cyclophosphamide)
VBC (vinblastine, bleomycin,
cisplatin)
VBD (vinblastine, bleomycin, DDP)
VBM (vincristine, bleomycin,
methotrexate)
VBMCP (vincristine, BCNU,

melphalan, cyclophosphamide,
prednisone)
VBMF (vincristine, bleomycin,
methotrexate, 5-fluorouracil)
VBP (vinblastine, bleomycin,
Platinol)
VC (VP-16, carboplatin)
VCAP (vincristine,
cyclophosphamide, Adriamycin,
prednisone)
VCAP-I (VP-16, cyclophosphamide,
Adriamycin, Platinol)
VCAP-III (VP-16–213,
cyclophosphamide, Adriamycin,
Platinol)
VCF (vincristine,
cyclophosphamide, 5-fluorouracil)
VCMP (vincristine,
cyclophosphamide, melphalan,
prednisone)
VCP (vincristine,
cyclophosphamide, prednisone)
VCP-1 (VP-16, cyclophosphamide,
Platinol)
VDP (vinblastine, dacarbazine,
Platinol)
VDP (vincristine, daunorubicin,
prednisone)
VEMP (vincristine, Endoxan,
6-mercaptopurine, prednisone)
VIC (vinblastine, ifosfamide, CCNU)
VIC (VP-16, ifosfamide,
carboplatin)
VIE (vincristine, ifosfamide,
etoposide)
VIP (VePesid, ifosfamide, Platinol)
VIP-B (VP-l6, ifosfamide, Platinol,
bleomycin)
VLP (vincristine, L-asparaginase,
prednisone)
VMAD (vincristine, methotrexate,
Adriamycin, actinomycin D)
VMC (VP-16, methotrexate,
citrovorum factor)
VMCP (vincristine, melphalan,
cyclophosphamide, prednisone)
VMP (VePesid, mitoxantrone,
prednimustine)
VOCA (VP-16, Oncovin,
cyclophosphamide, Adriamycin)
VOCAP (VP-16–213, Oncovin,
cyclophosphamide, Adriamycin,
Platinol)

ADDITIONAL TERMS

VP + A (vincristine, prednisone, asparaginase)
VPB (vinblastine, Platinol, bleomycin)
VPBCPr (vincristine, prednisone, vinblastine, chlorambucil, procarbazine)
VPCA (vincristine, prednisone, cyclophosphamide, ara-C)
VPCMF (vincristine, prednisone, cyclophosphamide, methotrexate, 5-fluorouracil)
VP-16 + DDP (etoposide, cisplatin)
VP + L-Asparaginase (vincristine, prednisone, L-asparaginase)
VP-16-P (VP-16, Platinol)
VPP (VePesid, Platinol)
VPVCP (vincristine, prednisone, vinblastine, chlorambucil, procarbazine)
Wayne State p. (cisplatin, 5-fluorouracil)
Protocult
protoheme
protohemin
protoleukocyte
proton
    beam, p.
    beam accelerator, p.
    beam boost, p.
    NMR (nuclear magnetic resonance) spectroscopy, p.
    -synchroton, p.
Proton Therapy Cooperative Group (PTCOG)
proto-oncogene
protoplasm
protoplasmic
    astrocytes, p.
Protoplast
protoporphyria
    erythrohepatic p.
    erythropoietic p.
protoporphyrin
protoporphyrinogen
    oxidase, p.
protropin
protothecosis
protozoa
protozoal
protozoan
protozoiasis
protransglutamase

Provera
proviral
provirus
Prower factor
proxicromil
proximal tubule cells
proximate carcinogen
Proximate intraluminal stapler
pruritic
pruritus
Prussian blue stain
PSA (prostate-specific antigen)
psammocarcinoma
psammoma
    bodies, p.
psammomatous
psammosarcoma
PSCH (peripheral stem cell harvest)
Pseudallescheria
    boydii, P.
pseudoactinomyocosis
pseudoagglutination
pseudoalleles
pseudoanemia
pseudoarthritis
pseudocapsule
pseudocarcinoma
pseudocyst
pseudoencapsulated
pseudoencapsulation
pseudoendometritis
pseudoeosinophil
pseudogene
pseudoglioma
pseudoglobulin
pseudohemagglutination
pseudohemophilia
pseudohemoptysis
pseudohermaphroditism
pseudohydronephrosis
pseudohypericin
pseudohyperkalemia
pseudohyponatremia
pseudohypoparathyroidism
pseudoicterus
pseudojaundice
pseudo-Kaposi sarcoma
pseudoleukemia
    cutis, p.
    gastrointestinalis, p.
    lymphatica, p.
    myelogenous p.
pseudoleukocythemia

ADDITIONAL TERMS

pseudolipoma
pseudolymphoma
    Spiegler-Fendt, p. of
pseudomalignancy
pseudomamma
pseudomelanoma
pseudomelanosis
pseudomembranous
    colitis, p.
    enteritis, p.
    enterocolitis, p.
pseudomonal
Pseudomonas
    acidovorans, P.
    aeruginosa, P.
    alcaligenes, P.
    cepacia, P.
    fluorescens, P.
    maltophilia, P.
    pickettii, P.
    polycolor, P.
    putida, P.
    pyocyanea, P.
    stutzeri, P.
    thomasii, P.
pseudomonas exotoxin
pseudomosaicism
pseudomucin
pseudomucinous
    cyst, p.
    cystadenocarcinoma, p.
    cystadenoma, p.
    tumor, p.
pseudomyxoma
    peritonei, p.
pseudoneoplasm
pseudoneuroma
pseudo-obstruction
pseudo-ovum
pseudoparalysis
pseudopolycythemia
pseudopolyp
pseudopolyposis
pseudoreaction
pseudoremission
pseudosarcoma
pseudosarcomatosis
pseudosarcomatous
    fasciitis, p.
pseudothrombocytopenia
pseudotuberculoma
    silicoticum, p.
pseudotuberculosis

pseudotumor
    cerebri, p.
    orbital p.
psicofuranine
PSIFT (platelet suspension
    immunofluorescence test)
psittacosis
psoralen
psoriasis
psoriatic
PSP (phenolsulfonphthalein)
PSS (progressive systemic sclerosis)
psychic
    surgery, p.
psychogenic
    alopecia, p.
    overlay, p.
    purpura, p.
psychoimmunology
psychoneuroimmunology
psycho-oncology
psychopharmacological
psychosexual
psychosocial
psychosurgery
psychotherapy
Psychotonin M
psychotropic
pT (pathologic assessment of primary
    tumor)
PT (prothrombin time)
PTA (plasma thromboplastin
    antecedent)
ptaquiloside
PTC (plasma thromboplastin
    component)
PTCOG (Proton Therapy Cooperative
    Group)
pteridine ring
Pteridium
    aquilinum, P.
pteroic
pteroyldiglutamic acid (PDGA)
pteroylglutamate
pteroylglutamic acid
PTF (plasma thromboplastin factor)
PTH (parathyroid hormone)
PTH (posttransfusion hepatitis)
PTHB (percutaneous transhepatic
    biopsy)
pTNM (pathologic TNM classification)
PTP-gamma
PTT (partial thromboplastin time)

ADDITIONAL TERMS

PTU (prophythiouracil)
ptyalocele
   sublingual p.
Pu (plutonium)
public antigens
Pulmo-Aide nebulizer
pulmonary
   anthrax, p.
   carcinosis, p.
   circulation, p.
   dead space, p.
   embolus, p.
   fibrosis, p.
   function studies, p.
   function test, p. (PFT)
   histiocytosis, p.
   infiltrate, p.
   lymphoid hyperplasia, p. (PLH)
   metastasis, p.
   nodule, p.
   pneumonia, p.
   shunting, p.
   sulcus, p.
   toxicity, p.
   tumor, p.
pulsatile
pulse
   analyzer, p.
   ionization chamber, p.
   therapy, p.
   VAC, p. (vincristine, actinomycin D,
     cyclophosphamide)
pulsed
   field gradient electrophoresis, p.
     (PFGE)
   chemotherapy, p.
   liquid phase protein sequencer, p.
   prednisone therapy, p.
pultaceous carcinoma
punch biopsy
pure red cell
   anemia, p.
   aplasia, p.
purge
purging
   bone marrow, p. of
purified protein derivative (PPD)
purine
   analogue, p.
   antimetabolites, p.
   biosynthesis, p.
   -nucleoside phosphorylase, p.
     (PNP)

-5'-nucleotidase, p.
nucleotide, p.
Purinethol (mercaptopurine)
Purkinje cell
puromycin
purpura
   allergic p.
   anaphylactoid p.
   annular telangiectatic p.
   annularis telangiectodes, p.
   autoimmune thrombocytopenic p.
   brain p.
   fibrinolytic p.
   fibrinolytica, p.
   fulminans, p.
   hemorrhagic p.
   hemorrhagica, p.
   Henoch p.
   Henoch-Schönlein p.
   hyperglobulinemica, p.
   idiopathic thrombocytopenic p.
     (ITP)
   Landouzy p.
   Majocchi p.
   malignant p.
   nervosa, p.
   newborn, p. of
   nonthrombocytopenic p.
   posttransfusion p.
   psychogenic p.
   rheumatica, p.
   Schonlein p.
   Schönlein-Henoch p.
   senile p.
   senilis, p.
   simplex, p.
   steroid p.
   thrombocytopenic p.
   thrombopenic p.
   thrombotic thrombocytopenic p.
purpuric
Purtillo lymphoproliferative syndrome
purulence
purulent
pus
pustular
pustule
pustulosis
pusy exudate
putative
Putnam-Dana syndrome
putrefaction
putrefy

ADDITIONAL TERMS

putrescence
putrescent
putrid
PUVA (psoralens, ultraviolet A)
PV (polycythemia vera)
PV (polyoma virus)
PVA (prednisone, vincristine,
    asparaginase)
PVB (Platinol, vinblastine, bleomycin)
PVDA (prednisone, vincristine,
    daunorubicin, asparaginase)
PVP (Platinol, VP-16)
PWA (person with AIDS)
PWM (pokeweed mitogen)
PXT (piroxantrone)
pycnemia
pyelogram
    dragon p.
pyelography
    intravenous p. (IVP)
    retrograde p.
pyelonephritis
pyeloscopy
pyemia
pyemic
pyesis
pyknemia
pyknocyte
pyknocytoma
pyknocytosis
pyknosis
pyknotic
    bodies, p.
pylorectomy
pyloric
    stenosis, p.
pyloristenosis
pylorectomy
pylorogastrectomy
pyloromyotomy
pyloroplasty
pyloroscopy
pylorus
pyocele
pyocolpocele
pyocyst
pyoderma
    gangrenosum, p.
pyogenic
pyomyoma
Pyopen
pyosepticemia

pyostomatitis
pyothorax
pyovarium
PYP (pyrophosphate scan)
pyramid
pyramidal
pyrantel pamoate
pyrazinamide (PZA)
pyrazine diazohydroxide (PZDH)
pyrazofurin
pyrazole
pyrazoloacridine
pyrectic
pyrenemia
pyretherapy
pyretic therapy
pyretogen
pyretogenesia
pyretogenesis
pyretogenic
pyretotherapy
pyridoxilated
    stroma-free hemoglobin, p. (SFGb)
    stroma-free hemoglobinuria, p.
pyridoxine
    -responsive anemia, p.
pyriform
pyrimethamine-sulfadoxine (Fansidar)
pyrimidine
    analogue, p.
    antagonist, p.
    biosynthesis, p.
    dimers, p.
pyrogen
    bacterial p.
    endogenous p.
    exogenous p's
    leukocytic p.
pyrogenic
pyroglobulin
pyroglobulinemia
pyrolysis
pyronin Y dye
pyronine
pyrophosphate (PYP)
    scan, p.
Pyrost
pyrrole
    cells, p.
    ring, p.
pyrroline
pyruvate kinase (PK)

ADDITIONAL TERMS

pyruvic acid
PZA (pyrazinamide)
PZDH (pyrazine diazohydroxide)

Q Q (quinacrine) banding
Q compound
Q-prep
Qa antigen
QCT (quantitative computed tomography)
QF (quality factor)
QM (quinacrine mustard)
QT6 cell line
quadrant
quadrantectomy
axillary dissection and radiotherapy, q. with (QUART)
quadrate
qualitative
clot retraction, q.
quality
factor, q. (QF)
life, q. of
quanta (pl. of quantum)
quantification
quantify
quantimeter
quanti-Pirquet
reaction, q.
test, q.
Quantisorb 125-I 4N diagnostic kit
quantitation
quantitative
autoradiography, q.
computed tomography, q. (QCT)
hepatobiliary scintigraphy, q.
quantization
quantum (pl. quanta)
mechanics, q.
number, q.
theory, q.
quark
QUART (quadrantectomy, axillary dissection, radiotherapy)
quelamycin
quellung reaction
quenching
fluorescence q.
quercetin
-3-rutinoside, q.
Quetelet index
Queyrat erythroplasia

Quick test
quid
quiescence
quiescent
Quimby
dosimetry, Q.
interstitial single-plane implant, Q.
planar implant table, Q.
quinacrine
banding, q. (Q-banding)
hydrochloride, q.
mustard, q. (QM)
quinine
quinolinium
quinone
quinonimine
Quinton suction biopsy instrument
Quinton Mahurkar dual-lumen catheter

R R (prefix used to identify recurrent tumors when staged after a disease-free interval)
R0 (no residual tumor)
R1 (microscopic residual tumor)
R2 (macroscopic residual tumor)
RX (presence of residual tumor at primary site cannot be assessed)
R (roentgen)
R-51211
R-64,633
R-75251
R banding (reverse banding)
R binder
R factor
R-loop
R-meter (roentgen meter)
R syndrome
Ra (radium)
RA (ragocyte)
cell, R.
RA (rheumatoid arthritis)
factor, R.
latex fixation test, R.
RAB (remote afterloading brachytherapy)
rabbit
-antidog thymus serum, r. (RADTS)
-antimouse thymocyte, r. (RAMT)
antirat lymphocyte serum, r. (RARLS)
antithymocyte globulin, r. (RATG)

ADDITIONAL TERMS

rabbit — *Continued*
  complement, r.
  fibroma virus, r.
  myxoma virus, r.
  papilloma virus, r.
  RABP (retinoic acid-binding protein)
  racemized protein
  racemose adenoma
  rachiodynia
  rachioplegia
  Rachromate-51
  racket amputation
  Racobalamin
    -57 kit, R.
  rad (radiation absorbed dose)
    increment, r.
    split-field, r.
    unit, r.
  RAD (roentgen administered dose)
  radiability
  radiable
  radial immunodiffusion (RID)
    assay, r. (RIDA)
  radial spreading
  radiant
  radiation
    adaptive r.
    alpha r.
    annihilation r.
    background r.
    beta r.
    braking r.
    Cerenkov r.
    corpuscular r.
    cosmic r.
    cyclotron r.
    direct r.
    dose-equivalent r.
    effective direct r. (EDR)
    electromagnetic r.
    environmental r.
    fractionated r.
    gamma r.
    hemibody r.
    heterogeneous r.
    homogeneous r.
    Huldshinsky r.
    infrared r.
    interstitial r.
    intracavitary r.
    ionization r.
    ionizing r.

  irritative r.
  leakage r.
  low-energy r.
  magnetic r.
  Markov r.
  Maxwell theory of r.
  megavoltage r.
  mitogenetic r.
  mitogenic r.
  monochromatic r.
  monoenergetic r.
  nonionizing r.
  nuclear r.
  occupational r.
  oncology r.
  orthovoltage r.
  palliative r.
  photochemical r.
  primary r.
  pyramidal r.
  recoil r.
  remnant r.
  Rollier r.
  scatter r.
  solar r.
  specific r.
  spontaneous r.
  supervoltage therapy r.
  terrestrial r.
  thermal r.
  total body r.
  ultraviolet r.
  white r.
  whole-body r.
  whole-brain r.
radiation absorbed dose (rad)
radiation absorption
radiation alopecia
radiation atom
radiation biology
radiation burn
radiation changes
radiation chimera
radiation colitis
radiation counter
radiation cystitis
radiation damage
radiation dermatitis
radiation desquamation
radiation detector
radiation diarrhea
radiation dose

ADDITIONAL TERMS

radiation dosimetry
radiation edema
radiation effect
Radiation Effects Research Foundation
  (RERF)
radiation energy
radiation enteritis
radiation enteropathy
radiation equivalent
radiation exposure
radiation exposure limit
radiation fallout
radiation fibrosis
radiation gastritis
radiation gingivitis
radiation grid
radiation hazard
radiation hepatitis
radiation-induced
  bone marrow suppression, r.
  carcinogenesis, r.
  ulceration, r.
radiation injury
radiation killing
radiation leakage
radiation leukemia virus (RadLV)
radiation management
radiation mantle techique
radiation marker
radiation monitor
radiation myelitis
radiation myelopathy
radiation necrosis
radiation neuritis
radiation neurosis
radiation odynophagia
radiation oncology
radiation osteitis
radiation penetration
radiation physics
radiation pigmentation
radiation pneumonia
radiation pneumonitis
radiation portals
radiation proctitis
radiation protection
radiation protection factor (RPF)
radiation psychosis
radiation pyrometer
radiation reaction
radiation release
radiation response

radiation seeds
radiation-sensitive
radiation sickness
radiation stent
radiation stomatitis
radiation surgery
radiation syndrome
radiation therapy (RT)
radiation tolerance
radiation treatment
radiation window
radical
  cure, r.
  cystectomy, r.
  cystoprostatectomy, r.
  excision, r.
  groin dissection, r.
  hip dissection, r.
  hysterectomy, r.
  jaw dissection, r.
  lymph node dissection, r.
  lymphadenectomy, r.
  mastectomy, r.
  neck dissection, r. (RND)
  pelvic dissection, r.
  procedure, r.
  prostatectomy, r.
  radiation therapy, r.
  retroperitoneal node dissection, r.
  surgery, r.
radicular
  pain, r.
  syndrome, r.
radiculitis
radioactinium
radioaction
radioactive
  albumin, r.
  applicator, r.
  balloon irradiation, r.
  camera, r.
  cobalt, r.
  colloidal gold, r. (Au 198)
  decay, r.
  disintegration, r.
  dust, r.
  effluents, r.
  element, r.
  equilibrium, r.
  fallout, r.
  gallium, r.
  gas, r.

ADDITIONAL TERMS

radioactive—*Continued*
  gold, r.
  half-life, r.
  implant, r.
  iodinated human serum albumin, r.
    (RIHSA)
  iodinated serum albumin, r. (RISA)
  iodine, r. (RAI)
  iodine uptake, r. (RAIU)
  iron, r.
  isotope, r.
  label, r.
  marker, r.
  microspheres, r.
  nuclide, r.
  patient, r.
  phosphorus, r.
  renogram, r.
  rod, r.
  seeds, r.
  series, r.
  source, r.
  strontium, r.
  tag, r.
  tagging, r.
  technetium, r.
  thorium, r.
  tracer, r.
  uptake, r. (RU)
  waste, r. (radwaste)
radioactivity
  artificial r.
  induced r.
  natural r.
radioactor
radioaerosol
radioallergosorbent
    test, r. (RAST)
radioanaphylaxis
radiobioassay
radiobiologic
radiobiological
radiobiology
radiocalcium
radiocarbon
    dating, r.
radiocarcinogenesis
radiochemical
    analysis, r.
radiochemistry
radiochemotherapy
radiochemy
radiochroism

radiochromatography
radiochrometer
radiocinematograph
radiocobalt
  -labeled vitamin B_{12}, r.
    (cyanocobalamin)
radiocolloid
radiocontrast
  -induced acute renal failure, r.
    (RCI-ARF)
radiocurable
radiocure
radiocyanocobalamin solution
radiocystitis
radiode
radiodense
radiodensity
radiodermatitis
radiodiagnosis
radiodiaphane
radiodilution
radioecology
radioelectroencephalogram (REEG)
radioelectroencephalography (REEG)
radioelement
radioenzymatic
    assay, r. (REA)
radioenzyme
radioepidermitis
radioepithelitis
radiofluoride
radiofluorine
radiofluoroscope
radiofluoroscopy
radiofrequency
radiogallium
radiogen
radiogenesis
radiogenic
radiogold (^{198}Au)
    seed, r.
    solution, r.
radiographic
    density, r.
    lesion, r.
    mass, r.
radiography
radioimmune
    precipitation assay, r. (RIPA)
radioimmunity
radioimmunoassay (RIA)
radioimmunoconjugate (RIC)
radioimmunodetection (RAID)

ADDITIONAL TERMS

radioimmunodiffusion
radioimmunoelectrophoresis
radioimmunoglobulin
radioimmunoprecipitation (RIP)
    assay, r. (RIPA)
radioimmunosorbent
    test, r. (RIST)
radioimmunotherapy
radioinduction
radioiodinated
    human serum albumin, r. (RIHSA)
    serum albumin, r. (RISA)
radioiodine (I 131)
radioiron
radioisotope
    carrier-free r.
radioisotope applicator
radioisotope bone scan
radioisotope camera
radioisotope cisternography
radioisotope-gated study
radioisotope liver scan
radioisotope liver/spleen scan
radioisotope nuclear scan
radioisotope scanning
radioisotope scintigraphy
radioisotope thyroid scan
radioisotopic
    medicine, r. (RIM)
radiokymography
radiolabeled
    antibodies, r.
    antiglobulin assay test, r.
    fibrinogen, r.
    ligand, r.
    probe, r.
radiolabeling
radiolead
radiolesion
radioligand
radiologic
radiological
    warfare, r.
radiologist
radiology
radiolucency
radiolucent
    defect, r.
    density, r.
radioluminescence
radioluminescent
radiometallography
radiometer

pastille r.
photographic r.
radiometric
    culture system, r.
radiomicrometer
radiomimetic
radiomutation
radion
radionecrosis
radioneuritis
radionics
radionitrogen
radionuclear
radionuclide
    bone scan, r.
    brain scan, r.
    cisternography, r.
    dosimetry, r.
    imaging, r.
    liver scan, r.
    lymphangiogram, r.
    scan, r.
radio-osteonecrosis
radiopacity
radiopaque
    contrast, r.
    contrast medium, r.
    density, r.
    marker, r.
    speculum, r.
radioparency
radioparent
radiopathology
radiopharmaceutical
radiopharmacy
radiophobia
radiophosphate
radiophosphorus
radiophotography
radiophylaxis
radiophysics
radiopotassium
radiopotential
radiopotentiation
radiopotentiator
radiopraxis
radioprotective
radioprotector
radiopulmonography
radioreaction
radioactive
radioreceptor
    assay, r. (RRA)

ADDITIONAL TERMS

radioresistance
radioresistant
radioresponsive
radioresponsiveness
radioscopy
radiosensibility
radiosensitive
radiosensitiveness
radiosensitivity
radiosensitization
radiosensitizer
radiosensitizing
radiosialography
radiosodium
radiostereoscopy
radiosterilization
radiostrontium
radiosulfur
radiosurgery
radiotelemetry
radiotellurium
radiothanatology
radiotherapeutics
radiotherapist
radiotherapy
    adjunctive r.
    adjuvant r.
    computerized r.
    interstitial r.
    intracavitary r.
    particle beam r.
radiothermy
radiothorium
radiotomy
radiotoxemia
radiotracer
radiotransparency
radiotransparent
radiotropic
radiotropism
Radithor
radium (Ra)
    application, r.
    applicator, r.
    beam therapy, r.
    bougie, r.
    bromide, r.
    capsule, r.
    dial, r.
    dosimetry, r.
    emanation, r. (RE)
    equivalent, r.
    -equivalent cesium 137, r.

implant, r.
insertion, r.
isotope, r.
necrosis, r.
needle, r.
pack, r.
paint, r.
seeds, r.
tandem, r.
therapy, r. (RT)
radiumize
RadLV (radiation leukemia virus)
radon (Rn)
    219, r.
    gas, r.
    seed, r.
    seed implant, r.
    seed inserter, r.
    seed insertion, r.
RADTS (rabbit-antidog thymus serum)
radwaste (radioactive waste)
RAE endotracheal tube
Raeder syndrome
raf oncogene
ragocyte (RA)
    cell, r.
ragsorters' disease
RAI (radioactive iodine)
Rai staging system
Rainey
    corpuscle, R.
    tube, R.
    tubule, R.
Rainier hemoglobin
RAIU (radioactive iodine uptake)
Raji cell
    assay, R.
ramollissement
RAMT (rabbit-antimouse thymocyte)
Randerath assay
random
    biopsies, r.
    controlled trial, r.
    sampling, r.
    trials, r.
randomization
randomize
randomized trials
Ranke complex
ranula
ranular
Ranvier node
RAP1 protein

ADDITIONAL TERMS

rapamycin
rapid infusion pump
Rappaport classification
RARE (retinoic acid response element)
RARLS (rabbit-antirat lymphocyte
 serum)
ras (rat sarcoma)
    H1 oncogene, r.
    k1 oncogene, r.
    k2 oncogene, r.
    n oncogene, r.
    -related, r.
Rasheed sarcoma virus
RAST (radioallergosorbent test)
rat
    antibody, r.
    sarcoma, r. (ras)
    sarcoma oncogene, r.
    thymus antiserum, r.
    unit, r. (RU)
RATG (rabbit antithymocyte globulin)
Rathke
    cleft, R.
    cleft cyst, R.
    pouch, R.
    pouch tumor, R.
ratio
    sensitizer enhancement r. (SER)
rationale
Rauscher leukemia virus
RAV (Rous-associated virus)
ray
    actinic r.
    alpha r's
    anode r.
    Becquerel r's
    beta r's
    Blondlot r's
    border r's
    canal r.
    cathode r's
    central r.
    chemical r's
    convergent r.
    cosmic r's
    delta r's
    direct r.
    divergent r's
    dynamic r's
    erythema-producing r's
    Finsen r's
    fluorescent r's
    gamma r's

glass r's
Goldstein r's
grenz r's
hard r's
indirect r's
infrared r's
infraroentgen r's
intermediate r's
J r's
Lenard r's
Lyman r's
Millikan r's
n r's
necrobiotic r's
paracathode r's
pigment-producing r's
positive r's
primary r's
roentgen r's
s r's
Sagnac r's
scattered r's
Schumann r's
secondary r's
soft r's
ultra x-r's
ultraviolet r's
W r's
x-r's
Rayleigh scattering law
Raymond-Cestan syndrome
Razoxane
Rb (rubidium)
Rb-1 allele
Rb gene
RBC (red blood cell)
RBC (red blood cell count)
RBC/hpf (red blood cells per high
 power field)
RBCIT (red blood cell iron turnover)
RBCM (red blood cell mass)
RBE (relative biological effectiveness)
RBCIT (red blood cell iron turnover)
RCC (red cell count)
RCC (renal cell carcinoma)
RCF (red cell folate)
RCIA (red cell immune adherence)
RCI-ARF (radiocontrast-induced acute
 renal failure)
RCIT (red cell iron turnover)
RCM (red cell mass)
RCU (red cell utilization)
RCV (red cell volume)

ADDITIONAL TERMS

rd (rutherford)
RDDP (RNA-dependent DNA
  polymerase)
RDE (receptor-destroying enzyme)
RDW (red cell distribution width)
RE (radium emanation)
RE (reticuloendothelial)
REA (radioenzymatic assay)
reabsorption
reactant
reaction
reactive
    systemic amyloidosis, r.
reactivity
reactor
    nuclear r.
reactor pile
reading
    frame, r.
    frameshift mutation, r.
reagent
reagin
reaginic
reanastomosed
reanastomosis
REB (roentgen-equivalent biological)
Rebuck skin window technique
recall
    antigen, r.
    phenomenon, r.
Recamier theory
Receptin (CD4)
receptor
    adrenergic r's
    B-cell antigen r's
    cholinergic r's
    complement r's
    -destroying enzyme, r. (RDE)
    epithelial growth factor r. (EGRF)
    Fc r's
    histamine r's (H1 and H2)
    IgE r's
    low-density lipoprotein r's
    sheep red blood cell r.
    T-cell antigen r's
    transferrin r.
recessive
    gene, r.
    trait, r.
recipient
reciprocal gene
reciprocation
Recklinghausen

    disease, R.
    tumor, R.
Recklinghausen-Applebaum disease
Reclus disease
recognin
recognition
recoil atom
recombinant
    alpha interferon, r.
    DNA, r.
    DNA gene splicing, r.
    growth hormone, r. (hGHr)
    HIV-1 latex agglutination test, r.
    human beta interferon, r.
    human erythropoietin, r. (rHuEPO)
    human granulocyte colony-
      stimulating factor, r. (rGM-CSF)
    human interleukin-3, r.
    human macrophage, r.
    immunoblot assay, r.
    interferon alpha, r. (rIFN-A)
    interferon gamma, r. (rIFN-G)
    granulocyte-macrophage colony-
      stimulating factor, r. (rmGM-CSF)
    soluble CD4, r. (T4)
    tissue plasminogen activator, r.
      (rt-PA)
recombination
    bacterial r.
recombinational germline theory
recombinogenic
Recombivax
recruitment
    factor, r.
rectal
    alimentation, r.
    biopsy, r.
    bleeding, r.
    cancer, r.
    carcinoma, r.
    fisting, r.
    intercourse, r.
    lesion, r.
    mass, r.
    penetration, r.
    polyp, r.
    rimming, r.
    shelf, r.
    tear, r.
    trauma, r.
rectectomy
rectocolitis
rectoscope

ADDITIONAL TERMS

rectoscopy
rectosigmoid
rectosigmoidectomy
rectourethral
rectouterine
rectovaginal
    fistula, r.
rectovesical
rectovulvar
rectum
recurrence
recurrent
    disease, r.
    tumor, r.
red blood cell (RBC)
    count, r. (RBC)
    diameter width, r. (RDW)
    iron turnover, r. (RBCIT)
    mass, r. (RBCM)
    transfusion, r.
red cell
    aplasia, r.
    casts, r.
    count, r. (RCC)
    distribution width, r. (RCDW)
    folate, r. (RCF)
    fragility, r.
    ghost, r.
    immune adherence, r. (RCIA)
    indices, r.
    mass, r. (RCM)
    morphology, r.
    sequestration, r.
    tagging, r.
    utilization, r. (RCU)
    volume, r. (RCV)
red helium neon laser
red marrow
Redisol
redistribution
red-man syndrome
redox
    -acyclovir, r.
    cycling, r.
    -penicillin G, r.
reducible
reducing
    agent, r.
reductase
Redy 2000 hemodialysis system
Reed cells
Reed-Sternberg cells
REEG (radioelectroencephalogram)

REEG (radioelectroencephalography)
Rees and Ecker fluid
Reese-Ellsworth classification, group I
    through V
Reference Man
reflex sympathetic dystrophy
refractoriness
refractory
    anemia, r.
    ascites, r.
    cytopenia, r.
    disease, r.
    leukemia, r.
    sideroblastic anemia, r.
Regan
    isoenzyme, R.
    lysozyme, R.
Regaud tumor
regenerative blood shift
regimen
regional
    enteritis, r.
    involvement, r.
    lymph node dissection, r. (RLND)
    lymph node involvement, r.
    lymph nodes, r. (RLN)
    metastases, r.
    recurrence, r.
    spread, r.
regioselectivity
Regnoli operation
regramostim
regress
regressed
regression
    disease, r. of
    tumor, r. of
regressive
regulator
    gene, r.
regulatory
Reilly
    bodies, R.
    granulations, R.
reinfusate
reinfusion
Reinke crystals
Reinsch test
reintervene
reintervention
Reiter
    arthritis, R.
    protein complement fixation, R.

ADDITIONAL TERMS

Reiter—*Continued*
    syndrome, R.
Reitman-Frankel test
rejection
    acute cellular r.
    cellular r.
    chronic r.
    graft r.
    hyperacute r.
rel oncogene
relapse
relapsing
relative
    biological effectiveness, r. (RBE)
    leukocytosis, r.
    polycythemia, r.
    risk, r. (RR)
    survival rates, r.
relaxation therapy
REM (roentgen equivalent-man)
remission
    induction, r.
remittent
remnant
    radiation, r.
REMP (roentgen equivalent-man period)
remote afterloading brachytherapy
  (RAB)
renal
    adenocarcinoma, r.
    cell carcinoma, r. (RCC)
    failure, r.
    insuffiency, r.
    papillary necrosis, r.
    paraneoplastic syndrome, r.
    plasma flow, r. (RPF)
    transplantation, r.
Rendu-Osler-Weber syndrome
renin substrate
renogram
renopathy
renoprival
Renotec Tc 99m iron ascorbate
renotropic
reovirus
reoxygenation
REP (roentgen-equivalent–physical)
reparative
replicase
replicate
replication
    DNA r.

    semiconservative r.
replication fork
replication pathway
replicative
replicon
replisome
repolarization
repolarize
reporter gene
repressed
    gene, r.
repression
repressor
    gene, r.
reprogramming therapy
reptilase
RERF (Radiation Effects Research
  Foundation)
RES (reticuloendothelial system)
rescue
    leucovorin r.
rescue process
resect
resectable
resectability
resection
resectoscope
reserve cell carcinoma
reservoir
residual
    disease, r.
    tumor, r.
resorbed
resorption
respiratory
    alkalosis, r.
    failure, r.
    support, r.
    syncytial virus, r. (RSV)
Respirgard II nebulizer
response
    anamnestic r.
    autoimmune r.
    booster r.
    effector r.
    IgM r.
    immune r.
    primary immune r.
    reticulocyte r.
    secondary immune r.
resting cell
restitope

ADDITIONAL TERMS

restriction
    major histocompatibility complex
        (MHC) r.
    MHC (major histocompatibility
        complex) r.
restriction analysis
restriction endonuclease
restriction enzymes
restriction fragment length
    polymorphism (RFLP)
RET (roentgen-equivalent–therapy)
retardation
retch
retching
retethelioma
retic (reticulocyte)
    count, r.
reticular cell
reticulation
reticulin
reticulocyte
    count, r.
    production index, r. (RPI)
reticulocytogenic
reticulocytopenia
reticulocytosis
reticuloendothelial (RE)
    blockade, r.
    cell, r.
    system, r. (RES)
reticuloendothelioma
reticuloendotheliosis
    leukemic r.
reticuloendothelium
reticulohistiocytic
    granuloma, r.
reticulohistiocytoma
reticulohistiocytosis
    multicentric r.
reticuloid
    actinic r.
reticuloma
reticulopenia
reticulosarcoma
Reticulose
reticulosis
    familial hemophagocytic r.
    familial histiocytic r.
    histiocytic medullary r.
    lipomelanic r.
    malignant r.
    pagetoid r.

polymorphic r.
reticulothelial
reticulum cell
    sarcoma, r.
Retin-A (tretinoin)
retinal-anlage tumor
retinaldehyde
retinitis
    cytomegalovirus r.
    metastatic r.
retinoblastoma
    protein, r. (pRb)
retinoic acid
    -binding protein, r. (RABP)
    receptor, r.
    response element, r. (RARE)
retinoid
retinopathy
    diabetic r.
    leukemic r.
    proliferative r.
    radiation r.
retreatment staging of tumor, nodes,
    and metastasis (rTNM)
retrofection
Retrogen
retrograde
    cancer, r.
retromolar
    trigone, r.
retroperfusion
retroperitoneal
    lymph node, r.
    lymph node dissection, r. (RLND)
    lymphoma, r.
    neoplasm, r.
    space, r.
retropharyngeal
    lymph node, r.
    space, r.
retroposon
retropubic
    prevesical prostatectomy, r.
    prostatectomy, r.
retrorectal
    lymph node, r.
    tumor, r.
retrospective study
retrosternal
retrovesical
Retrovir
retroviral

ADDITIONAL TERMS

retrovirus
rev (regulator of expression virion
  proteins) gene
reverse
    banding, r.
    genetics, r.
    isolation, r.
    polarity, r.
    transcriptase, r.
    transcriptase-polymerase chain
      reaction (RT-PCR) technique, r.
reversible
    antigenic r.
Revici cancer control
rf (rutherfordium)
RF (rheumatoid factor)
RFLP (restriction fragment length
  polymorphism)
RG 12915
RG 83894
rGM-CSF (recombinant human
  granulocyte colony-stimulating factor)
rgpl 60
Rh (Rhesus)
    agglutination, R.
    antibody, R.
    antigen, R.
    antiserum, R.
    blood group, R.
    compatibility, R.
    factor, R.
    genes, R.
    immune globulin, R.
    incompatibility, R.
    isoantigen, R.
    isoimmunization, R.
    monkey kidney, R. (RhMK)
    -negative, R.
    -null syndrome, R.
    positive, R.
    sensitization, R.
rhabdocyte
rhabdoid
rhabdomyoblastoma
rhabdomyochondroma
rhabdomyolysis
rhabdomyoma
rhabdomyomyxoma
rhabdomyosarcoma
    alveolar r.
    embryonal r.
    pleiomorphic r.
rhabdosarcoma

rhabdovirus
rhagiocrine cell
rHb1.1 (recombinant hemoglobin)
Rheinberg microscope
RheothRx Copolymer
rhestocythemia
Rhesus (Rh)
    factor, R.
    macaque, R.
    monkey, R.
    monkey kidney, R. (RhMK)
rheumatic
rheumatoid
    arthritis, r. (RA)
    degeneration, r.
    factor, r. (RF)
    pneumoconiosis, r.
Rheumatrex (methotrexate)
rhGM-CSF (recombinant human
  granulocyte-macrophage colony-
  stimulating factor)
rhinopharyngocele
rhinophycomyocosis
rhinophyma
rhinovirus
RhMK (Rhesus monkey kidney)
rho particle
Rho(D) immune globulin
rhodamine 123
rhodopsin
RhoGAM immune globulin
rhomboid crystal
rhopheocytosis
rHuEPO (recombinant human
  erythropoietin)
Ri-80 antigen
RIA (radioimmunoassay)
RIA-DA (radioimmunoassay-double
  antibody) test
RIBA-HIV
ribavirin
Ribbert theory
ribbon
    iridium r.
    radioactive r.
ribbon stools
riboflavin
ribonuclear protein (RNP)
ribonuclease (RNase)
ribonucleic acid (RNA)
    heterogenous nuclear r. (hnRNA)
    messenger r. (mRNA)
    ribosomal r. (rRNA)

ADDITIONAL TERMS

transfer r. (tRNA)
ribonucleoprotein
ribonucleoside
    diphosphate reductase, r.
ribonucleotide
    reductase, r.
riboprine
ribose
    nucleic acid, r.
    -5-phosphate isomerase, r.
    -phosphate pyrophosphokinase, r.
ribosomal
ribosome
ribothymidine
ribozyme
RIC (radioimmunoconjugate)
Richter syndrome
ricin
    -A, r.
    anti-B4-blocked r.
    chain, r.
    conjugate, r.
Ricinus
    communis, R.
Rickham reservoir
RID (radial immunodiffusion)
RIDA (radial immunodiffusion assay)
Ridaura
RIDD (recombinant interleukin-2,
    dacarbazine, DDP)
Ridell operation
Ridley factor
Riechert-Mundinger (RM) stereotactic
    system
Riedel
    struma, R.
    thyroiditis, R.
Rieder
    cell, R.
    cell leukemia, R.
    lymphocyte, R.
Riehl melanosis
Riesman pneumonia
Rifabutin
rifabutine
Rifadin
Rifamate
rifampicin
rifampin
rifamycin
Rifater V
rIFN-A (recombinant interferon alpha)
rIFN-G (recombinant interferon gamma)

right shift
RIHSA (radioactive iodinated human
    serum albumin)
Riley-Day syndrome
Riley-Smith syndrome
RIM (radioisotopic medicine)
rim resection
Rimactane
Rimactane/INH
rimantadine
Rimifon
rimming
Rindfleisch cell
Ringer lactate
RIP (radioimmunoprecipitation)
RIPA (radioimmunoprecipitation assay)
RISA (radioactive iodinated serum
    albumin)
risk
    -benefit ratio, r.
    factor, r.
risky sex
RIST (radioimmunosorbent test)
ristianol phosphate
ristocetin cofactor test
RIT 4237
RLN (regional lymph nodes)
RLND (regional lymph node dissection)
RM (Riechert/Mundinger) stereotactic
    system
rmGM-CSF (recombinant murine
    granulocyte-macrophage colony-
    stimulating factor)
Rn (radon)
RNA (ribonucleic acid)
    -dependent DNA polymerase, R.
     (RDDP)
    -directed DNA polymerase, R.
    -directed RNA polymerase, R.
    nucleotidyltransferase, R.
    polymerase, R.
    retrovirus, R.
    splicing, R.
    transcription, R.
    virus, R.
RNase (ribonuclease)
RND (radical neck dissection)
RNP (ribonuclear protein)
RO-24-2027
RO-24-7429
ROAP (Rubidazone, Oncovin, ara-C,
    prednisone)
Robb-Smith reticulosis

ADDITIONAL TERMS

Robengatope
robenidine hydrochloride
Robson staging of renal cancer, grades
  I through IV
Rochon-Duvigneau syndrome
rocket immunoelectrophoresis
Rocky Flats nuclear site
rodent
    antibodies, r.
    -human chimeric antibodies, r.
    ulcer, r.
roentgen (R)
    administered dose, r. (RAD)
    -equivalent–man, r. (REM)
    -equivalent–biological, r.
      (REB)
    -equivalent–man period, r.
      (REMP)
    -equivalent–physical, r. (REP)
    -equivalent–therapy, r. (RET)
    keratosis, r.
    knife, r.
    meter, r. (R-meter)
    radiation, r.
    ray, r.
    unit, r. (RU)
roentgenogram
roentgenography
roentgenologist
roentgenology
roentgenolucent
roentgenometer
roentgenometry
roentgenopaque
roentgenoparent
roentgenoscope
roentgenoscopy
roentgenotherapy
roentgentherapy
Roferon-A (interferon alfa-2a)
Roger
    antigen, R.
    syndrome, R.
rogletimide
Rohl marginal corpuscles
Rokitansky tumor
rolled edge
Rollet stroma
Rollier radiation
rolling circle
    DNA replication, r.
    DNA synthesis, r.
roll-tube culture

Romanowsky
    dye, R.
    stain, R.
Romer test
Rommelaere sign
Romunda factor
ronidazole
roof of mouth
root
    lung, r. of
    tongue, r. of
ropy
    blood, r.
    tumor, r.
roquinimex
ros oncogene
rosacea
    granulomatous r.
    lupoid r.
    papular r.
rose bengal
    scintigraphy, r.
    sodium I 131, r.
Rose-Waaler test
Rosenmüller node
Rosenthal
    fibers, R.
    syndrome, R.
rosette
    E (erythrocyte) r.
    EAC (erythrocyte antibody
      complement) r.
    Homer-Wright r's
    sheep erythrocyte r.
rosette cell
rosetting
Rosewater syndrome
Rosomoff cordotomy
Rotalex test
rotamase
rotating anode
rotational
    arcs, r.
    electron beam dosimetry, r.
    fields, r.
    flap, r.
    x-ray beam dosimetry, r.
rotavirus
Rotazyme
Rothmund-Thomson syndrome
Ro-Thyroxine
Rotrim T
Rotter node

ADDITIONAL TERMS

roughage
rouleau (pl. rouleaux)
rouleaux (pl. of rouleau)
    formation, r.
round cell
    myxoid, r.
    sarcoma, r.
Rourke-Ernstein sedimentation rate
Rous
    -associated virus, R. (RAV)
    Prague strain of R. sarcoma virus
    sarcoma, R.
    sarcoma virus, R. (RSV)
    Schmidt-Ruppin strain R. sarcoma
      virus
    test, R.
Roux gastroenterostomy
Roux-en-Y
    anastomosis, R.
    limb, R.
    procedure, R.
Roux-Y chimney
rovamycin
Rovamycine
Rovighi sign
Rowasa
Roxanol
    CII, R.
    Rescudose, R.
roxarsone
Roxicet
Roxicodone
Roxilox
roxithyromycin
RPF (radiation protection factor)
RPF (renal plasma flow)
rpg 160
RPI (reticulocyte production index)
RPR (rapid plasma reagin)
RR (relative risk)
RRA (radioreceptor assay)
RS-47
rsCD4 (recombinant soluble CD4 or
  Receptin)
RSU 1069 compound
RSU 1164 compound
RSV (respiratory syncytial virus)
RSV (Roux sarcoma virus)
RT (radiation therapy)
rTNM (retreatment staging of tumor,
  nodes, and metastasis)
rt-PA (recombinant tissue plasminogen
  activator)

RT-PCR (reverse transcriptase-
  polymerase chain reaction)
Ru (ruthenium)
RU (radioactive uptake)
RU (rat unit)
RU (roentgen unit)
RU 486 (mifepristone)
RU-23908
Rubesol-1000
rubidazone
rubidium chloride Rb 86
rubidomycin
Rubin tube
Rubramin PC
Rubratope
    -57, R.
    -60, R.
Rubrex (doxorubicin)
rubriblast
rubricyte
ruby laser
rufocromomycin
Rumpel-Leede test
Runeberg
    anemia, R.
    disease, R.
    formula, R.
    type, R.
Russell
    bodies, R.
    viper, R.
    viper test, R.
    viper venom, R.
Rust
    phenomenon, R.
    syndrome, R.
ruthenium (Ru)
rutherford (rd)
Rutherford
    atom, R.
    theory, R.
Rutherford-Geiger counter
rutherfordium (Rf)
R-verapamil
RWJ 21757 (loxoribine)
RWJ 25213
RX (presence of residual tumor
  at primary site cannot be
  assessed)
R-Y (Roux-en-Y)
Rydberg number
Rye histopathologic
  classification

ADDITIONAL TERMS

S 10036 (fotemustine)
S cell
S factor
S-phase
-specific cytoxic chemotherapy, S.
tumor, S.
S100 protein
SA85–1 antigen
S1509a sarcoma
Sabin-Feldman dye test
Sabourad plate
saccate
Saccharomyces
cerevisiae, S.
sacciform
sacculated
sacculation
sacrococcygeal tumor
SAD (source-to-axis distance)
-opposed fields, S.
SADBE (squaric acid dibutyl ester)
S-adenosylmethionine
carcinoma, S.
deficiency, S.
Sadowsky hook wire
safe sex
sago spleen
Sahli
desmoid test, S.
method, S.
SAIDS (simian AIDS)
St. John's Wort
St. Jude Research Children's Hospital
protocol, S.
staging system, S.
salcatonin
salinazid
saline
agglutination test, s.
agglutinin, s.
-washing process, s.
saliva
blot test, s.
screening, s.
spot test, s.
Saliva substitute
salivant
salivary
-based assay, s.
corpuscle, s.
gland, s.
salivation

salivatory
salmon
calcitonin, s.
patch, s.
Salmonella
choleraesuis, s.
enteritidis, S.
paratyphi, S.
schottmülleri, S.
typhi, S.
typhimurium, S.
salmonella agglutinins
salmonella proctitis
salmonellal
salmonellosis
Salomon test
salpingectomy
salpinges (pl. of salpinx)
salpingo-oophorectomy
salpingo-ovariectomy
salpinx (pl. salpinges)
salt-losing syndrome
salvage
chemotherapy, s.
procedure, s.
therapy, s.
SAM (streptozocin, Adriamycin, methyl-CCNU)
samarium (Sm)
[153]samarium-EDTMP
sampling of node
Sampson cyst
Samuels casual therapy
sanamycin
sanctuary therapy
sand tumor
Sanders treatment
Sandhoff disease
Sandimmune
Sandoglobulin
Sandostatin (octreotide or SSTN)
sandwich
system, s.
technique, s.
Sanger sequencing
sanguicolous
sanguinaria
sanguine
sanguineous
sanguinopoietic
sanguinopurulent
sanguinoserous
San Joaquin Valley fever

ADDITIONAL TERMS

Santorini
   duct, S.
   fissure, S.
Santyl
saperconazole
sarcoadenoma
sarcoblast
sarcocarcinoma
sarcocele
sarcoenchondroma
sarcogenic
sarcohydrocele
sarcoid
   Boeck s.
   Darier-Roussy s.
   Schaumann s.
   Spiegler-Fendt s.
sarcoidosis
   Boeck s.
   cordis, s.
   Schaumann s.
sarcolemma
sarcolemmic
L-sarcolysin
sarcoma (pl. sarcomata)
   Abernethy s.
   acinous s.
   adipose s.
   alveolar soft part s.
   ameloblastic s.
   botryoid s.
   botryoides, s.
   chloromatous s.
   chondroblastic s.
   clear cell s.
   colli uteri hydropicum papillare, s.
   colloid s.
   deciduocellular s.
   embryonal s.
   endometrial stromal s.
   epithelial s.
   epithelioid s.
   Ewing s.
   fascial s.
   fascicular s.
   fibroblastic s.
   giant cell s.
   granulocytic s.
   Hodgkin s.
   idiopathic multiple pigmented
     hemorrhagic s.
   immunoblastic s. of B cells
   immunoblastic s. of T cells

   Jensen s.
   Kaposi s.
   Kirsten s.
   Kupffer cell s.
   leukocytic s.
   lymphatic s.
   melanotic s.
   mixed cell s.
   monomorphic s.
   monstrocellular s.
   M5076 ovarian reticulum cell s.
   multiple idiopathic hemorrhagic s.
   myelogenic s.
   myeloid s.
   neurogenic s.
   orbital granulocytic s.
   osteoblastic s.
   osteogenic s.
   osteoid s.
   osteolytic s.
   Parodi-Irgens s.
   parosteal s.
   pleiomorphic s.
   polymorphous s.
   postirradiation s.
   pseudo-Kaposi s.
   reticulocytic s.
   reticuloendothelial s.
   reticulum cell s.
   retothelial s.
   rhabdoid s.
   round cell s.
   Rous s.
   S1509a s.
   Schmidt-Ruppin strain Rous s.
   serocystic s.
   small cell s.
   spheroid cell s.
   spindle cell s.
   stromal s.
   synovial s.
   telangiectatic s.
   teratoid s.
   Walker s.
sarcoma virus (SV)
sarcomagenic
sarcomata (pl. of sarcoma)
sarcomatoid
sarcomatosis
   cutis, s.
   general s.
sarcomatous
   osteitis, s.

ADDITIONAL TERMS

sarcomphalocele
sarcoplasm
sarcoplasmic
sarcoplast
sarcopoietic
sarcosis
sarcosporidian cyst
sarcotic
sargramostim (GM-CSF or Leukine or leukopoietin or Prokine)
sarin
Sarkosyl extract
sarmoxicillin
satellite
    cell, s.
    lesion, s.
    tumor, s.
satelliting
saturation
    point, s.
saturnism
saucerization
saucerize
SBE (self breast examination)
SCA (sickle-cell anemia)
SCAB (streptozocin, CCNU, Adriamycin, bleomycin)
scalene
    fat pad, s.
    lymph node, s.
    node biopsy, s.
scaler
scalloping of vertebrae
scalp
    hypothermia, s.
    tourniquet, s.
Scanlon mastectomy
scanned
scanner
scanning
    radioisotope s.
    radionuclide s.
scanning electron microscopy, s. (SEM)
scanography
scansion
scapulectomy
scar
    carcinoma, s.
scarification
scarred-down
scarring
SCAT (sheep cell agglutination test)

Scatchard analysis
scatoma
scatter
    gate, s.
scatterdiagram
scattered radiation
scattergram
scattering
    Compton s.
    Rayleigh s.
    Thompson s.
scatterplot
scavenger cell
SCBC (small-cell bronchogenic carcinoma)
SCC (small-cell carcinoma)
SCC (squamous cell carcinoma)
SCCHN (squamous cell carcinoma of head and neck)
SCE (secretory carcinoma of endometrium)
SCH 39304
SCH 42427
Schaedler blood agar
Schalfijew test
Schatzki ring
Schaumann
    bodies, S.
    disease, S.
    sarcoid, S.
    sarcoidosis, S.
    syndrome, S.
Schauta operation
Schede operation
Scheie disease
Scherer secondary structure
Schick test
Schiff test
Schilder
    disease, S.
    encephalitis, S.
Schiller test
Schilling
    blood count, S.
    classification, S.
    leukemia, S.
    test, S.
Schimmelbusch disease
Schirmer test
schistocyte
schistocytosis
Schistosoma
    haematobium, S.

ADDITIONAL TERMS

japonicum, S.
mansoni, S.
schistosomal
schistosomiasis
schizocyte
Schizosaccharomyces
  pombe, S.
Schlesinger solution
Schmidt
  factor, S.
  syndrome, S.
Schmidt-Ruppin strain Rous sarcoma
  virus
Schmincke tumor
Schmitz bacillus
Schmorl
  bacillus, S.
  disease, S.
  node, S.
schneiderian
  carcinoma, s.
Scholz disease
Schönbein operation
Schonlein
  disease, S.
  purpura, S.
Schönlein-Henoch purpura
Schrodinger
  atom, S.
  theory, S.
Schuco nebulizer
Schuffner
  dots, S.
  stippling, S.
Schüller disease
Schultz
  syndrome, S.
  triad of S.
Schultze
  cell, S.
  granule masses, S.
Schumm test
Schwachman syndrome
Schwachman-Diamond syndrome
Schwann
  cell, S.
  cell tumor, S.
  membrane, S.
  substance, S.
schwannian
schwannoglioma
schwannoma
  granular cell s.

schwannosis
Schwartz leukemia virus
Schwartz-Bartter syndrome
Schwartzman reaction
SCID (severe combined
  immunodeficiency disease)
  -hu mouse, S.
scintigram
scintigraphic
scintigraphy
  thyroidal lymph node s.
scintillascope
scintillascopy
scintillation
  camera, s.
  counter, s.
  counting technique, s.
scintillometer
scintiphotograph
scintiphotography
scintiscan
scintiscanner
scirrhoid
scirrhoma
  caminianorum, s.
scirrhous
  adenocarcinoma, s.
  cancer, s.
  carcinoma, s.
  lesion, s.
  tumor, s.
scirrophthalmia
scirrhus
scissile
scission
Sclavo serum
Sclavotest-PPD
SCLC (small-cell lung cancer)
sclerema
scleroderma
scleroma
  respiratorium, s.
scleromyxedema
sclerosant
sclerosarcoma
sclerose
sclerosing
  agent, s.
sclerosis
sclerotherapy
SCOOP 1 and 2 (transtracheal oxygen
  catheters)
scorbutic anemia

ADDITIONAL TERMS

scout film
screening mammography
screen-wall counter
Scribner shunt
scrofula
scrofuloderma
scrotal
scrotectomy
scrotum
Scully classification
scythropasmus
SD (serodefined)
    antigens, S.
SD (serologically defined)
    antigens, S.
SD (streptodornase)
SDC-28
SDS-PAGE (sodium dodecyl sulfate-
    polyacrylamide gel electrophoresis)
SDZ MSL-109
Se (selenium)
SE (spin echo)
sea
    algae extract, s. (SEA)
    -blue histiocyte syndrome, s.
    fan, s.
    fronds, s.
SEA (sea algae extract)
SEA (sheep erythrocyte agglutination)
SEA (side-entry access) port
Seabright bantam syndrome
Seattle hemoglobin
sebaceous
    adenoma, s.
    carcinoma, s.
    cyst, s.
    gland, s.
Sebileau classification
seborrhea
seborrheic
    dermatitis, s.
    keratosis, s.
sec18 gene
secondary
    anemia, s.
    buffering, s.
    cancer, s.
    tumor, s.
second-look procedure
second-set
    phenomenon, s.
    rejection, s.
secretin

secretion
secretor
secretory
    carcinoma, s.
    carcinoma of endometrium, s.
        (SCE)
    endometrium, s.
    IgA, s.
section
    frozen s.
    paraffin s.
    permanent s.
sectioned
SED (skin erythema dose)
sed rate (sedimentation rate)
Sedamine
Sedillot operation
sedimentation
    coefficient, s.
    rate, s.
seed
    radiogold (^{198}Au) s.
    radon s.
seed implantation
seed vs. soil hypothesis
seeding of tumor
SEER (Surveillance, Epidemiology, and
    End Results) Program
segmental
    resection, s.
    washings, s.
segmentary syndrome
segmentation
segmentectomy
segmented
    cell, s.
    eosinophils, s.
    neutrophils, s.
segmenter
segs (segmented neutrophils)
selectin
selective
    decontamination, s.
    excitation, s.
    excitation irradiation, s.
    irradiation, s.
Selectomycin
Selectron afterloading system
selenium
selenoid cell
selenomethionine (Se 75)
self
    antigen, s.

ADDITIONAL TERMS

-aspirating cut-biopsy needle, s.
breast examination, s.
-differentiation, s.
-healing squamous epithelioma, s.
-infection, s.
-limiting, s.
-quenched counter, s.
-tolerance, s.
-wise, s.
SEM (scanning electron microscope)
semelincident
semen
seminal
cyst, s.
vesicle, s.
seminoma
ovarian s.
seminoma cell
semipermeable
Semliki Forest virus
Semon sign
semustine (MeCCNU or methyl-CCNU)
Sendoxan
Senear-Usher syndrome
senescence
senescent
Sengstaken-Blakemore tube
senograph
senography
sense strand
sensitization
sensitize
sensitizer
enhancement ratio, s. (SER)
sensitizing
antibody, s.
sensitometer
sensitometry
sensorimotor
sentinel
gland, s.
node, s.
separation gel
sepiapterin reductase
sepsis
Septacin
septic
anemia, s.
arthritis, s.
fever, s.
shock, s.
septicemia
septicemic

septicopyemia
septicopyemic
Septra
Sequamycin
sequela (pl. sequelae)
sequelae (pl. of sequela)
sequence
flanking s.
intervening s.
nearest neighbor s.
sequence mapping
Sequence Multiple Analyzer (SMA)
sequence-specific
sequence-specificity
sequence-tagged site (STS)
mapping, s.
sequencing
sequential
analysis, s.
blockade, s.
determinant, s.
sequestration
sequestrectomy
sequestrum
SER (sensitizer enhancement ratio)
sera (pl. of serum)
Serc
serendipitous
serendipity
series
aliphatic s.
basophilic s.
eosinophilic s.
erythrocytic s.
granulocytic s.
Hofmeister s.
homologous s.
leukocytic s.
lymphocytic s.
monocytic s.
myelocytic s.
myeloid s.
neutrophilic s.
plasmacytic s.
thrombocytic s.
serine
carboxypeptidase, s.
protease, s.
proteinase, s.
-threonine protein kinase, s.
seroconversion
seroconvert
seroconverted

ADDITIONAL TERMS

seroconverter
seroculture
serocyst
serocystadenoma
serocystic
serodefined (SD)
serodiagnosis
seroepidemiology
serofast
seroflocculation
seroglobulin
serogroup
serohepatitis
seroimmunity
serolipase
serologic
serologically defined (SD)
serology
serolysin
serolysis
seroma (pl. seromata)
Seroma-Cath
seromata (pl. of seroma)
Seromycin
seronegative
seronegativity
seropneumothorax
seropositive
seropositivity
seroprevalence
seroprevalent
seroprophylaxis
seroreaction
seroreactive
seroresistance
seroresistant
seroreversal
seroreversion
seroreverter
serosanguineous
serositis
serostatus
serosurvey
serotherapy
serotonin
    type-3 receptor antagonists, s.
serotype
serous
    cavity, s.
    cyst, s.
    cystadenocarcinoma, s.
    cystadenoma, s.
    effusion, s.

    exudate, s.
    tumor, s.
serovaccination
serovar
serozyme
serpin
Serratia
    liquifaciens, S.
    marcescens, S.
    marcescens extract, S.
    plymuthica, S.
    proteamaculans, S.
Sertoli cell
    tumor, S.
Sertoli-Leydig cell
    tumor, S.
serum (pl. sera)
    anticomplementary s.
    antilymphocyte s. (ALS)
    antiplatelet s.
    antireticular cytotoxic s.
    antithymocyte s.
    blood grouping s's
    cytotrophic s.
    despeciated s.
    endotheliolytic s.
    hyperimmune s.
    immune s.
    leukocytolytic s.
    Löffler s.
    lymphatolytic s.
    monovalent s.
    nephrotoxic s.
    polyvalent s.
    pooled s.
    pregnancy s.
    pregnant mare's s.
    Sclavo s.
    thyrotoxic s.
serum acid phosphatase
serum albumin
serum alkaline phosphatase
serum chemistry
serum electrolytes
serum electrophoresis
serum ferritin
serum folate
serum globulin
serum glutamic-oxaloacetic
    transaminase (SGOT)
serum glutamic-pyruvic transaminase
    (SGPT)
serum hepatitis (SH)

ADDITIONAL TERMS

serum hepatitis antigen
serum iron (SI)
serum M component
serum osmolality
serum P24 antigen concentration
serum precipitable iodine
serum protein
serum protein electrophoresis (SPEP)
serum protein-bound iodine (SPBI)
serum prothrombin conversion
  accelerator (SPCA)
serum testosterone
serum thrombotic accelerator
serumal
Servox Electrolarynx
sesquiterpene
  dilactone, s.
sessile
  polyp, s.
  lesion, s.
Sethotope
severe combined immunodeficiency
  (SCID)
  -hu mouse, s.
sex
  chromosome, s.
  -conditioned, s.
  cord-stromal germ cell tumor, s.
  -limited, s.
  -linked, s.
  -specific, s.
sexually transmitted disease (STD)
Sézary
  cell, S.
  erythroderma, S.
  syndrome, S.
SFHb (stroma-free hemoglobin)
SFV (simian foamy virus)
7S gamma autoantibody
SGOT (serum glutamic-oxaloacetic
  transaminase)
SGPT (serum glutamic-pyruvic
  transaminase)
SH (serum hepatitis)
  antigen, S.
shadow
  -casting, s.
  cell, s.
shaggy
  endometrium, s.
  tumor, s.
  ulcer, s.
shake culture

shared needle
shark-jaw biopsy needle
shave biopsy
shedded
shedding
Sheehan syndrome
sheep
  cell agglutination test, s. (SCAT)
  erythrocyte agglutination, s. (SEA)
  erythrocyte rosette, s.
  red blood cell, s. (SRBC)
sheet sign
shelled out
shield
  gonad s.
  lead s.
  phallic s.
shielding
shift to the left
shift to the right
shifting dullness on percussion
shig (Shigella)
Shigella
  alkalescens, S.
  ambigua, S.
  arabinotarda type A, S.
  arabinotarda type B, S.
  boydii, S.
  ceylonensis, S.
  dispar, S.
  dysenteriae, S.
  etousae, S.
  flexneri, S.
  madampensis, S.
  newcastle, S.
  paradysenteriae, S.
  parashigae, S.
  schmitzii, S.
  shigae, S.
  sonnei, S.
shigella dysentery
shigellosis
shiitake
  extract, s.
  mushrooms, s.
Shimada
  grading system, S.
  terminology, S.
Shine-Dalgarno sequence
shingles
Shinya maneuver
shock wave
Shohl solution

ADDITIONAL TERMS

shoot up
shooting gallery
shotty nodes
shoulder-hand syndrome
shrinkage
    tumor, s. of
shrinking field technique
shunt
shunted
shunting
Shwachman syndrome
Shwachman-Diamond syndrome
Swartzman reaction
SI (serum iron)
SI (stimulation index)
Sia test
SIADH (syndrome of inappropriate
  antidiuretic hormone)
sialaden
sialadenitis
sialadenoncus
sialic acid
sialidase
sialidosis
sialitis
sialoadenectomy
sialocele
sialogenous
sialoglycoprotein
sialogogue
sialogram
sialography
sialometaplasia
    necrotizing s.
sialoncus
sialophorin
sialoschesis
sialtransferase
sialyated
sibling
    donor, s.
    marrow grafting, s.
Sicard syndrome
Sicard-Collet syndrome
sicca syndrome
sickle cell
    anemia, s. (SCA)
    crisis, s.
    disease, s.
    gene, s.
    -hemoglobin C disease, s.
    -hemoglobin D disease, s.

    -persistent fetal hemoglobin
      syndrome, s.
    thalassemia, s.
    trait, s.
Sickledex
sicklemia
sicklemic
sickling
SID (source-to-image distance)
Sid blood group system
side
    -chain, s.
    -chain theory, s.
    effect, s.
    entry access, s. (SEA)
sideroachrestic
    anemia, s.
sideroblast
sideroblastic
    anemia, s.
siderocyte
sideroderma
siderofibrosis
siderogenous
sideropenia
sideropenic
    anemia, s.
    dysphagia, s.
siderophage
siderophil
siderophilin
siderophilous
siderophore
siderosis
siderotic
sievert (Sv)
sigma
    particle, s.
    receptor, s.
    S tumor marker, s.
Sigma method
sigmoid
    colectomy, s.
    colon, s.
    lymph node, s.
sigmoidectomy
sigmoidoproctectomy
sigmoidoproctostomy
sigmoidoscope
sigmoidoscoped
sigmoidoscopy
sigmoidosigmoidostomy

ADDITIONAL TERMS

sigmoidostomy
sigmoidovesical
Sigmund glands
signal
    node, s.
    sequence, s.
    transduction, s.
    tumors concept, s.
signet-ring
    carcinoma, s.
    cell, s.
    pattern, s.
SIL (squamous intraepithelial lesion)
Silastic
    implant, S.
    prosthesis, S.
silent gene
silica
    colloidal s.
silicatosis
silicoanthracosis
silicon
silicone
    gel, s.
    implant, s.
    prosthesis, s.
silicosiderosis
silicosis
silicotic
silicotuberculosis
Silverman needle
SIMAL—pilot (ara-C, hydrocortisone, mesna, prednisone, VP-16, leucovorin)
SIMAL—2nd induction/maintenance (prednisone, L-asparaginase, daunomycin, VM-26, methotrexate, ara-C, VP-16, leucovorin)
SIMAL-BMT (ara-C, methotrexate, prednisone)
simian
    acquired immunodeficiency syndrome, s. (SAIDS)
    adenovirus, s.
    AIDS, s. (SAIDS)
    foamy virus, s. (SFV)
    immunodeficiency virus, s. (SIV)
    sarcoma virus, s. (SSV)
    T-cell leukemia virus, s. (STLV)
    type D retrovirus, s.
    virus, s. (SV)
Simmonds syndrome
Simon septic factor

Simonton method
Simplastin
simple
    achlorhydric anemia, s.
    mastectomy, s.
Simplified ANTI-GENES
simtrazene
simulate
simulation
simulator
simvastatin
Singer-Blom
    electrolarynx prosthesis, S.
    method, S.
    valve, S.
single
    -agent chemotherapy, s.
    -arm phase, s.
    -arm study, s.
    blind, s.
    -hit theory, s.
    -stranded, s.
    -stranded DNA, s. (ssDNA)
    -stranded RNA, s. (ssRNA)
    unit diagnostic system, s. (SUDS)
sinography
sinus
sinusitis
sinusoid
SIOP (Société Internationale d'Oncologie Pédiatrique or International Society of Pediatric Oncology)
siphonoma
Sipple syndrome
SIRD (source-to-image-receptor distance)
SIRS (soluble immune response suppressor)
sis oncogene
sisomicin sulfate
Sisson voice prosthesis
sissorexia
sister chromatid exchange
Sister Mary Joseph
    node, S.
    nodule, S.
site
    active s.
    allosteric s.
    antigen-binding s.
    antigen-combining s.

ADDITIONAL TERMS

site—*Continued*
  binding s's
  combining s.
  immunologically privileged s's
  restriction s.
sitogluside
B-sitosterolemia
sitotherapy
SIV (simian immunodeficiency virus)
Sjögren syndrome (SS)
  antigen A, S. (SS-A)
  antigen B, S. (SS-B)
SK (streptokinase)
SK-39–39 (HIV-1 specific primer pair)
sk 1 oncogene
SK (Sloan-Kettering) protocol
SK 770 virus
skeletal
  metastases, s.
  neoplasm, s.
skeocytosis
skiagraphy
skiameter
skiascopy
skimming
  plasma s.
skin
  appendage cancer, s.
  breakdown, s.
  cancer, s.
  disuse syndrome, s.
  dose, s. (SD)
  erythema dose, s. (SED)
  flap, s.
  reaction, s.
  reactive factor, s. (SRF)
  retraction, s.
  test dose, s. (STD)
  -to-tumor distance, s. (STD)
  unit dose, s. (SUD)
skinning
  colpectomy, s.
  vaginectomy, s.
  vulvectomy, s.
  vulvovaginectomy, s.
skinny needle
skip
  lesion, s.
  metastases, s.
Skoda sign
SKSD (streptokinase-streptodornase)
SKY epidural pain control system
SL (streptolysin)

slaty anemia
SLE (systemic lupus erythematosus)
sleeve
  lobectomy, s.
  pneumonectomy, s.
slim disease
Sloan-Kettering (SK) protocol
slot-blot technique
slow
  hemoglobin, s.
  pile, s.
slough
sloughed
sloughing
sludged blood
sludging of blood
Sm (samarium)
SM (Smith) antigen
SMA (sequential multiple analyzer)
  profile, S.
SMAC (sequential multiple analyzer
  computerized)
  profile, S.
SMAF (specific macrophage arming
  factor)
small-cell
  bronchogenic carcinoma, s. (SCBC)
  carcinoma, s. (SCC)
  lung cancer, s. (SCLC)
  osteosarcoma, s.
  tumor, s.
smear
  Pap (Papanicolaou) s.
  Papanicolaou s.
  peripheral s.
smegma
SMF (streptozocin, mitomycin-C,
  5-fluorouracil)
Smith (SM)
  antigen, S.
  disease, S.
smog
smoke
  inhaled s.
  second-hand s.
smokeless tobacco (snuff)
smoker's
  cancer, s.
  cough, s.
  palate, s.
  patches, s.
  tongue, s.
smoking

ADDITIONAL TERMS

active s.
   passive s.
smoking cessation
smoking history
smoldering leukemia
smooth muscle tumor
smudge cells
SMX (sulfamethoxazole)
SMX/TMP (sulfamethoxazole/
  trimethoprim)
Sn (stannum)
snapback DNA
SNOMED (Systematized Nomenclature
  of Medicine)
snort (inhale drugs nasally)
snuff
   cancer, s.
   dipping, s.
   tumor, s.
soap-bubble hemangioma
SOD (source-to-object distance)
sodium (Na)
   butyrate, s.
   cacodylate, s.
   chromate, s.
   diethyldithiocarbamate, s. (DTC)
   dodecyl sulfate, s. (SDS)
   dodecyl sulfate gel electrophoresis,
    s.
   hydroxybutyrate, s.
   iodide I 125 solution, s.
   iodide I 131 solution, s. (Iodotope)
   levothyroxine, s.
   liothyronine, s.
   orthovanadate, s.
   pertechnetate, s.
   phosphate P 32 solution, s.
   phytate, s.
   -potassium adenosine triphosphate,
    s.
   radioiodide solution, s.
   radiophosphate solution, s.
   rose bengal I 131, s.
   -2-mercapto-ethanesulfonate, s.
    (Mesna)
   phosphate P 32, s.
   succinate, s.
   tetradecyl sulfate, s.
   thiosulfate, s.
   valproate, s.
sodomist
sodomize
sodomy

soft
   applicator, s.
   cancer, s.
   copper seeds, s.
   palate cancer, s.
   rays, s.
   sore, s.
   tissue density, s.
   tissue mass, s.
   tissue necrosis, s.
   tissue sarcoma, s.
solanoid cancer
solanoma
solar
   gamma ray counter, s.
   keratosis, s.
   physics, s.
   radiation, s.
   rays, s.
   x-ray counter, s.
Solatene
solemona
solid
   lesion, s.
   mass, s.
   organ, s.
   -phase immunoabsorbent assay, s.
    (SPIA)
   -phase immunoassay, s. (SPIA)
   -state physics, s.
   tumor, s.
solitary
   bone cyst, s.
   lesion, s.
   myeloma, s.
   nodule, s.
   pulmonary nodule, s. (SPN)
   tumor, s.
soluble
   CD4, s.
   immune response suppressor, s.
    (SIRS)
   T4, s.
Soluset
somatic
   agglutinin, s.
   antigen, s.
   cell hybridization, s.
somatogenesis
somatogenetic
somatomammotropin
somatomedin
somatostatin

ADDITIONAL TERMS

somatostatin—*Continued*
analogue, s.
somatostatinoma
somatotropic hormone (STH)
somatotropin
-releasing hormone, s. (SRH)
somatuline
somnolence syndrome
Somogyi phenomenon
sonogram
sonography
sonolucency
sonolucent
soot
cancer, s.
wart, s.
sorcin
sor gene
sorter
cell s.
fluorescence-activated cell s.
(FACS)
source
-to-axis distance, s. (SAD)
-to-image distance, s. (SID)
-to-image-receptor distance, s.
(SIRD)
-to-object distance, s. (SOD)
-to-skin distance, s. (SSD)
-to-surface distance, s. (SSD)
Southern
blot test, S.
blotting, S.
hybridization, S.
hybridization analysis, S.
transfer analysis, S.
Southwest Oncology Group (SWOG)
Souttar tube
space
lattice, s.
-occupying lesion, s.
spacer gel
Sparcifloxacin
sparfloxacin
sparfosate sodium
spark chamber
sparking
sparsomycin
spatial
analysis, s.
encoding, s.
SPBI (serum protein-bound iodine)

SPCA (serum prothrombin conversion
activator)
specialized blocking procedure
species-specific
specific
macrophage arming factor, s.
(SMAF)
-pathogen free, s. (SPF)
soluble substance, s. (SSS)
suppressor cells, s.
specificity
specificness
SPECT (single photon emission
computed tomography)
spectinomycin
spectra (pl. of spectrum)
spectral
analysis, s.
array, s.
spectrin
spectrofluorometer
spectrograph
spectrometer
beta-ray s.
Bragg s.
gamma-ray s.
mass s.
Mossbauer s.
scintillation s.
x-ray s.
spectrometry
spectrophotofluorometer
spectrophotometer
absorption s.
spectrophotometry
spectropyrheliometer
spectroradiometer
spectroradiometry
Spectroscaler
spectroscope
spectroscopic
analysis, s.
spectroscopy
spectrum (pl. spectra)
absorption s.
action s.
chemical s.
diffraction s.
electromagnetic s.
invisible s.
solar s.
thermal s.

ADDITIONAL TERMS

x-ray s.
spectrum analysis
spectrum emission
speech synthesizer
Spengler fragment
SPEP (serum protein electrophoresis)
sperm
    bank, s.
    banking, s.
spermatocele
spermatocelectomy
spermatocystectomy
spermatocytoma
spermatogenesis
spermectomy
spermine
    phosphate, s.
spermocytoma
SPF (specific-pathogen free)
SPF (sunscreen protective factor)
sphacelate
sphacelation
sphacelism
sphaceloderma
sphenoid
    ridge meningioma, s.
spherocyte
spherocytic
    anemia, s.
spherocytosis
    hereditary s.
spheroidal cell
    carcinoma, s.
spheroma
spheroplast
Spherulin
sphincter
    implantation, s.
    -saving procedure, s.
    -sparing procedure, s.
sphincterectomy
sphincterotomy
sphingogalactoside
sphingoglycolipid
sphingolipid
sphingolipidosis
sphingolipodystrophy
sphingomyelin
    phosphodiesterase, s.
sphingomyelinase
    deficiency, s.
sphingomyelinosis

sphingophospholipid
sphingosine
SPIA (solid-phase immunoabsorbent
  assay)
SPIA (solid-phase immunoassay)
spiculated
spiculed red cell
spider
    cell, s.
    telangiectasia, s.
Spiegler-Fendt
    pseudolymphoma, S.
    sarcoid, S.
Spielmeyer-Sjögren syndrome
spinal axis
    tumor, s.
spinal cord
    compression, s.
    neurofibroma, s.
    stenosis, s.
    tumor, s.
spinal fluid
spindle cell
    carcinoma, s.
    lipoma, s.
    thymoma, s.
spindling
spinthariscope
spintherometer
Spiractone
spiradenoma
    cylindromatous s.
    eccrine s.
spiramycin
spiritual
    pain, s.
    therapy, s.
Spiro-32 (spirogermanium
  hydrochloride)
spirochete
spirochetemia
spirochetosis
spirogermanium hydrochloride
  (Spiro-32)
spiroma
spirometer
spirometry
spiromustine
Spironazide
spironolactone
spiroplatin
Spiroptera carcinoma

ADDITIONAL TERMS

Spitz nevus
splanchnicectomy
spleen
  accessory s.
  bacon s.
  enlarged s.
  flecked s. of Feitis
  Gandy-Gamna s.
  hard-baked s.
  lardaceous s.
  porphyry s.
  sago s.
  speckled s.
  waxy s.
splenadenoma
splenauxe
splenculus
splenectasia
splenectasis
splenectomize
splenectomy
splenectopia
splenectopy
splenelcosis
splenemia
splenic
  anemia, s.
  flexure, s.
  irradiation, s.
  lymph nodes, s.
  sequestration, s.
splenicterus
splenoblast
splenocaval shunt
splenocele
splenocyte
splenogenic
splenogenous
splenogram
splenography
splenohemia
splenohepatomegaly
splenoid
splenolymph nodes
splenolymphatic
splenolysin
splenolysis
splenolytic
splenoma
splenomalacia
splenomedullary
splenomegalia
splenomegalic

splenomegaly
  congestive s.
  Egyptian s.
  Gaucher s.
  hematogenous s.
  hemolytic s.
  infective s.
  infectious s.
  myelophthisis s.
  siderotic s.
  spodogenous s.
  thrombophlebitic s.
  tropical s.
splenometry
splenomyelogenous
splenomyelomalacia
splenoncus
splenonephric
splenopancreatic
splenoparectasis
splenopathy
splenoportography
splenorenal
splenorrhagia
splenosis
splenotoxic
splenotoxin
splenulus
splenunculus
splice junction mutation
spliceosome
splicing
  gene s.
split-course
  irradiation, s.
  radiation, s.
  technique, s.
split products
SPN (solitary pulmonary nodule)
spodogram
spodography
spodophagous
Spodoptera
  frugiperda, S.
spongioblast
spongioblastoma
  multiforme, s.
  unipolare, s.
spongiocyte
spongiocytoma
spontaneous
  fracture, s.
  regression, s.

ADDITIONAL TERMS

remission, s.
spoon nail
Sporanox (itraconazole)
sporotrichin
sporotrichosis
SP-PG
Sprague-Dawley rats
spread
    disease, s. of
    metastatic s.
spreading
    radial s.
    superficial s.
sprue
    celiac s.
    nontropical s.
    tropical s.
spruelike syndrome
spur cell
    anemia, s.
spurious
    polycythemia, s.
sputa (pl. of sputum)
sputum (pl. sputa)
    blood-tinged s.
    bloody s.
    brown s.
    green s.
    hemorrhagic s.
    nummular s.
    prune juice s.
    rusty s.
    septicemia s.
    yellow s.
sputum collection
sputum cytology
sputum induction
sputum production
squama (pl. squamae)
squamae (pl. of squama)
squamate
squamatization
squame
squamocellular
squamocolumnar
squamosal
squamous
    carcinoma, s.
    cell carcinoma, s. (SCC)
    differentiation, s.
    epithelial cells, s.
    epithelium, s.
    intraepithelial lesion, s. (SIL)

metaplasia, s.
squaric acid dibutyl ester (SADBE)
Sr (strontium)
    applicator, S.
    isotope, S.
SR (stimulation rate)
SR-2508 (etanidazole)
SR-4233
SR-44163
SRBC (sheep red blood cell)
src oncogene
SRF (skin reactive factor)
SRF (somatotropin-releasing factor)
SRH (somatotropin-releasing hormone)
SRIF (somatotropin-releasing inhibiting
    factor)
SS (Sjögren syndrome)
    antigen, S.
SS-A (Sjögren syndrome antigen A)
SS-B (Sjögren syndrome antigen B)
SSD (source-to-skin distance)
    -opposed fields, S.
SSD (source-to-surface distance)
ssDNA (single-stranded DNA)
SSM (superficial spreading melanoma)
ssRNA (single-stranded RNA)
SSS (specific soluble substance)
SSTN (octreotide or Sandostatin)
SSV (simian sarcoma virus)
stab (stabnuclear neutrophil)
    cell, s.
stabnuclear neutrophil
Stadol NS
Staffieri voice prosthesis
stage
    grouping, s. (stage O, I, II, III, IV
        subdivided into stage IIA, IIB,
        etc.)
staged
staging
    autopsy s.
    retreatment s.
    TNM (tumor, necrosis, metastasis)
        s.
    surgical s.
    tumor s.
    tumor, necrosis, metastasis (TNM)
        s.
staging criteria
staging of disease
staging laparotomy
staging lymphadenectomy
staging system

ADDITIONAL TERMS

Stahr gland
stain
staining
Stamm gastrostomy
Stammler reaction
STAMP (Solid Tumor Autologous Bone
  Marrow Program)
    protocol, S.
    regimen, S.
Stanford
    protocol, S.
    regimen, S.
stanolone
stanozolol
Stanton disease
staph (Staphylococcus)
staphylocoagulase
staphylococcal
staphylococcemia
Staphylococcus
    albus, S.
    aureus, S.
    epidermidis, S.
    hemolyticus, S.
    hominis, S.
    pyogenes, S.
    saprophyticus, S.
    simulans, S.
staphylodermatitis
staphylolysin
staphyloma
staphyloncus
staphylotomy
staphylotoxin
starch microsphere
Starling hypothesis
starry-sky pattern
statics
stationary
    beam, s.
    disease, s.
    gantry, s.
statolon
staurosporine
stave cells
stavudine (d4T or
  didehydrodideoxythymidine)
STD (sexually transmitted disease)
STD (skin test dose)
STD (source-to-tumor distance)
steal syndrome
steatadenoma
steatocele

steatocystoma
    multiplex, s.
steatoma
steatomatosis
steatonecrosis
steerable biopsy brush
Stein-Leventhal syndrome
Steiner tumor
Steinthal
    classification, S.
    grouping, S.
stellarator
stellate
    ganglion, s.
    incision, s.
Stellwag sign
stem cell
    assay, s.
    leukemia, s.
    lymphoma, s.
    marrow harvesting, s.
    rescue, s.
Stemphyllium
Stensen duct
stent
STEPA (thiotepa)
stercoroma
Stercyt
stereochemical
stereochemistry
stereofluorography
stereofluoroscopy
stereomicroradiography
stereophotomicrography
stereophysics
stereoradiography
stereoroentgenography
stereoroentgenometry
stereoscopic x-ray
stereospecificity
stereotactic
    automated large-core biopsy, s.
    brachytherapy, s.
    craniotomy, s.
    radiotherapy, s.
stereotaxic
stereotaxis
stereotaxy
sternal marrow aspiration
Sternberg
    disease, S.
    giant cells, S.
Sternberg-Reed cells

ADDITIONAL TERMS

Sterneedle test
sternodynia
sternum
steroid
-dependence, s.
-dependent, s.
psychosis, s.
steroidogenesis
Stevens-Johnson syndrome
Stewart-Treves syndrome
STH (somatotropic hormone)
stibamine glucoside
stibocaptate
stibophen
stiff-man syndrome
stigma (pl. stigmata)
stigmata (pl. of stigma)
stilbamidine
stilbestrol
Still disease
Stilphostrol (diethylstilbestrol)
Stimate
stimulation
index, s. (SI)
rate, s. (SR)
stimulator
human thyroid adenylate cyclase
s's (HTACS)
long-acting thyroid s's (LATS)
stipple cells
stippled
stippling
St. John's Wort
St. Jude Research Children's Hospital
protocol, S.
staging system, S.
STLV (simian T-cell leukemia virus)
sTNM (surgical staging of tumor, nodes, metastasis)
stochastic
Stockholm
box method, S.
radium application, S.
Stoltzfus blood group system
stoma (pl. stomata)
button, s.
site, s.
Stomahesive
stomal
adhesive, s.
bag, s.
stomata (pl. of stoma)
stomatitides (pl. of stomatitis)

stomatitis (pl. stomatitides)
aphthous s.
herpetic s.
mycotic s.
necrotizing ulcerative s.
parasitica, s.
ulcerative s.
vesicular s.
Vincent s.
stomatocace
stomatocyte
stomatocytosis
stomatodynia
stomatoglossitis
stomatomycosis
stomatonecrosis
stomatonoma
stomatopathy
Stomeasure
Stones factor
stool
bloody s.
melenic s.
mucous s.
pipe-stem s.
ribbon s.
silver s.
tarry s.
stool guaiac
STOP protein
stop
codon, s.
gene, S.
protein, S.
storage pool disease
storiform
histiocytoma, s.
Storm Von Leeuwen chamber
Stormby brush
Storz surgical instruments
stoss
stosstherapy
Stout fibromatosis
Stoxil
straight (heterosexual)
strange particle
stratification
stratified
Strauchen classification system
strawberry
hemangioma, s.
mark, s.
Streptase

ADDITIONAL TERMS

streptavidin
-coupled enzyme, s.
strepticemia
streptococcal
streptococci (pl. of streptococcus)
  anhemolytic s.
  group A through T s.
  hemolytic s.
  indifferent s.
  nonhemolytic s.
Streptococcus
  anginosus, S.
  erysipelatis, S.
  faecalis, S.
  hemolyticus, S.
  pneumoniae, S.
  pyogenes, S.
  salivarius, S.
  viridans, S.
streptococcus (pl. streptococci)
  MG, s.
streptodornase (SD)
  streptokinase-s. (SKSD)
streptoduocin
streptohydrazid
streptokinase (SK)
  -streptodornase, s. (SKSD)
streptoleukocidin
streptolysin (SL)
  O, s.
  S, s.
Streptomyces
  agrillaceus, S.
  ambofaciens, S.
  caespitosis, S.
  flocculus, S.
  hygroscopicus, S.
  leuteogriseus, S.
  malayensis, S.
  peucetius, S.
  plicatus, S.
  somaliensis, S.
  staurosporine, S.
  tanashiensis, S.
  tsukubaensis, S.
  variabilis, S.
  viridochromogenes, S.
streptomycin
streptomycosis
streptomycylidene isonicotinyl
  hydrazine sulfate
streptonicozid
streptonigrin

streptosepticemia
streptothricosis
streptovaricin
streptozocin (Zanosar)
streptozotocin
Streptozyme
stress
  alopecia, s.
  factor, s.
  fracture, s.
  -induced immune suppression, s.
  polycythemia, s.
stria (pl. striae)
striae (pl. of stria)
striated
striation
striatonigral
stricture
structuring
string carcinoma
stripped atom
stroma (pl. stromata)
  -free hemoglobin, s. (SFHb)
stromal
  adenomyosis, s.
  cells, s.
  desmoplasia, s.
  tumor, s.
stromata (pl. of stroma)
stromatin
stromatogenous
stromatolysis
stromatosis
Strongyloides
  intestinalis, S.
  stercoralis, S.
strongyloidiasis
strongyloidosis
strongylosis
Stronscan-85
strontium (Sr)
  85, s.
  87m generator, s.
  90 beta applicator, s.
  -yttrium applicator, s. (^{90}Sr/^{90}Y
  applicator)
strontiuresis
strontiuretic
Strotope
ST1-RTA immunotoxin
structural
  anomaly, s.
  gene, s.

ADDITIONAL TERMS

lesion, s.
struma
    aberranta, s.
    calculosa, s.
    cast iron s.
    colloides, s.
    fibrosa, s.
    follicularis, s.
    gelatinosa, s.
    Hashimoto s.
    ligneous s.
    lipomatodes aberrata renis, s.
    lymphatica, s.
    lymphomatosa, s.
    maligna, s.
    nodosa, s.
    ovarii, s.
    parenchymatosa, s.
    Riedel s.
    thymus s.
strumal
strumectomy
    median s.
strumiprivous
strumitis
STS (sequence-tagged site)
    mapping, S.
Stuart factor
Stuart-Prower factor
stucco keratosis
studded
studding
    tumor s.
Student t test
stump
    carcinoma, s.
    pain, s.
Sturge-Weber syndrome
Stypven time test
subalimentation
subatomic
subcarinal
subclass
subclinical
subclone
subcutaneous
    mastectomy, s.
    metastasis, s.
    tumor, s.
subdiaphragmatic
    fields, s.
    involvement, s.
    irradiation therapy, s.

subdigastric
    lymph nodes, s.
subdural
subependymoma
subfamily
subglottic
subgroup
subhepatic
sublesional
sublethal
    dose, s.
    gene, s.
subleukemic
    leukemia, s.
subline
sublingual
sublocus
sublymphemia
submammary
submandibular
submaxillary
submucosal
subperiosteal
    amputation, s.
subpopulation
Sub-Q-Set
subsegmental
subserosal
subset
subshell
substance P
substernal
    goiter, s.
    thyroid, s.
substrate
    analogue, s.
substratum
subtotal
    colectomy, s.
    cystectomy, s.
    gastrectomy, s.
    hysterectomy, s.
    orbital exenteration, s.
    pancreatectomy, s.
    resection, s.
    thyroidectomy, s.
subtraction cloning
subtractive hybridization
subtype
subungual
subunit
suburethral
subxiphoid

ADDITIONAL TERMS

succinyl-CoA
   synthetase, s.
succinylated
sucralfate
sucrose lysis test
SUD (skin unit dose)
Sudan black B fat stain
Sudeck critical point
SUDS (single unit diagnostic system)
suicidal risk
sulci (pl. of sulcus)
sulcus (pl. sulci)
   tumor, s.
sulfabenz
sulfadiazine
sulfadozine
   -pyrimethamine (Fansidar)
sulfaguanidine
sulfamethoxazole (SMX)
   -trimethoprim, s. (SMX/TMP)
sulfation factor
sulfhemoglobin
sulfhemoglobinemia
sulfinpyrazone
sulfmethemoglobin
sulfamethoxypyridazine
sulfapyridine
sulfinpyrazone
sulfobromophthalein
sulfolipid
Sulfolobus
   solfataricus, S.
sulforaphone
sulfoxone sodium
sulfur
   35, s.
   colloid, s.
   mustard, s.
sulindac
sulisobenzone
sulmarin
sulnidazole
sulofenur
Sulzberger-Garbe syndrome
Sumamed
Sumatriptan
sunburn
sunburst hemangioma
sunscreen
   protective factor, s. (SPF)
   protective factor index, s.
suntan
superantigen

super-CM regimen (cyclophosphamide,
   methotrexate, 5-fluorouracil)
supercoiled plasmid
superficial spreading melanoma (SSM)
superhelical
superhelix
superinfection
superior
   sulcus tumor syndrome, s.
   vena cava syndrome, s.
supernatant
supernate
superradical mastectomy
Superscript enzyme
supersoft
supervascularity
supervascularization
supervoltage
supplementary gene
supportive treatment
suppressant
suppression
   bone marrow s.
suppressive
   therapy, s.
suppressor
   cells, s.
   cytotoxic T-cells, s.
   gene, s.
suppurate
suppuration
suppurative
supraclavicular
supraglottic
   carcinoma, s.
   laryngectomy, s.
suprahyoid
   neck dissection, s.
supralethal
supramohyoid
   neck dissection, s.
suprapubic
   prostatectomy, s.
suprarenal
suprarenalectomy
suprarenoma
suprasellar
   cyst, s.
   mass, s.
suralimentation
suramin (Fourneau 309 or Germanin or
   Moranyl or Naganol or Naphuride or
   SUR)

ADDITIONAL TERMS

sodium, s.
surface immunoglobulin
surfactant
surgical
  absence, s.
  adjuvant chemotherapy, s.
  debulking, s.
  excision, s.
  intervention, s.
  resection, s.
  risk, s.
  staging, s.
surgically absent
Surgitron
surrogate
  marker, s.
surveillance
  immune s.
  immunological s.
surveilled
survival
  curve, s.
  functions, s.
  rate, s.
  tail, s.
  trends, s.
susceptibility
susceptible
suspension intracavitary irradiation
Sutter factor
Sutton
  disease, S.
  nevus, S.
suture line cancer
Sv (sievert)
SV (sarcoma virus)
SV (simian virus)
  40, S.
  40 virus vector system, S.
Svedberg
  flotation unit, S.
  unit, S.
Swan-Ganz catheter
Sweet syndrome
swish-and-swallow
  method, s.
  mouthwash, s.
Swiss nu/nu mouse
Swiss-type
  agammaglobulinemia, S.
  hypogammaglobulinemia, S.
SWOG (Southwest Oncology Group)
  CMFVP, S. (cyclophosphamide,

methotrexate, 5-fluorouracil,
  vincristine, prednisone)
  protocol, S.
sycoma
Syed
  implant, S.
  radium applicator, S.
  template, S.
Syed-Neblett
  implant, S.
  template, S.
sylvian aqueduct syndrome
Symadine
Syme amputation
Symmer disease
sympathectomy
sympathicoblast
sympathicoblastoma
sympathicogonioma
sympathoblast
sympathoblastoma
sympathoglioblastoma
sympathogonioma
sympathoma
sympathomimetic
symplex
symptosis
synalgia
synchondrectomy
synchrocyclotron
SynchroMed
  Infusion System, S.
  programmable pump, S.
synchroton
syncytial
syncytioma
  benignum, s.
  malignum, s.
syncytium
syncytoid
syndesmoma
syndrome
syndromic
synergism
synergist
synergistic
synergy
syngeneic
  transplantation, s.
syngenesioplastic
syngenesioplasty
syngenesious
synovectomy

ADDITIONAL TERMS

synovectomy—*Continued*
  radioisotope s.
synovial cell
  carcinoma, s.
  sarcoma, s.
synovialoma
synovioma
synoviosarcoma
synovitis
syntenic
synteny
synterectic
synteresis
synteretic
syntexis
syntheses (pl. of synthesis)
synthesis (pl. syntheses)
synthesize
synthesizer
synthetase
synthetic
  organic chemistry, s.
  protein chemistry, s.
syphilis
syphilitic
syphiloma
Syrian gold hamster
syringoadenoma
syringocarcinoma
syringocystadenoma
syringocystoma
syringoma
System 22 Mizer nebulizer
Systematized Nomenclature of Medicine
  (SNOMED)
systemic
  blood flow, s.
  candidiasis, s.
  cancer, s.
  chemotherapy, s.
  lesion, s.
  lupus erythematosus, s. (SLE)
systemoid
Sytobex

T T (prefix used to identify
       primary tumor)
            T0 (no evidence of primary
              tumor)
       T1, T2, T3, T4 (increasing size
         and/or local extent of primary
         tumor)

TX (primary tumor cannot be
  assessed)
T (tumor)
2,4,5-T (2,4,5-trichlorophenoxyacetic
  acid)
T2 protocol (dactinomycin, Adriamycin,
  vincristine, cyclophosphamide,
  radiation)
T3 (triiodothyronine)
  resin uptake, T.
  RIA (radioimmunoassay), T.
T4 (thyroxine)
  RIA (radioimmunoassay), T.
  surface marker, T.
T-1824 (Evans blue)
T agglutination
T agglutinin
T antigens (tumor antigens)
T-banding (terminal banding)
T (thymus-dependent) cell
  acute lymphoblastic leukemia, T.
    (TALL)
  antigen, T.
  antigen receptors, T.
  chronic lymphocytic leukemia, T.
    (TCC)
  depletion, T
  growth factor, T. (TCGF)
  helper cells, T.
  leukemia, T.
  lymphocytes, T.
  marker, T.
  -mediated immunity, T. (TCMI)
  mitogen, T.
  proliferation, T.
  -replacing factor, T. (TRF)
  -subset phenotype, T.
T4 cells
T8 cells
T-cytotoxic cell
T-dependent antigen
T factor
T-helper cell
T-independent antigen
T-inducer cells (T-IND cells)
T-locus
T-lymphocyte
  subset ratio, T.
T-lymphotrophic human retrovirus
  (HLTV)
T-piece
T3 RIA (radioimmunoassay)
T4 RIA (radioimmunoassay)

ADDITIONAL TERMS

T3 RIABead
T-suppressor cell
T-tube
Ta (tantalum)
    182 isotope, T.
TA (thoracoabdominal)
    stapler, T.
TAA (transfusion-associated AIDS)
TAA (tumor-associated antibody)
TAA (tumor-associated antigen)
TA-AIDS (transfusion-associated AIDS)
tabac nodules
tabacism
tabacosis
tabacum
tabagism
tabella
tabetic
    bladder, t.
tabun
TAC (total abdominal colectomy)
Tac antigen
Tacaribe virus
TACE (chlorotrianisene)
tachyalimentation
tachyphylaxis
tachysterol
TAD (6-thioguanine, ara-C,
    daunomycin)
TAF (tumor angiogenesis factor)
tag
    radioactive t.
TAG 72 antigen
tagged
    atom, t.
    red blood cells, t.
tagging
TAH (total abdominal hysterectomy)
TAH/BSO (total abdominal
    hysterectomy and bilateral salpingo-
    oophorectomy)
taheebo tea
tail
    axillary t.
    breast, t. of
    pancreas, t. of
    Spence, t. of
takedown
    anastomosis, t.
    colostomy, t.
TAL (thymic alymphoplasia)
talcosis
talisomycin

talking tracheostomy tube
T-ALL (T-cell acute lymphoblastic
    leukemia)
Talwin
TAM (tamoxifen)
Tamiami virus
Tamofen
tamoxifen citrate (Nolvadex or TAM or
    TMX)
tan (suntan)
tandem
    insertion, t.
    needle, t.
    ovoids, t. and (T&O)
tangent
    screen testing, t.
tangential
    fields, t.
    portals, t.
    ports, t.
Tangier disease
TANI (total axial node irradiation)
tanned
    red cells, t. (TRC)
    skin, t.
Tanner-Roux-19 procedure
tannin
tanning
    bed, t.
    salon, t.
tantalum (Ta)
    bronchogram, t.
    mesh, t.
    ophthalmic applicator, t.
    plate, t.
    powder, t.
    prosthesis, t.
    ring, t.
    wire, t.
tap
tapping
    ascitic fluid, t. of
    chest, t. of
    lung, t. of
    spinal fluid, t. of
Taq polymerase
tar cancer
Tar symptom
TAR (thrombocytopenia-absent radius)
    syndrome
TARA (tumor-associated rejection
    antigen)
target

ADDITIONAL TERMS

target—*Continued*
　area, t.
　cell, t.
　lesion, t.
　organ, t.
　-oval cell anemia, t.
　selection, t.
　selectivity, t.
　sequence, t.
　-skin distance, t. (TSD)
　site, t.
　theory, t.
targeting agent
tarry
　cyst, t.
　stools, t.
tarsophyma
TART (tumorectomy, axillary
　dissection, radiotherapy)
tart cells
tartrate-resistant acid phosphatase
　(TRAP)
tas gene
TASA (tumor-associated surface
　antigen)
tat (transactivator)
　gene, t.
　-1 gene, t.
　inhibitor, t.
TAT (thromboplastin activation test)
TATA (tumor-associated transplantation
　antigen)
　box, T.
　sequence, T.
tattoo
tattooed
tattooing
tau-meson
taurine
Taussig-Bing anomaly
tautomer
tautomerism
tax gene
taxis
taxofere
taxol
Tay-Sachs disease (TSD)
TBG (thyroid-binding globulin)
TBG (thyroxine-binding globulin)
TBI (thyroxine-binding index)
TBI (total body irradiation)
TBII (thyroid-binding inhibitory
　immunoglobulin)

TBII (TSH-binding inhibitory
　immunoglobulin)
TBP (thyroxine-binding protein)
TBPA (thyroxine-binding prealbumin)
TBSA (total body surface area)
T&C (type and crossmatch)
Tc (technetium)
　99 colloid, T.
　DMSA, T. (technetium 99
　　dimercaptosuccinic acid)
　HIDA, T. (technetium hepato-
　　iminodiacetic acid)
　99m, T. (technetium pertechnetate)
　99m MAA, T. (technetium 99
　　macroaggregated albumin)
　99m medronate scan, T.
　99m-SC, T. (technetium-sulfur
　　colloid)
TC (thioguanine, cytarabine)
3TC
T-CAP (Baker Antifol,
　cyclophosphamide, Adriamycin,
　Platinol)
T-CAP III (triazinate,
　cyclophosphamide, Adriamycin,
　Platinol)
TCC (transitional cell cancer)
TCCB (transitional cell cancer of
　bladder)
TCDD (dioxin)
TCE (trichloroethylene)
TCGF (T-cell growth factor)
TCID (tissue culture infective dose)
TCMI (T-cell mediated immunity)
TCN-P (triciribine phosphate)
TcR gene
tcRNA (translation control RNA)
TD (tumor dose)
TDA (TSH-displacing antibody)
TDD (thoracic duct drainage)
TDF (tumor dose fractionation)
TDR (thymidine deoxyriboside)
T65DR (tentative 1965 radiation dose)
TdT (terminal deoxynucleotidal
　transferase)
Tdth cells
TDx Thyroxine
TDx Total T3
TEA (thromboendarterectomy)
tea
　ginseng t.
　green t.
　herbal t.

ADDITIONAL TERMS

teardrop
    cell, t.
    poikilocytosis, t.
TEC (Thiotepa, etoposide, carboplatin)
TEC (transient erythroblastopenia of childhood)
TECA (technetium albumin) study
teceleukin (recombinant interleukin-2)
TechneColl
technetium (Tc)
    99m, t.
    99m aggregated albumin, t.
    99m disofenin, t.
    99m etidronate, t.
    99m medronate, t.
    99m pertechnetate, t.
    99m polyphosphate, t.
    albumin, t. (TECA)
    diphosphonate, t.
    stannous pyrophosphate, t. (TSPP)
    stannous pyrophosphate rectilinear bone scan, t.
    sulfur colloid, t. (99mTc-SC)
Technetope II
TechniScan MAA kit
TED (threshold erythema dose)
TED (thromboembolic disease)
Teebazone
tegafur
Tegagel
tegmental syndrome
Teichmann crystals
teichoic acid
Teilum tumor
teknocyte
telangiectasia
    generalized essential t.
    hereditary hemorrhagic t.
    lymphatica, t.
    macularis eruptiva perstans, t.
    spider t.
    unilateral nevoid t.
telangiectasis
telangiectatic
    glioma, t.
    sarcoma, t.
    wart, t.
telangiectodes
telangioma
telecobalt
telecurietherapy
telefluoroscopy
teleocidin toxin

teleology
teleradiography
teleradiology
teleradium
teleroentgenogram
teleroentgenography
teleroentgentherapy
telescoping method of classification
teletherapy
Teletrast
telogen
    effluvium, t.
telomere
telophase
telosynapsis
TEM (transanal endoscopic microsurgery)
TEM (transmission electron microscope)
TEM (triethylenemelamine)
    Cathetron afterloader, T.
temafloxacin
Temin theory
TEMP (tamoxifen, etoposide, mitoxantrone, Platinol)
template
    Syed t.
    Syed-Neblitt t.
    x-ray t.
template applicator
template theory
TEN (total enteral nutrition)
tenacity
tenacious
teniposide (VM-26)
tenontophyma
tentorial meningioma
TEPP (tetraethylpyrophosphate)
tense ascites
Tensilon test
tensin
ter (terminator)
    sequence, t.
teratoblastoma
teratocarcinogenesis
teratocarcinoma
teratogen
teratogenic
teratogenicity
teratogenous
teratoid
    tumor, t.
teratoma (pl. teratomata)
    benign cystic t.

ADDITIONAL TERMS

teratoma—*Continued*
   calvarial t.
   cystic t.
   immature t.
   malignant t.
   mature t.
   nasopharyngeal t.
   ovarian t.
   sacrococcygeal t.
   solid t.
   testicular t.
   trophoblastic malignant t.
teratomata (pl. of teratoma)
teratomatous
terebinthinism
terminal
   addition enzyme, t.
   cancer, t.
   carcinoma, t.
   care, t.
   colostomy, t.
   condition, t.
   deoxynucleotidal transferase, t.
    (TdT)
   disease, t.
   illness, t.
   leukocytosis, t.
   patient, t.
   state, t.
   transferase, t.
terminality
terminator (ter)
   sequence, t.
terminus
teroxalene hydrochloride
teroxirone (alpha-TGI)
Ter-Pogossian cervical applicator
terrestrial
   radiation, t.
Tersavid
tertiary
Terumo dialyzer
tesla
Teslac (testolactone)
TESPA (triethylenethiophosphoramide
  or Thiotepa)
Testamone (testosterone)
Testaqua (testosterone)
testectomy
testes (pl. of testis)
test-estrin timed action (TETA)
Testex (testosterone)
testicle

testicular
   adenocarcinoma, t.
   cancer, t.
   carcinoma, t.
   choriocarcinoma, t.
   feminization, t.
   germ cell, t.
   leukemia, t.
   lymphoma, t.
   neoplasm, t.
   nonseminoma, t.
   prosthesis, t.
   relapse, t.
   self-examination, t.
   teratoma, t.
   tumor, t.
testiculi (pl. of testiculus)
testiculoma
   ovarii, t.
testiculus (pl. testiculi)
testis (pl. testes)
testoid
testolactone (Teslac)
Testone (testosterone)
testopathy
testosterone
   cyclopentylpropionate, t.
   cypionate, t.
   enanthate, t.
   heptanoate, t.
   ketolaurate, t.
   phenylacetate, t.
   propionate, t.
TestPackChlamydia
Testred (testosterone)
Testrin (testosterone)
Testroject (testosterone)
Testryl
Tesuloid
TETA (test-estrin timed action)
tetanus
   antitoxin, t.
   immune globulin, t.
   toxoid, t.
Tetrabead
tetrabromofluorescein
tetrachloroplatinum
tetrad
tetraethylpyrophosphate (TEPP)
tetrahydrocannabinol (THC)
tetrahydrofuran
tetrahydroimidazobenzodiazepine
  (TIBO)

ADDITIONAL TERMS

tetraiodothyronine (T4)
tetrapeptide
tetraplatin
tetraploid
tetraploidy
tetratomic
tetrazolium
textoblastic
TF (transfer factor)
TFP3 gene
TFT (thyroid function test)
TFT (trifluorothymidine)
6-TG (6-thioguanine)
TGD (tumor growth delay)
TGF (transforming growth factor)
    -beta, T.
6-TGR (thioguanine riboside)
TGT (thromboplastin generation test)
TGT (thromboplastin generation time)
Th (thorium)
Thal procedure
thalamectomy
thalamencephalon
thalamic
thalamotomy
thalamus
thalassanemia
thalassemia
    alpha t.
    beta t.
    beta-intermedia t.
    delta t.
    delta-beta t.
    gamma t.
    gamma-delta-beta t.
    hemoglobin C t.
    hemoglobin E t.
    hemoglobin Q-alpha t.
    hemoglobin S t.
    hemoglobin SC-alpha t.
    heterozygous t.
    homozygous t.
    intermedia, t.
    major, t.
    minor, t.
    mixed t.
    neonatal t.
    nondeletion delta-beta t.
    sickle cell t.
thalassemia gene
thalassemia trait
thalassemia-sickle cell disease
thalassemic

thallitoxicosis
thallium (Tl)
    201, t.
    chloride, t.
    sulfate, t.
thallous chloride Tl 201
Thayer-Doisy unit
THC (tetrahydrocannabinol)
theca
    cell, t.
    cell tumor, t.
    -lutein cyst, t.
thecal cell
    tumor, t.
    whitlow, t.
thecofibroma
thecoma
    -fibroma, t.
thecomatosis
theliolymphocyte
theloncus
theoretical physics
theory
Theovent
TheraCys (BCG)
therapeutic
    touch, t.
therapy
    adjuvant t.
    anticoagulant t.
    antiemetic t.
    antilymphocyte globulin t.
    autoserum t.
    beam t.
    biological t.
    blood disease t.
    cancer t.
    Chaoul t.
    chelation t.
    consolidation t.
    Curie t.
    deep roentgen-ray t.
    deleading t.
    diathermic t.
    drug t.
    duplex t.
    electron beam radiation t.
    emanation t.
    endocrine t.
    estrogen t.
    factor replacement t.
    fast neutron radiation t.
    fever t.

ADDITIONAL TERMS

therapy—*Continued*
  fibrinolytic t.
  filter t.
  fixed-field t.
  grid t.
  heat particle t.
  helium ion t.
  high-voltage roentgen t.
  hormonal t.
  immunization t.
  immunosuppressive t.
  inhalation t.
  interstitial t.
  intracavitary t.
  intraoperative electron beam t.
    (IOEBT)
  intraoperative radiation t. (IORT)
  intraosseous t.
  intraperitoneal t.
  intrathecal t.
  intravesical t.
  iron chelation t.
  irradiation t.
  laser t.
  light t.
  local t.
  malaria t. for Lyme disease
  medication t.
  megavolt t.
  multiple drug t.
  neoadjuvant t.
  neutron beam t.
  nucleotherapy
  occupational t.
  opsonic t.
  photodynamic t.
  physical t.
  primary t.
  proton beam t.
  radiation t.
  radiotherapy t.
  radium t.
  radium beam t.
  rotation t.
  salvage t.
  sanctuary t.
  secondary t.
  short wave t.
  sieve t.
  speech t.
  supervoltage t.
  tertiary t.
  thrombolytic t.

  trimodality t.
  vocational t.
  x-ray t.
therapy field
TheraSeed implant
Theratron-80
thermacogenesis
thermacogenetic
thermal
  agent, t.
  blast, t.
  burn, t.
  dose, t.
  effect, t.
  equilibrium, t.
  imaging, t.
  luminescent dosimetry, t. (TLD)
  neutrons, t.
  radiation, t.
  spectrum, t.
thermatology
thermionic
thermoagglutination
thermochemistry
thermochemotherapy
thermocoagulation
thermodynamics
thermoelectron
thermoexcitory
thermogenesis
thermogenetic
thermogenic
thermogenous
thermogram
thermograph
  continuous scan t.
thermographic
thermography
thermogravimeter
thermoluminescent
  dose, t.
  dosimetry, t. (TLD)
thermomastography
thermometry
thermonuclear
  effect, t.
  fusion, t.
  reaction, t.
  reactor, t.
  war, t.
thermopenetration
thermoradiotherapy
thermoresistance

ADDITIONAL TERMS

thermoresistant
thermostabile
thermostability
thermotherapeutics
thermotherapy
thermotolerance
thermotolerant
Thermus
    aquaticus, T.
theta antigen
THF (tetrohydrofolic acid)
THF (thymic humoral factor)
THI (transient hypogammaglobulinemia
    of infancy)
thiacetazone
thiaminase
thiamine
thiamiprine
thianamycin
thiarubrine-A
thiazole blue
thiemia
thiethylene thiophosphoramide
thiethylperazine
    maleate, t.
thin
    -layer chromatography, t.
    -section CT scanning, t.
    -section immunoelectron
        microscopy, t.
thinned
thinning
ThinPrep system
thiocarbamide
thiocarbanidin
thiocarlide
thioester
thioflavin
thioguanine (Lanvis or 6-TG or
    6-thioguanine)
6-thioguanine (6-TG or thioguanine)
thioisonicotamide
thiokinase
thiolase
thiolester
thioneine
thionin
thiophosphate
Thioprine
thioredoxin
thiosulfate
thiotepa (STEPA or TESPA or
    ThioTEPA or TTPA)

2-thiouracil
thiourea
ThO_2 (thorium dioxide)
Thom flap
Thoma-Zeiss counting
    chamber
Thomson
    atom, T.
    hypothesis, T.
thoracectomy
thoracentesis
thoraces (pl. of thorax)
thoracopathy
thoracoplasty
Thora-Port
thorascope
thorascopy
thoracostomy
thoracotomy
thorax (pl. thoraces)
thoriagram
thorium (Th)
    D, t.
    dioxide, t. (ThO_2)
    nitrate, t.
    sodium t.
    tartrate, t.
    X, t.
Thorn
    syndrome, T.
    test, T.
thoron
three
    -arm study, t.
    -phase bone scan, t.
    -step theory, t.
Three Mile Island
threonine
threshold
    dose, t.
    erythema, t.
    erythema dose, t. (TED)
thrombapheresis
thrombase
thrombasthenia
    Glanzmann t.
Thrombate III
thrombectomy
thrombi (pl. of thrombus)
thrombin
Thrombinar
thrombinogen
thromboagglutinin

ADDITIONAL TERMS

thromboangiitis
   obliterans, t.
thromboarteritis
   purulenta, t.
thromboclasis
thromboclastic
thrombocytapheresis
thrombocyte
thrombocythemia
   essential t.
   hemorrhagic t.
   idiopathic t.
   primary t.
thrombocytic
thrombocytin
thrombocytocrit
thrombocytolysis
thrombocytolytic
thrombocytopathia
thrombocytopathic
thrombocytopathy
   constitutional t.
thrombocytopenia
   -absent radius (TAR) syn-
      drome, t.
   acquired t.
   congenital t.
   drug-induced t.
   essential t.
   HIV-associated t.
   hypersplenic t.
   hypoplastic t.
   immune t.
   malignant t.
   neonatal t.
   rebound t.
   splenomegalic t.
   spurious t.
   viral t.
thrombocytopenia-absent radius (TAR)
   syndrome
thrombocytopenic
   purpura, t.
thrombocytopoiesis
thrombocytopoietic
thrombocytosis
thromboelastogram
thromboelastograph
thromboelastography
thromboembolia
thromboembolic
   disease, t. (TED)
thromboembolism

thromboendarterectomy (TEA)
thromboendarteritis
thrombogenesis
thrombogenic
thromboid
thrombokinase
thrombokinesis
thrombokinetics
thrombolymphangitis
Thrombolysin
thrombolysis
thrombolytic
thrombon
thrombo-occlusive
thrombopathia
thrombopathy
thrombopenia
   essential t.
thrombopenic
thrombophilia
thrombophlebitis
thromboplastic
thromboplastid
thromboplastin
   extrinsic t.
   intrinsic t.
   tissue t.
thromboplastin activation test (TAT)
thromboplastin generation test (TGT)
thromboplastinogen
thrombopoiesis
thrombopoietic
thrombopoietin
thrombosed
thrombosis
thrombospondin
thrombostasis
Thrombostat
thrombosthenin
thrombotest
thrombotic
   thrombocytopenic purpura, t.
      (TTP)
thrombotonin
thromboxane
thrombus (pl. thrombi)
   agonal t.
   annular t.
   antemortem t.
   ball t.
   blood plate t.
   blood platelet t.
   coral t.

ADDITIONAL TERMS

currant jelly t.
hyaline t.
Laennec t.
laminated t.
lateral t.
milk t.
mural t.
obstructing t.
occluding t.
organized t.
parietal t.
phagocytic t.
plate t.
platelet t.
progressive t.
propagated t.
red t.
stratified t.
white t.
thrush
thulium (Tm)
    chloride, t.
thumbprinting
Thy (thymosin)
    1 antigen, T.
    1 epitope, T.
    fraction 5, T.
thymectomize
thymectomy
thymelcosis
thymic
    alymphoplasia, t. (TAL)
    aplasia, t.
    differentiation antigen, t.
    dysplasia, t.
    humoral factor, t. (THF)
    humoral hormone, t. (thymosin)
    hypoplasia, t.
    neoplasm, t.
    nodule, t.
    -parathyroid aplasia, t.
    peptide, t.
    polypeptide, t.
    tumor, t.
thymicolymphatic
thymidine
    deoxyriboside, t. (TDR)
    diphosphate, t.
    kinase, t.
    -labeling index, t.
    monophosphate, t.
    triphosphate, t. (TTP)
thymidylate synthase

thymine dimer
thyminic acid
thymitis
thymocyte
    mitogenic factor, t. (TMF)
thymogenic
thymokesis
thymokinetic
thymol
    iodide, t.
    turbidity test, t.
Thymolin
thymolipoma
thymolysis
thymolytic
thymoma
thymometastasis
thymonucleic acid
thymopathic
thymopathy
thymopentin (Timunox)
thymopoietin
thymoprivic
thymoprivous
thymosin (Thy)
    alpha-1, t.
    fraction 5, t. (Thy fr 5)
thymostimuline (TP-1)
thymotoxic
thymotoxin
thymotrinin (TP3)
thymotrophic
thymulin
thymus
    cell, t. (T-cell)
    -dependent, t.
    -independent, t.
    gland, t.
    leukemia, t. (TL)
    leukemia antigen, t.
    lymphoma, t. (TL)
    nucleic acid, t.
    nurse cell, t.
    -replacing factor, t. (TRF)
thymusectomy
Thyrar
thyreoplasia
Thyrimeter
thyroactive
thyroadenitis
thyroaplasia
thyrocalcitonin
thyrocele

ADDITIONAL TERMS

thyrocolloid
thyrofissure
thyrogenic
thyrogenous
thyroglobulin
thyroglossal
   duct, t.
   duct cyst, t.
thyroid
   ablation, t.
   adenoma, t.
   bed, t.
   -binding inhibitory
     immunoglobulins, t. (TBII)
   body, t.
   cachexia, t.
   cancer, t.
   carcinoma, t.
   cartilage, t.
   collar, t.
   crisis, t.
   extract, t.
   function, t.
   function test, t. (TFT)
   gland, t.
   hormone, t.
   imaging, t.
   insufficiency, t.
   isthmectomy, t.
   isthmus, t.
   neoplasia, t.
   nodule, t.
   scan, t.
   peroxidase, t.
   radioisotope assay, t. (TyRIA)
   -releasing factor, t. (TRF)
   replacement therapy, t.
   scan, t.
   -stimulating hormone, t. (TSH)
   -stimulating hormone-releasing
     factor, t. (TSH-RF)
   -stimulating immunoglobulins, t.
     (TSI)
   storm, t.
   tumor, t.
   uptake, t.
thyroidal
thyroidea
   accessoria, t.
   ima, t.
thyroidectomize
thyroidectomy

thyroidism
thyroiditis
   acute t.
   autoimmune t.
   chronic fibrous t.
   chronic lymphadenoid t.
   chronic lymphocytic t.
   creeping t.
   de Quervain t.
   focal t.
   giant cell t.
   giant follicular t.
   granulomatous t.
   Hashimoto t.
   invasive t.
   ligneous t.
   lymphocytic t.
   lymphoid t.
   pseudotuberculous t.
   Reidel t.
   silent t.
   subacute granulomatous t.
   subacute lymphocytic t.
   woody t.
thyroidization
thyroidotoxin
thyrointoxication
Thyrolar
Thyrolute
thyrolytic
thyromegaly
thyromimetic
thyronucleoalbumin
thyro-oxyindole
thyroparathyroidectomy
thyroparathyroprivic
thyropathy
thyropenia
thyroplasia
thyroprival
thyroprivia
thyrosis
thyrotherapy
thyrotomy
thyrotoxemia
thyrotoxic
thyrotoxicosis
thyrotoxin
thyrotroph
thyrotropic
thyrotropin
   receptors, t.

ADDITIONAL TERMS

-releasing factor, t. (TRF)
-releasing hormone, t. (TRH)
thyroxine (T4)
 -binding globulin, t. (TBG)
 -binding index, t. (TBI)
 -binding prealbumin, t. (TBPA)
 -binding protein, t. (TBP)
 radioisotope assay, t. (T2RIA)
Thyrozyme-II A
Thytropar
Ti (titanium)
TI-23 monoclonal antibody
tian hau fen (Compound Q)
tiazofurin
 -adenine dinucleotide, t.
tiazuril
TIBC (total iron-binding capacity)
TIBO
 (tetrahydroimidazobenzodiazepine)
 derivative, T.
ticarcillin
Tice (intravesical BCG)
tick-borne
ticlopidine hydrochloride
Tigan
Tikhoff-Lindberg procedure
TIL (tumor-infiltrating lymphocytes)
Tilden method
Tillaux disease
tilomisole
tilorone hydrochloride
TIM (transgenic immunodeficient
 mouse)
time
 bleeding t.
 coagulation t.
 doubling t.
 partial thromboplastin t. (PTT)
 prothrombin t. (PT or pro time)
time trends
Timentin
Timunox (thymopentin)
T-IND cells (T-inducer cells)
tint B
Tis (carcinoma in situ)
Tiselius apparatus
tissue
 activator, t.
 bank, t.
 biopsy, t.
 cryopreservation, t.
 culture, t.

culture infective dose, t. (TCID)
culture medium, t.
dose, t.
-equivalent detector, t.
factor, t.
graft, t.
immunity, t.
macrophage, t.
plasminogen activator, t. (t-PA)
polypeptide antigen, t. (TPA)
rejection, t.
RNA, t.
sampling, t.
-specific antigen, t.
tolerance dose, t. (TTD)
turgor, t.
typing, t.
Tissue Tek medium
tissular
titanium (Ti)
 capsule, t.
 dioxide, t.
titer
 agglutination t.
 whole complement t.
titrate
titration
titrimetric
titrimetry
TKO (to keep open)
 -type I.V., T.
Tl (thallium)
TL (thymus-leukemia)
 antigen, T.
TL (thymus lymphoma)
 antigen, T.
TLC G-65
TLD (thermoluminescent dosimetry)
TLD (tumor lethal dose)
T4+Leu3a+ cells
T8+Leu2a+ cells
TLI (total lymphoid irradiation)
Tm (thulium)
Tm antigen
Tmax (time of maximum concentration)
TMCA
TMF (thymocyte mitogenic factor)
TMGF (transformed mesothelial growth
 factor)
TMNG (toxic multinodular goiter)
T-MOP (6-thioguanine, methotrexate,
 Oncovin, prednisone)

ADDITIONAL TERMS

TMP (trimethoprim)
TMP/SMA (trimethoprim/
  sulfamethoxazole or Bactrim/Septra)
TMP/SMX (trimethoprim/
  sulfamethoxazole or Bactrim/Septra)
TMQ (trimetrexate)
TMTX (trimetrexate)
TMV (tobacco mosaic virus)
TMX (tamoxifen)
T4N5
Tn antigen
TNB (Tru-Cut needle biopsy)
TNF (tumor necrosis factor)
TNI (total nodal irradiation)
TNM (tumor, nodes, metastases)
  T size/extent of primary tumor
  N lymph node involvement
  M distant metastasis absent or
    present
TNM classification
TNM Committee of AJCC
TNM Committee of the International
  Union Against Cancer (UICC)
TNM system
T&O (tandem and ovoids)
TOAP (thioguanine, Oncovin, cytosine
  arabinoside, prednisone)
tobacco
  abuse, t.
  addiction, t.
  chewing, t.
  habit, t.
  history, t.
  mosaic virus, t. (TMV)
  smoke, t.
  smoking, t.
tobaccoism
Tocantins bone marrow needle
Todd
  paralysis, T.
  unit, T.
Todd-Wells guide
togavirus
Toison solution
Tokyo pneumatic speech aid
tolerance
  acquired t.
  adoptive t.
  crossed t.
  high-dose t.
  high-zone t.
  immunologic t.
  low-dose t.

  low-zone t.
  skin t.
  split t.
  tissue t.
tolerance dose
tolerogen
tolerogenesis
tolerogenic
tolonium chloride
toluidine
  blue O, t.
  blue stain, t.
tomogram
tomograph
tomography
  computed t.
  computerized axial t. (CAT)
  emission computer t.
  hypercycloidal t.
  hypocycloidal t.
  polycycloidal t.
  positron emission t. (PET)
  positron emission transverse t.
    (PETT)
  quantitative computed t.
  radionuclide emission t.
  single-photon emission t. (SPECT)
  ultrasonic t.
tonsillar invasive tongue lesion
topholipoma
topo (topoisomerase)
  gene, t.
topoisomerase
  II, t.
  III, t.
  gene, t.
topotecan
Toradol
TORCH (toxoplasmosis, rubella,
  cytomegalovirus, congenital herpes)
  screening, T.
  syndrome, T.
  titer, T.
toremifene citrate
torr
Torres syndrome
Torula
  histolytica, T.
toruloma
Torulopsis
  glabrata, T.
torulosis
total

ADDITIONAL TERMS

abdominal colectomy, t. (TAC)
abdominal hysterectomy, t. (TAH)
abdominal hysterectomy with
  bilateral salpingo-
  oophorectomy, t. (TAH-BSOO)
administered dose, t. (TAD)
axial node irradiation, t. (TANI)
bladder resection, t.
blood granulocyte pool, t.
blood volume, t.
body irradiation, t. (TBI)
body surface area, t. (TBSA)
complement assay, t.
enteral nutrition, t. (TEN)
gastrectomy, t.
hysterectomy, t.
iron-binding capacity, t. (TIBC)
laryngectomy, t.
laryngectomy with radical neck
  dissection, t.
lymphoid irradiation, t. (TLI)
mastectomy, t.
nodal field, t.
nodal irradiation, t. (TNI)
pancreatectomy, t.
parenteral alimentation, t. (TPA)
parenteral nutrition, t. (TPN)
pelvic exenteration, t.
peripheral parenteral nutrition, t.
  (TPPN)
pneumonectomy, t.
protected environment, t. (TPE)
renal blood flow, t. (TRBF)
rosette-forming cell, t. (TRFC)
totipotency
totipotential
Touton giant cell
toxanemia
toxemia
toxic
  -allergic syndrome, t.
  -antitoxin, t.
  appearance, t.
  chemical, t.
  dose, t.
  dump, t.
  dust, t.
  effect, t.
  erythema, t.
  fumes, t.
  gas, t.
  goiter, t.
  granulation, t.

hemolytic anemia, t.
leukocytosis, t.
multinodular goiter, t. (TMNG)
shock syndrome, t.
smoke, t.
spill, t.
substance, t.
unit, t. (TU)
waste, t.
toxicity
toxicology
  testing, t.
toxin
toxogenin
toxoid
toxolysin
toxometabolic
Toxoplasma
  cuniculi, T.
  gondii, T.
toxoplasmin
toxoplasmosis
TP-1 (thymostimuline)
TP3 (thymotrinin)
TP-5
TP-40
t-PA (tissue plasminogen activator)
TPA (12-O-tetradecanoyl-phorbol
  13-acetate)
TPA (tissue polypeptide antigen)
TPA (total parental alimentation)
TPDCV (thioguanine, procarbazine,
  DBC, CCNU, vincristine)
TPE (total protected environment)
TPHA (Treponema pallidum
  hemagglutination assay)
TPI (Treponema pallidum
  immobilization)
TPN (total parenteral nutrition)
TPPN (total peripheral parenteral
  nutrition)
TRA (trans-retinoic acid or tretinoin)
trace element
tracer
  radioactive t.
tracer atom
trachea
tracheal
  deviation, t.
  stoma, t.
tracheitis
trachelectomy
trachelematoma

ADDITIONAL TERMS

trachelotomy
tracheobronchial
tracheobronchoscopy
tracheoesophageal
tracheolaryngotomy
tracheomegaly
tracheoscopy
tracheostoma
tracheostomy
tracheotomize
tracheotomy
TRAIDS (transfusion-related AIDS)
trait
    sickle cell t.
TRAM (transverse rectus abdominis
  musculocutaneous)
    flap, T.
    procedure, T.
trans
    -acting, t.
    -activation response, t.
    -dominant, t.
    -factor, t.
    -rotamer, t.
transactivator
transaminase
    glutamic-oxaloacetic t. (GOT)
    glutamic-pyruvic t. (GPT)
transanal endoscopic microsurgery
  (TEM)
transaxillary
transbronchial
transcatheter
    irradiation, t.
transcobalamin
transcortin
transcribed genes
transcript
    primary t.
transcriptase
    reverse t.
transcription
transdermal
    infusion system, t.
transducer
transduction
transesophageal biopsy
transexamic acid
transfect
transfectant
transfection
transfectoma
transfer
    factor, t. (TF)

    RNA, t. (tRNA)
transferase
transferrin
transformed
    mesothelial growth factor, t.
    (TMGF)
transformation
    zone, t.
transforming
    agent, t.
    gene, t.
    growth factor, t. (TGF)
transfuse
transfusion
    autologous t.
    blood t.
    cadaver t.
    direct t.
    exchange t.
    exsanguination t.
    fetomaternal t.
    immediate t.
    indirect t.
    intraperitoneal t.
    leukocyte t.
    packed red cell t.
    platelet t.
    replacement t.
    single-unit t.
    substitution t.
    washed red cell t.
    whole blood t.
transfusion-associated AIDS (TAA or
  TA-AIDS)
transfusion reaction
transfusion-related AIDS (TRAIDS)
transfusion syndrome
transgene
transgenic
    cells, t.
    expression, t.
    immunodeficient mouse, t. (TIM)
    Mov mouse, t.
    organism, t.
    rat, t.
transglutaminase
Transgrow
transhepatic
transient
    erythroblastopenia of childhood, t.
    (TEC)
    hypogammaglobulinemia of
    infancy, t. (THI)
transit

ADDITIONAL TERMS

transition zone
transitional cell carcinoma (TCC)
    stages A, B1, B2, C, D1, D2, t.
transitional leukocyte
transitional tumor
transitional zone
transjugular liver biopsy
translation
    chromosomal t.
translocase
translocation
translumbar
    hemicorporectomy, t.
transmembrane
    protein, t.
transmigration
transmissible
transmission
    electron microscope, t. (TEM)
transorbital lobotomy
transperineal
    needle biopsy, t.
transplacental
    antiviral drug therapy, t.
transplantation
    allogeneic t.
    autologous t.
    autoplastic t.
    bone marrow t.
    heteroplastic t.
    heterotopic t.
    homoplastic t.
    homotopic t.
    organ t.
    orthopic t.
    syngeneic t.
    syngenesioplastic t.
    tenoplastic t.
transplantation antigen
transplantation biology
transplantation rejection
transport
transposition
transposon
transrectal
    perineal needle biopsy, t.
    prostatic biopsy, t.
    ultrasonography, t. (TRUS)
transretinoic acid
transsphincteric surgery
transthermia
transthoracic
transthoracotomy
transtracheal

transudate
transudation
transudative
    ascites, t.
transuranium
transurethral
    perineal biopsy, t.
    prostatectomy, t.
    resection, t. (TUR)
    resection of bladder, t. (TURB)
    resection of bladder tumor, t.
        (TURBT)
    resection of prostate, t. (TURP)
transvaginal
    biopsy, t.
    cone, t.
transvector
tranylcypromine
Travenol
    biopsy needle, T.
    dialyzer, T.
    infusor device, T.
transverse rectus abdominis
    musculocutaneous (TRAM)
    flap, t.
    procedure, t.
TRAP (tartrate-resistant acid
    phosphatase)
TRAP (thioguanine, rubidomycin, ara-C,
    prednisone)
traumatic
    herpes, t.
    proctitis, t.
traumatized tissue
Travenol infuser
TRBF (total renal blood flow)
TRC (tanned red cell)
    titer, T.
TRE (true radiation emission)
treating distance (TD)
treatment
    Beard t.
    Bell t.
    choline t.
    Coffey-Humber t.
    conservative t.
    curative t.
    eventration t.
    fever t.
    Fichera t.
    Guinard t.
    high-frequency t.
    holistic t.
    IND (investigational new drug) t.

ADDITIONAL TERMS

treatment—*Continued*
    ionizing radiation t.
    Koga t.
    Koranyi t.
    light t.
    Minot-Murphy t.
    palliative t.
    radium t.
    sanctuary t.
    supportive t.
    teleradium t.
Trecator SC
trenimon
Treponema pallidum
    hemagglutination assay, T. (TPHA)
    immobilization, T. (TPI)
treponemal
trestolone acetate
tretamine
tretinoin (all-trans-retinoic acid or
  Retin-A)
Trexan
TRF (T-cell replacing factor)
TRF (thymus-replacing factor)
TRF (thyroid-releasing factor)
TRFC (total rosette-forming cell)
TRH (thyrotropin-releasing hormone)
triad
trial
    clinical t.
    crossover t.
trialistic theory
triaminotriphenylmethane nuclear dye
triatomic
triazinate (TZT)
triaziquone
tributyrin
2,4,5-trichlorophenoxyacetic acid
  (2,4,5-T)
trichobasalioma hyalinicum
trichoepithelioma
    papillosum multiplex, t.
tricholeukocyte
Trichosanthes
    kirilowii, T.
trichosanthin (compound Q)
Trichosporin
    beigelii, T.
    cutaneum, T.
    giganteum, T.
triciribine phosphate (TCN-P)
tricyclic
tridermoma

triester
    method, t.
triethanomelamine
triethylene melamine
triethylenemelamine (TEM)
triethylenethiophosphoramide (thiotepa
  or TSPA or TESPA or TTPA)
trifluoperazine
trifluorothymidine (TFT)
triflupromazine
trifluridine
trigger
    point, t.
    substance, t.
trigone
trigonectomy
triiodothyronine (T3)
    red cell uptake test, t.
    resin uptake, t.
trilostane
Trimadeau sign
trimellitic anhydride
trimer
trimethoprim (TMP)
    -sulfamethoxazole, t. (Bactrim/
    Septra or TMP/SMX)
trimetrexate (TMTX)
    gluconate, t.
    glucuronate, t.
trimodality therapy (heat, radiation, and
  chemotherapy)
Trimox
Trimpex
trimustine
Triniad (isoniazid)
Trinsicon
trinucleotide
Triobead-125
triolein (I 131)
triosephosphate
    dehydrogenase, t.
    isomerase, t.
tripe palm
tripeptide
triphosphate
triphthemia
Tripier amputation
triple
    antibody sandwich technique, t.
    blind, t.
triptorelin
triradiation
Tris buffer

ADDITIONAL TERMS

trisaccharide
    A, t.
    B, t.
trisodium phosphoformate (Foscarnet)
trisomy
trisulfapyrimidine
tritiated
    thymidine, t.
    water, t.
tritiation
tritium
triton
Triton X
tRNA (transfer ribonucleic acid)
Trobicin
troche
trochiscus
Troisier
    node, T.
    sign, T.
    syndrome, T.
trophoblast
trophoblastic
trophoblastoma
trophocyte
trophotherapy
tropical
    anemia, t.
    eosinophilia, t.
    macrocytic anemia, t.
    spastic paraparesis, t.
    splenomegaly syndrome, t.
    sprue, t.
tropism
Trousseau syndrome
Trousseau-Lallemand bodies
Tru-Arc trachea tube
Tru-Cut
    biopsy needle, T.
    needle biopsy, T. (TNB)
true radiation emission (TRE)
truncal rhabdomyosarcoma
TruQuant
    RIA, T.
    tumor marker, T.
TRUS (transrectal ultrasonography)
Trypanosoma
    cruzi, T.
trypanosomal
trypanosomiasis
    American t.
trypsin
    crystallized t.

trypsinized
trypsinogen
Tryptar
tryptophan
T/S (thyroid/serum iodine ratio)
Tsa (a virus mutant)
TSA (tumor-specific antigen)
TSC (technetium sulfur colloid)
TSD (target-skin distance)
TSH (thyroid-stimulating hormone)
    -binding inhibitory
      immunoglobulin, T. (TBII)
    -displacing antibody, T. (TDA)
    -RF, T. (thyroid-stimulating
      hormone-releasing factor)
    -RH, T. (thyroid-stimulating
      hormone-releasing hormone)
TSI (thyroid-stimulating
  immunoglobulin)
TSPA (thiotepa)
TSPP (technetium stannous
  pyrophosphate)
    rectilinear bone scan, T.
TSTA (tumor-specific transplantation
  antigen)
T4:T8 ratio
TTA (all-trans-retinoic acid)
TTD (tissue tolerance dose)
TTP (thrombotic thrombocytopenic
  purpura)
TTP (thymidine triphosphate)
TTPA (thiotepa)
TTPA (triethylenethiophosphoramide)
TU (toxic unit)
tube feeding
tubed flap
tubercle
tubercular
tuberculigenous
tuberculid
tuberculin
    zymoplastiche, t. (TZ)
tuberculization
tuberculoma
    en plaque, t.
tuberculosilicosis
tuberculosis
    aerogenic t.
    anthracotic t.
    atypical t.
    basal t.
    bones and joints, t. of
    cerebral t.

ADDITIONAL TERMS

tuberculosis—*Continued*
   cestodic t.
   colliquativa, t.
   cutis, t.
   disseminated t.
   exudative t.
   genital t.
   genitourinary t.
   hematogenous t.
   hilus t.
   indurativa, t.
   inhalation t.
   lichenoides, t.
   miliaris disseminata, t.
   miliary t.
   open t.
   oral t.
   orificial t.
   papulonecrotic t.
   postprimary t.
   primary t.
   productive t.
   pulmonary t.
   reinfection t.
   surgical t.
   tracheobronchial t.
   ulcerosa, t.
   verrucosa cutis, t.
   warty t.
tuberculosis chemotherapy
tuberculostatic
tuberculostearic acid
tuberculotic
tuberculous
tuberculum
   sellae meningioma, t.
tuberous
   arthritis, t.
   carcinoma, t.
   sclerosis, t.
tubo-ovariotomy
tubular
   adenoma, t.
   carcinoma, t.
   necrosis, t.
tubule
tubulin
tubulodermoid
tubuloreticular
tubulovillous
   adenoma, t.
   polyp, t.
tubulozole hydrochloride

tuftsin
tularemia
tumefacient
tumefaction
tumeur
   perlee, t.
   pileuse, t.
tumor
   Abrikosov t.
   Abrikossoff t.
   acoustic nerve t.
   acute splenic t.
   adenoid t.
   adenomatoid t.
   adipose t.
   adrenal rest t.
   albus, t.
   albus pyogenes, t.
   ameloblastic adenomatoid t.
   amyloid t.
   aniline t.
   Askin t.
   benign t.
   biliary t.
   blood t.
   Brenner t.
   Brigham brain t.
   Brooke t.
   brown t.
   Brown-Pearce t.
   Burkitt t.
   Burkitt-like t.
   Buschke-Löwenstein t.
   butyroid t.
   carcinoid t. of bronchus
   carcinomatous t.
   carotid body t.
   cartilaginous t.
   cavernous t.
   cellular t.
   C3H mammary t.
   chromaffin-cell t.
   Codman t.
   colli, t.
   collision t.
   colloid t.
   connective-tissue t.
   craniopharyngeal duct t.
   Cruveilhier t.
   cystic t.
   dermoid t.
   desmoid t.
   doubling t.

ADDITIONAL TERMS

dumbbell t.
eccrine sweat gland t.
E1C-negative breast t.
eiloid t.
embryonal t.
embryoplastic t.
encysted t.
epithelial t.
Erdheim t.
erectile t.
Ewing t.
extragonadal germ cell t.
false t.
fatty t.
fecal t.
fibrocellular t.
fibroid t.
fibro-osseous t.
fibroplastic t.
functioning t.
fungating t.
gastric glomus t.
gelatinous t.
germ cell t.
germinal t.
gestational t.
giant cell t.
glomus t.
glomus jugulare t.
glomus tympanicum t.
Godwin t.
granular cell t.
granulation t.
granulosa t.
granulosa cell t.
granulosa-theca cell t.
Grawitz t.
Gubler t.
gummy t.
heterologous t.
heterotypic t.
hilar cell t.
hilus cell t.
histioid t.
homoiotypic t.
homologous t.
Hortega cell t.
hourglass t.
Hürthle cell t.
Hutter t.
iceberg t.
infiltrating t.
innocent t.

interstitial cell t.
intra-axial brain t.
islet cell t.
ivory-like t.
Jensen t.
Keashy t.
Koenen t.
Klatskin t.
Krompecher t.
Krukenberg t.
lacteal t.
Leydig cell t.
lienis, t.
Lindau t.
lipid cell ovarian t.
lipoid cell t. of ovary
luteinized granulosa-theca cell t.
malignant t.
malignant mixed t.
malignant mixed müllerian t.
march t.
margaroid t.
mast cell t.
melanotic neuroectodermal t.
Merkel cell t.
mesenchymal mixed t.
mesodermal t.
mesonephroid t.
metastatic t.
Middeldorph t.
migrated t.
migratory t.
mixed t.
mixed germ cell t.
mucinous t.
mucoepidermoid t.
mucous t.
müllerian t.
muscular t.
Nelaton t.
Nelson t.
neuroectodermal t.
neuroepithelial t.
neurogenic t.
nonseminomatous germ cell t.
oozing t.
organoid t.
oxyphil cell t.
Pancoast t.
papillary t.
paraffin t.
pearl t.
pearly t.

ADDITIONAL TERMS

tumor—*Continued*
Perlmann t.
phantom t.
5-phase t.
phyllodes, t.
Pindborg t.
plasma cell t.
plasmacytic t.
polycystic t.
postirradiation t.
potato t.
Pott puffy t.
pregnancy t.
premalignant fibroepithelial t.
primary t.
pseudointraligamentous t.
pulmonary sulcus t.
Rathke t.
Rathke pouch t.
Recklinghausen t.
recurring digital fibrous t's of
childhood
Regaud t.
retinal anlage t.
sacrococcygeal germ cell t.
salivary gland t.
sand t.
Schmincke t.
Schwann cell t.
serous t.
Sertoli cell t.
Sertoli-Leydig cell t.
sex cord–stromal germ cell t.
sheath t.
S-phase t.
Steiner t's
stercoral t.
sulcus t.
superior sulcus t.
Teilum t.
teratoid t.
testicular germ cell t.
theca cell t.
transition t.
tridermic t.
true t.
turban t.
ulcerogenic t.
Vanek t.
vanishing t.
varicose t.
vascular t.

vermian t.
villous t.
virilizing t.
Warthin t.
white t.
Wilms t.
yolk sac t.
Zollinger-Ellison t.
tumor activity
tumor angiogenesis factor (TAF)
tumor antigen
tumor-associated antibody (TAA)
tumor-associated antigen (TAA)
tumor-associated surface antigen
(TASA)
tumor-associated transplantation
antigen (TATA)
tumor autocrine motility factor
tumor-bearing area
tumor bed
tumor biology
tumor biopsy
tumor blush
Tumor Board
tumor boost
tumor burden
tumor cell
tumor cell-host bone relationship
tumor cell line
tumor characteristic
tumor-cloning assay
tumor cloud
tumor defect
tumor deposit
tumor depth
tumor destruction
tumor dose (TD)
tumor dose fractionation (TDF)
tumor doubling time
tumor embolism
tumor growth delay (TGD)
tumor implant
tumor-infiltrating lymphocytes (TIL)
tumor infiltration
tumor invasion
tumor lethal dose (TLD)
tumor-limiting factor
tumor localization
tumor lysis syndrome
tumor marker
tumor mass
tumor metabolism

ADDITIONAL TERMS

tumor necrosis factor (TNF)
tumor nests
tumor persistence
tumor pH
tumor plop
tumor progression
tumor progression gene
tumor promoter
Tumor Registry
tumor regression
tumor screw
tumor seeding
tumor shrinkage
tumor site
tumor-specific
tumor-specific antigen (TSA)
tumor-specific glycoprotein
tumor-specific transplantation antigen
  (TSTA)
tumor spread
tumor staging
tumor stain
tumor suppressant
tumor suppression
tumor vaccine
tumor virus
tumor volume
tumoraffin
tumoral
tumorectomy
tumoricidal
tumorigenesis
tumorigenic
tumorigenicity
tumorlet
tumorous
tungsten target
TUR (transurethral resection)
turacoporphyrin
TURB (transurethral resection of
  bladder)
turbid
turbidimeter
turbidimetry
turbidity
TURBT (transurethral resection of
  bladder tumor)
Turcot syndrome
Türk
    cell, T.
    irritation leukocyte, T.
Turnbull staging system

Turnbull-Cutait operation
turnover
    erythrocyte iron t.
    plasma iron t.
    red blood cell iron t.
TURP (transurethral resection of
  prostate)
Turrissi regimen
Tus protein
TWiST (time without symptoms or
  toxicity)
two
    -dimensional gel analysis, t.
    -dimensional
      immunoelectrophoresis, t.
    -tailed test, t.
Tworek bone marrow aspirating
  needle
TX (primary tumor cannot be assessed)
tylectomy
tylosis
tyloxapol
type and crossmatch (T&C)
Type I and II interferon
typhlectomy
typing
    bacteriophage t.
    blood t.
    crossmatching, t. and
    HLA t.
    phage t.
    primed lymphocyte t. (PLT)
    tissue t.
tyramine
TyRIA (thyroid radioimmunoassay)
TyRIA (thyroid radioisotope assay)
tyroma
tyromatosis
tyrosinase
tyrosine
    527, t.
    aminotransferase, t.
    aminotransferase deficiency, t.
    phosphorylation, t.
    protein kinase, t.
tyrosinemia
tyrosis
TZ (tuberculin zymoplastiche)
Tzanck
    cell, T.
    test, T.
TZT (triazinate)

ADDITIONAL TERMS

U (uranium)
U-8344
U (undefined) cell
  lymphoma, U.
U9379 histiocytic lymphoma cells
UA001
UBI (ultraviolet blood irradiation)
ubiquinol
    -cytochrome c reductase, u.
    dehydrogenase, u.
ubiquinone
UCHL-1 (T-cell marker)
UDP (uridine diphosphate)
UDPG (uridine diphosphate glucose)
UDPGA (uridine diphosphoglucuronic
  acid)
UDPgalactose-4-epimerase
UDPglucose-4-epimerase
U-87201E
Uendex
UHBI (upper hemibody irradiation)
U937/HIV-1 cell line
UIBC (unsaturated iron-binding
  capacity)
UICC (Union Internationale Contre
  Cancer or Committee of the
  International Union Against
  Cancer)
    staging, U.
UK-49,858
UL13 gene
UL9 protein (origin-binding protein)
ulca (pl. of ulcus)
ulcer
    amputating u.
    anastomotic u.
    aphthous u.
    atheromatous u.
    burrowing phagedenic u.
    Buruli u.
    callus u.
    chronic leg u.
    Curling u.
    decubitus u.
    diabetic u.
    follicular u.
    fungus u.
    gouty u.
    Hunner u.
    indolent u.
    Jacob u.
    Malabar u.
    Marjolin u.

penetrating u.
perambulating u.
phagedenic u.
rodent u.
serpiginous u.
stasis u.
stercoral u.
sump u.
trophic u.
tropical phagedenic u.
varicose u.
venereal u.
ulcer bed
ulcer crater
ulcerate
ulcerated
ulcerating
    adenocarcinoma, u.
    granuloma, u.
    lesion, u.
ulceration
ulcerative
    cancer, u.
    colitis, u.
    gingivitis, u.
    lesion, u.
ulcerogangrenous
ulcerogenic
    drug, u.
    tumor, u.
ulcerogranuloma
ulceromembranous
ulcus (pl. ulca)
    cancrosum, u.
    induratum, u.
    vulvae acutum, u.
ulectomy
uletic
ulitis
ulocace
ulocarcinoma
uloglossitis
uloncus
ultimate carcinogen
ultracentrifuge
ultrafilter
ultrafiltration
ultraisolation
ultramicron
ultramicroscope
ultramicroscopy
ultramicrotome
ultraradian rhythm

ADDITIONAL TERMS

ultrasonic
    nebulizer, u.
ultrasonics
ultrasonogram
ultrasonographic
ultrasonography
    A-mode u.
    B-mode u.
    Doppler u.
    endoscopic u.
    gray-scale u.
    M-mode u.
    real-time u.
ultrasound
ultrastructure
Ultra-TechneKow
ultraviolet (UV)
    far u.
    near u.
ultraviolet blood irradiation (UBI)
ultraviolet fluorescent dose
ultraviolet fluorescent dosimetry
ultraviolet light
ultraviolet radiation (UVR)
ultraviolet rays
ultraviolet therapy
ultraviolet wave
ultravirus
ultravisible
umbelliferone
umber
    mutation, u.
umbilicated
umbilicus
umbrella filter
UMP (uridine monophosphate)
uncinate
    fits, u.
    gyrus, u.
uncomplemented
unconjugated
understaging
undifferentiated
    adenocarcinoma, u.
    carcinoma, u.
    cell leukemia, u.
    lymphoma, u.
    sarcoma, u.
undifferentiation
Undritz anomaly
unfixed human salivary gland
  immunofluorescence test
Uniad

Unilab Surgibone
Unimist
uninhibited neurogenic bladder
uninuclear
uninucleated
uninvolved
un-ionized hemoglobin
unipotential
unit
    activation u.
    amboceptor u.
    Angstrom u.
    Ansbacher u.
    antigen u.
    antitoxic u.
    atomic mass u.
    atomic weight u.
    Behnken u.
    Bethesda u.
    Bodansky u.
    burst-forming u.
    colony-forming u.
    complement u.
    curie u.
    electromagnetic u's
    electrostatic u's
    gray-scale u.
    half-life u.
    Hampson u.
    hemolytic u.
    Hounsfield u.
    immunizing u.
    Kienböck u.
    Mache u.
    Magnetrode cervical u.
    map u.
    megacurie u.
    membrane attack u.
    microcurie u.
    millicurie u.
    mouse u.
    multicurie u.
    Phillips contact therapy u.
    quantum u.
    rat u.
    recognition u.
    roentgen u. (RU)
    Svedberg u.
    Svedberg flotation u.
    Thayer-Doisy u.
    Todd u.
    uranium u.
    x-ray u.

ADDITIONAL TERMS

unit skin dose
unitarian
    hypothesis, u.
    theory, u.
univalent
univariant analysis
universal
    donor, u.
    recipient, u.
University of Illinois marrow needle
unknown primary
Unna
    alkaline methylene blue stain, U.
    boot, U.
    nevus, U.
    wrap, U.
Unna-Pappenheimer stain
unresectable
unroofed
unroofing
unsaturated iron-binding capacity
  (UIBC)
unstable hemoglobin
up-modulated
upper hemibody irradiation (UHBI)
up-regulated
UPPP (uvulopalatopharyngoplasty)
uptake
UR2 sarcoma virus
uracil mustard
uramustine
uranium (U)
    unit, u.
uranyl lead staining
urate nephropathy
UR2AV-induced lymphoma
urea
    frost, u.
    nitrogen, u.
Ureaplasma
    urealyticum, U.
uredepa
uremia
uremic
uremigenic
ureterectasis
ureterectomy
ureteritis
ureterocele
ureterocelectomy
ureterocolostomy
ureteroileostomy
ureteroneocystostomy

ureteronephrectomy
ureteropelvioplasty
ureteroproctostomy
ureteropyeloneostomy
ureteropyelostomy
ureteropyelonephrostomy
ureterorectal
ureterorectoneostomy
ureterosigmoidostomy
ureterostoma
ureterostomy
    cutaneous u.
ureterotrigonenterostomy
ureterotrigonosigmoidostomy
ureteroureteral
ureteroureterostomy
ureterouterine
ureterovaginal
ureterovesical
urethan
urethra
urethral
urethrectomy
urethremphraxis
urethritis
urethrocystitis
urethrocystography
urethrography
urethroperineoscrotal
urethrophyma
urethroplasty
urethroprostatic
urethrorectal
urethroscope
urethroscopy
urethrostomy
urethrovaginal
urethrovesical
uric acid
    nephropathy, u.
uridine
    diphosphate, u. (UDP)
    diphosphate glucose, u. (UDPG)
    diphosphoglucuronic acid, u.
     (UDPGA)
    monosphate, u. (UMP)
    rescue, u.
    triphosphate, u.
urinary
    incontinence, u.
    retention, u.
    tract, u.
urine

ADDITIONAL TERMS

urinoma
Urocyte diagnostic cytometry system
urogastrone
urogenital
urogram
urography
urohematoporphyrin
urokinase
    protocol, u.
urokymography
urologic
urology
uropathy
uroporphyria
    erythropoietic u.
uroporphyrin
uroporphyrinogen
    I, u.
    decarboxylase, u.
    III synthetase, u.
uroradiology
urorectal
urostomy
    pouch, u.
urothelial
urothelium
urticaria
urticarial
urticariogenic
uta
uterectomy
uteri (pl. of uterus)
    adenomyosis u.
    fibromyomata u.
    leiomyoma u.
    myomata u.
uterine
    biopsy, u.
    carcinoma, u.
    cavity, u.
    cervix, u.
    corpus, u.
    curettage, u.
    curettings, u.
    fibroid, u.
    fibroidectomy, u.
    fibroma, u.
    fundus, u.
    leiomyosarcoma, u.
    myoma, u.
    myomectomy, u.
    radium insertion, u.
    sarcoma, u.

uterocervical
uterography
utero-ovarian
uteroplasty
uterorectal
uterosacral
uterovaginal
uterovesical
uterus (pl. uteri)
UV (ultraviolet)
    -induced squamous cell carcinoma,
      U.
    radiation carcinogenesis, U.
uvea
uveal
    melanoma, u.
    staphyloma, u.
uveitis
uviolize
uviometer
uvioresistant
uviosensitive
UVR (ultraviolet radiation)
uvula
uvulectomy
uvulopalatopharyngoplasty (UPPP)

V V (assessment of tumor
    involvement within veins)
      V0 (veins do not contain
      tumor)
    V1 (efferent veins contain tumor)
    V2 (afferent veins contain tumor)
    VX (venous invasion cannot be
      assessed)
V (vanadium)
V (volt)
V antigen
V-2 carcinoma
V factor
V genes
V-particle
V region
VA (vincristine, Adriamycin)
VA factor
VAAP (vincristine, asparaginase,
    Adriamycin, prednisone)
VAB 1 (vinblastine, actinomycin D,
    bleomycin)
VAB 2 (vinblastine, actinomycin D,
    bleomycin, cisplatin)
VAB 3 (vinblastine, actinomycin D,

ADDITIONAL TERMS

VAB 3—*Continued*
  bleomycin, cisplatin, chlorambucil,
    cyclophosphamide)
VAB 4 (vinblastine, actinomycin D,
  bleomycin, cisplatin,
  cyclophosphamide)
VAB 5 (vinblastine, actinomycin D,
  bleomycin, cisplatin,
  cyclophosphamide)
VAB 6 (cyclophosphamide,
  dactinomycin, vinblastine, bleomycin,
  cisplatin)
VABCD (vinblastine, Adriamycin,
  bleomycin, CCNU, DTIC)
VAC (vincristine, actinomycin D,
  cyclophosphamide)
VAC (vincristine, Adriamycin,
  cyclophosphamide)
VAC pulse (vincristine, actinomycin D,
  cyclophosphamide) administered
  periodically
VAC standard (vincristine, actinomycin
  D, cyclophosphamide) administered
  daily
VACA (vincristine, actinomycin D,
  cyclophosphamide, Adriamycin)
VACAD (vincristine, Adriamycin,
  cyclophosphamide, actinomycin D,
  dacarbazine)
vaccinate
vaccination
vaccine
vaccinia
    fetal v.
    gangrenosa, v.
    generalized v.
    progressive v.
vaccinia immune globulin (VIG)
vaccinia virus
VACP (VePesid, Adriamycin,
  cyclophosphamide, Platinol)
vacuolating
vacuolation
vacuum phenomenon
VAD (vincristine, Adriamycin,
  dexamethasone)
VAD/V (vincristine, Adriamycin,
  dexamethasone, verapamil)
VAFAC (vincristine, amethopterin,
  5-fluorouracil, Adriamycin,
  cyclophosphamide)
vagina
vaginal

    candle, v.
    carcinoma, v.
    condom, v.
    cuff, v.
    hysterectomy, v.
    intraepithelial neoplasia, v. (VIN)
    radium insertion, v.
    reconstruction, v.
    vault, v.
    warts, v.
vaginal, cervical, endometrial (VCE)
    smears, v.
vaginalectomy
vaginectomy
vaginitis
vaginocutaneous
vaginogram
vaginography
vaginomycosis
vaginoperineoplasty
vaginoperineotomy
vaginoplasty
vaginoscope
vaginoscopy
vaginovesical
vaginovulvar
VAHS (virus-associated hemophagocytic
  syndrome)
VAI (vincristine, actinomycin D,
  ifosfamide)
valence
    shell, v.
valency
Valergen (estradiol)
valine
valinemia
Valtrac
VAM (VP-16–213, Adriamycin,
  methotrexate)
VAMP (vincristine, Adriamycin,
  methotrexate, prednisone)
VAMP (vincristine, amethopterin,
  6-mercaptopurine, prednisone)
vanadate
vanadium (V)
vanadiumism
van Bogaert
    disease, v.
    sclerosing leukoencephalitis, v.
Van de Graaff generator
van den Bergh
    technique, v.
    test, v.

ADDITIONAL TERMS

Vancocin
vancomycin hydrochloride
Vanek tumor
Vanguard Study
vanillylmandelic acid (VMA)
vanishing tumor
Vansil
vanSonnenberg biopsy needle
van't Hoff rule
VAP (vincristine, Adriamycin,
    procarbazine)
VAP (vincristine, asparaginase,
    prednisone)
VAP-II (vinblastine, actinomycin D,
    Platinol)
VAPA program
Vapo-Iso
vapreotide
Vaquez disease
Vaquez-Osler disease
variability
variable
Varian
    accelerator, V.
    simulator, V.
variant
    surface glycoprotein, v. (VSG)
variation
variceal
varicella
    gangrenosa, v.
varicella-zoster (VZ)
    immune globulin, v. (VZIG)
    virus, v. (VZV)
varicelliform
varicelloid
varices (pl. of varix)
varicocele
varicoid carcinoma
varicomphalus
varicose
    veins, v.
    ulcers, v.
varix (pl. varices)
vascular
    hemophilia, v.
    leiomyoma, v.
    tumor, v.
vasculitic
vasculitis
    allergic v.
    hypersensitivity v.
    leukocytoclastic v.

    necrotizing v.
vasculolymphatic
vasectomize
vasectomy
vasoactive
    intestinal peptides, v. (VIP)
vasoepididymography
vaso-occlusive disease
vasopressin
vasotocin
vasovesiculectomy
VAT (vinblastine, Adriamycin, thiotepa)
VAT (vincristine, ara-A, 6-thioguanine)
VATD (vincristine, ara-C, 6-thioguanine,
    daunorubicin)
VATH (vinblastine, Adriamycin,
    thiotepa, Halotestin)
VAV (VP-16-213, Adriamycin,
    vincristine)
Vaxsyn HIV-1 vaccine
VBA (vincristine, BCNU, Adriamycin)
VBAP (vincristine, BCNU, Adriamycin,
    prednisone)
VBC (VePesid, BCNU,
    cyclophosphamide)
VBC (vinblastine, bleomycin, cisplatin)
VBD (vinblastine, bleomycin, DDP)
VBL (vinblastine)
VBM (vincristine, bleomycin,
    methotrexate)
VBMCP (vincristine, BCNU, melphalan,
    cyclophosphamide, prednisone)
VBMF (vincristine, bleomycin,
    methotrexate, 5-fluorouracil)
VBP (vinblastine, bleomycin, Platinol)
VC (vincristine)
VC (VP-16, carboplatin)
VCA (viral capsid antigen)
VCAP (vincristine, cyclophosphamide,
    Adriamycin, prednisone)
VCAP-I (VP-16, cyclophosphamide,
    Adriamycin, Platinol)
VCAP-III (VP-16-213,
    cyclophosphamide, Adriamycin,
    Platinol)
VCE (vaginal, cervical, endometrial)
    smears, V.
VCF (vincristine, cyclophosphamide,
    5-fluorouracil)
VCMP (vincristine, cyclophosphamide,
    melphalan, prednisone)
VCP (vincristine, cyclophosphamide,
    prednisone)

ADDITIONAL TERMS

VCP-1 (VP-16, cyclophosphamide, Platinol)
VCR (vincristine)
VD (venereal disease)
VDP (vinblastine, dacarbazine, Platinol)
VDP (vincristine, daunorubicin, prednisone)
VDS (vindesine)
VDT (video display terminal)
Vectastain kit
vection
vector
    biological v.
    cloning v.
    insect v.
    recombinant v.
vegetable
    calomel, v.
    fibrin, v.
vegetation
vegetative
veil cells
veiled cells
Vel blood group system
Velban (vinblastine sulfate)
Velbe
Velsar (vinblastine sulfate)
VEMP (vincristine, Endoxan, 6-mercaptopurine, prednisone)
Ven factor
venereal
    bubo, v.
    collar, v.
    disease, v. (VD)
    sore, v.
    urethritis, v.
    wart, v.
venipuncture
venogram
venography
veno-occlusive disease (VOD)
Venoglobulin-I
venom
    Russell viper v.
venothrombotic
venous
    invasion, v.
    stasis, v.
    thrombosis, v.
ventricular
    shunt, v.
ventriculography
ventriculoperitoneal (VP)

shunt, v.
Venuglobin I
venule
VePesid (etoposide or VP-16)
verapamil (R-verapamil or VPAM)
verazide
Vercyte (pipobroman)
verdohemin
verdohemochromogen
verdohemoglobin
verdoperoxidase
Veress needle
Verhoeff-van Gieson stain
vermian tumor
vermilionectomy
Vermox
Versene
Verner-Morrison syndrome
Vernet syndrome
Verneuil neuroma
vernolepin
Verocay bodies
verruca (pl. verrucae)
    acuminata, v.
    digitata, v.
    filiformis, v.
    plana, v.
    plantaris, v.
    vulgaris, v.
verrucae (pl. of verruca)
verruciform
verrucose
verrucosis
verrucous
    carcinoma, v.
    lesion, v.
    vegetation, v.
    wart, v.
VersaPulse holmium laser
vertebral
    body, v.
    collapse, v.
    disintegration, v.
vertiginous
vertigo
very high-density lipoproteins (VHDL)
very late-appearing antigen
very low-density lipoproteins (VLDL)
vesical
vesicle
vesicocolonic
vesicoperineal
vesicoprostatic

ADDITIONAL TERMS

vesicorectal
vesicostomy
vesicourethral
vesicouterine
vesicovaginal
vesicular
    stomatitis virus, v. (VSV)
vesiculobullous
vesiculopapular
VESP.2 antibody
VESP8.2 antibody
vestibulectomy
vestige
vestigial
veto
    cells, v.
    phenomenon, v.
v-fms gene
VH (viral hepatitis)
VHDL (very high-density lipoproteins)
VHL (von Hippel-Lindau) disease
Vi
    agglutination, V.
    agglutinin, V.
    antigen, V.
vibrio (pl. vibriones)
    NAG (nonagglutinating) v.
    nonagglutinating (NAG) v.
vibrion
    septique, v.
vibriones (pl. of vibrio)
vibriosis
VIC (vinblastine, ifosfamide, CCNU)
VIC (VP-16, ifosfamide, carboplatin)
Victoreen
    dosimeter, V.
    R-meter, V.
vidarabine (ara-A or Vira-A)
video display terminal (VDT)
Videx (didanosine or dideoxyinosine or
    ddI)
VIE (vincristine, ifosfamide, etoposide)
vif (virion infectivity factor)
VIG (vaccinia immune globulin)
Vigilon
Viliva
Villaret syndrome
villiform
villoadenoma
villoglandular
villoma
villonodular
    adenoma, v.

villose
villous
    adenoma, v.
    cancer, v.
    polyp, v.
villusectomy
vilona (inosine pranobex)
vimentin
VIMRxyn (hypericin)
Vim-Silverman needle
VIN (vaginal intraepithelial neoplasia)
VIN (vulvar intraepithelial neoplasia)
vinblastine sulfate (Alkaban-AQ or VBL
    or Velban or Velsar)
vinca
    alkaloid, v.
Vinca
    rosea Linn, v.
vincaleukoblastine (vinblastine)
Vincasar PFS (vincristine)
Vincent
    angina, V.
    infection, V.
    stomatitis, V.
vincristine sulfate (Oncovin or VC or
    VCR or Vincasar PFS)
vindesine sulfate (DAVA or Eldesine or
    VDS)
vinepidine sulfate
vinglycinate sulfate
vinleurosine sulfate
vinpocetine
vinorelbine (VOB)
vinrosidine sulfate
vinyl
    chloride, v.
    cyanide, v.
vinzolidine sulfate
viocid
violaceous
VIP (vasoactive intestinal peptides)
VIP (VePesid, ifosfamide, Platinol)
VIP chemotherapy pump
VIP-B (VP-16, ifosfamide, Platinol,
    bleomycin)
viper
    Russell v.
    Russell v. venom
vipoma (vasoactive intestinal
    polypeptide-secreting tumor)
    syndrome, v.
Vira-A (vidarabine)
viral

ADDITIONAL TERMS

viral—*Continued*
  budding, v.
  capsid antigen, v. (VCA)
  DNA, v.
  envelope protein, v.
  hepatitis, v. (VH)
  inactivation, v.
  neutralization, v.
  oncogenes, v. (v-onc)
  precursor, v.
  replication, v.
  ribonucleic acid, v. (VRNA)
  transcription, v.
ViraPap
viratyping
Virazole
Virchow
  cell, V.
  law, V.
  node, V.
viremia
virgin B-cell
virginium
viricidal
viricide
virile
virilism
virility
virilization
virilizing tumor
virion
  assembly, v.
  RNA, v.
Virogen test
virogene
virogenetic
viroid
virology
Vironostika ELISA AIDS screening test
Viroptic
virosis
virostatic
viroxime
Virozyme Injection
virulence
virulent
virulicidal
virus
  Abelson v.
  adeno-associated v.
  AIDS-associated v.
  arbor v.

  attenuated v.
  avian v.
  avian erythroblastosis v.
  avian leukosis v.
  avian myeloblastosis v.
  bacterial v.
  Bittner v.
  bovine leukemia v.
  C v.
  cancer-inducing v.
  Cas-Br-E v.
  CID (cytomegalic inclusion disease)
    v.
  coxsackie-v.
  cytomegalic v. (CMV)
  cytomegalic inclusion disease (CID)
    v.
  defective v.
  dengue v.
  DNA v.
  EB (Epstein-Barr) v.
  ECHO (enteric cytopathogenic
    human orphan) v.
  enteric v.
  enteric cytopathogenic human
    orphan (ECHO) v.
  enteric orphan v.
  Epstein-Barr (EB) v.
  FBJ osteosarcoma v.
  feline leukemia v.
  feline sarcoma v.
  filterable v.
  filtrable v.
  fixed v.
  Friend murine v.
  gibbon ape lymphosarcoma v.
    (GALV)
  granulosis v.
  Harvey sarcoma v.
  helper v.
  hemadsorption v. type I and II
  hemagglutinating v.
  hepatitis A v. (HAV)
  hepatitis B v. (HBV)
  hepatitis C v. (HCV)
  hepatitis delta v.
  hepatitis E v.
  herpes simplex v.
  herpes zoster v.
  HIV (human immunodeficiency) v.
  human immunodeficiency v. (HIV)
  human mammary tumor v.

ADDITIONAL TERMS

human T-cell leukemia v. (HLTV)
human T-cell lymphoma v. (HLTV)
human T-cell lymphotrophic v.
 (HLTV)
infectious wart v.
influenza v.
JC v.
Kirsten sarcoma v.
latent v.
Latino v.
LAV (lymphadenopathy-associated)
 v.
Lucké v.
lymphadenopathy-associated v.
 (LAV)
lytic v.
M-25 v.
mammary tumor v.
Marburg v.
masked v.
Mason Pfizer monkey v.
MC29 myelocytomatosis v.
McKrae strain herpes-v.
MH2 v.
Moloney sarcoma v.
Mossuril v.
mouse mammary tumor v.
murine leukemia v.
murine sarcoma v.
neurotropic v.
non-A hepatitis v.
non-B hepatitis v.
nononcogenic v.
Norwalk v.
oncogenic v.
orphan v's
papilloma v.
parainfluenza v.
polyoma v.
Rauscher leukemia v.
respiratory syncytial v. (RSV)
retro-v.
RNA v.
rota-v.
Rous-associated v. (RAV)
Rous sarcoma v. (RSV)
St. Louis encephalitis v.
salivary gland v.
sarcoma v.
Schwartz leukemia v.
simian v.
simian 40 v's (SV 40)

simian AIDS v.
simian foamy v. (SFV)
simian immunodeficiency v.
simian sarcoma v.
slow v.
T-cell lymphotropic v.
tick-borne v.
tobacco mosaic v.
tumor v.
vacuolating v.
varicella-zoster v. (VZV)
vesicular stomatitis v.
visnamaedi v.
wart v.
Yamaguchi sarcoma v.
virus-associated hemophagocytic
 syndrome (VAHS)
virus-induced interferon
virus-like infectious agent (VLIA)
virus-like particle (VLP)
virus-specific
virustatic
viscera (pl. of viscus)
visceral
viscerography
visceromegaly
viscid
viscosimeter
viscosimetry
viscosity
viscous
Viscum
 album, V.
viscus (pl. viscera)
Visidex
visnamaedi virus
visor flap
visual analogue scale
visualization
Vita Carn
vital status of patient (alive, dead, or
 unknown)
vitamin
 deficiency, v.
vitrification
vitrogen
vividialysis
vividiffusion
Vivonex
v-kit gene
Vladimiroff-Mikulicz amputation
VLB (vinblastine)

ADDITIONAL TERMS

VLDL (very low-density lipoproteins)
VLIA (virus-like infectious agent)
VLP (virus-like particle)
VLP (vincristine, L-asparaginase, prednisone)
VM-26 (teniposide)
VM-26 (epidophyllotoxin)
VMA (vanillylmandelic acid)
VMAD (vincristine, methotrexate, Adriamycin, actinomycin D)
Vmax (maximum velocity)
VMC (VP-16, methotrexate, citrovorum factor)
VMCP (vincristine, melphalan, cyclophosphamide, prednisone)
v-mil gene
VMP (VePesid, mitoxantrone, prednimustine)
VOB (vinorelbine)
VOCA (VP-16, Oncovin, cyclophosphamide, Adriamycin)
vocal
    cords, v.
    cordectomy, v.
VOCAP (VP-16–213, Oncovin, cyclophosphamide, Adriamycin, Platinol)
VOD (veno-occlusive disease)
Voges-Proskauer test
voice
    button, v.
    prosthesis, v.
Voicebak
Volidan
Vollmer test
volt (V)
    gigaelectron v. (GeV)
    kiloelectron v. (keV)
    megaelectron v. (MeV)
voltage
Voltoline sign
volume dose
volumetric pump
Volutrol
vomit
vomiting
    anticipatory v.
    delayed v.
    intractable v.
vomiturition
vomitus
von Gierke disease
von Haberer

gastrectomy, v.
gastroenterostomy, v.
von Haberer-Aquirre gastrectomy
von Haberer-Finney anastomosis
von Hippel-Lindau (VHL) disease
von Jaksch
    anemia, v.
    disease, v.
von Meyenburg complex
von Recklinghausen
    disease, v.
    neurofibromatosis, v.
    tumor, v.
von Willebrand
    antigen, v.
    disease, v.
    factor, v. (vWF)
von Zeynek and Mencki test
VP (ventriculoperitoneal)
    shunt, V.
VP (vincristine, prednisone)
VP-16 (VePesid or etoposide)
VP-16 + DDP (etoposide, cisplatin)
VP-16-P (VP-16, Platinol)
VP-16213 or VP-16-213 (VP-16)
VP + A (vincristine, prednisone, L-asparaginase)
VPAM (verapamil)
VPB (vinblastine, Platinol, bleomycin)
VPBCPr (vincristine, prednisone, vinblastine, chlorambucil, procarbazine)
VPCA (vincristine, prednisone, cyclophosphamide, ara-C)
VPCMF (vincristine, prednisone, cyclophosphamide, methotrexate, 5-fluorouracil)
VPL (ventro-posterolateral)
    thalamic electrode, V.
VP + L-Asparaginase (vincristine, prednisone, L-asparaginase)
VPP (VePesid, Platinol)
vpr (viral protein r)
vpu (viral protein u)
VPVCP (vincristine, prednisone, vinblastine, chlorambucil, procarbazine)
Vr antigen
VRNA (viral ribonucleic acid)
Vs antigen
VSG (variant surface glycoprotein)
    gene, V.
v-src gene

ADDITIONAL TERMS

VSV (vesicular stomatitis virus)
VTF factor
vulva
vulvar
>   biopsy, v.
>   carcinoma, v.
>   condylomata, v.
>   intraepithelial neoplasia, v. (VIN)
>   leukoplakia, v.
>   vestibulitis syndrome, v.
vulvectomy
>   skinning v.
vulvitis
>   gangrenous v.
>   leukoplakic v.
>   mycotic v.
vulvorectal
vulvouterine
vulvovaginal
vulvovaginectomy
vulvovaginitis
Vumon
vWF (von Willebrand factor)
VX (venous invasion cannot be assessed)
VZ (varicella zoster)
VZIG (varicella-zoster immune globulin)
VZV (varicella-zoster virus)

W

W (tungsten or wehnelt)
W factor
Waaler-Rose test
Wagner test
WAK (wearable artificial kidney)
Waldenström macroglobulinemia
Waldeyer ring
Walker
>   carcinoma, W.
>   carcinoma cell, W.
>   carcinosarcoma 256, W.
>   sarcoma, W.
Wallhouser and Whitehead method
Walthard
>   inclusions, W.
>   islets, W.
wandering
>   abscess, w.
>   cells, w.
war gases
Warburg
>   apparatus, W.
>   effect, W.
warfarin

potassium, w.
sodium, w.
Waring blender syndrome
warm
>   agglutination, w.
>   agglutinins, w.
>   antibody, w.
>   hemagglutinin, w.
>   -reactive antibody, w.
Warren splenorenal shunt
wart
>   fig w.
>   genital w.
>   pitch w's
>   soot w.
>   vaginal w's
>   venereal w.
wart virus
Wartenberg symptom
Warthin
>   cell, W.
>   tumor, W.
Warthin-Finkeldey cells
Warthin-Starry stain
warty
WAS (Wiskott-Aldrich syndrome)
washed
>   platelets, w.
>   red blood cells, w. (WRBC)
>   red cells, w. (WRC)
washings
>   bronchial w.
>   gastric w.
>   nasopharyngeal w.
>   peritoneal w.
wasted appearance
wasting
>   disease, w.
>   syndrome, w.
watery diarrhea
Watson-Crick
>   helix, W.
>   pairing, W.
Watson-Ehrlich reaction
Watson-Schwartz test
wave mechanics
wavelength
>   effective w.
>   equivalent w.
>   minimum w.
waxy
>   degeneration, w.
>   spleen, w.

ADDITIONAL TERMS

Wayne State protocol
WBC (white blood cells)
WBC (white blood count)
WBC/hpf (white blood cells per high power field)
WBF (whole blood folate)
WBH (whole blood hematocrit)
WBH (whole-body hyperthermia)
WBR (whole-body radiation)
WBS (whole-body scan)
WC (white cell)
WCC (white cell count)
WDHA (watery diarrhea, hypokalemia, achlorhydria) syndrome
WDLL (well-differentiated lymphocytic lymphoma)
weaned off
wearable artificial kidney (WAK)
Weber syndrome
wedge
    isodose angle w.
    liver biopsy w.
    port w.
    step w.
wedge biopsy
wedge filter
wedge resection
wedged
    field, w.
    lateral portals, w.
    pair, w.
wedging
Wegener
    granulomatosis, W.
    syndrome, W.
WEHI-3 cell line
wehnelt (W)
Weibel-Palade body
Weigert iron hematoxylin stain
Weil syndrome
Weingarten syndrome
Welcker method
well
    -circumscribed, w.
    -collimated megavoltage radiation beam, w.
    -defined, w.
    -demarcated, w.
    -differentiated, w.
    -differentiated lymphocytic lymphoma, w. (WDLL)
    -epithelialized, w.
    -marginated, w.

Well counter calibration source
Well-Cogen test
Wellcovorin (leucovorin)
Wellferon (interferon alfa-n1)
Werlhof disease
Wermer syndrome
Werner syndrome
Wernicke encephalopathy
Wertheim radical hysterectomy
Westergren
    method, W.
    sedimentation rate, W.
Westermark sign
Western
    blot test, W.
    blotting, W.
Western Electric Electrolarynx
Westhroid
wet colostomy
Wharton
    duct, W.
    tumor, W.
wheat germ agglutinin
Wheeless method
whey
    protein concentrate, w.
Whipple
    disease, W.
    procedure, W.
    triad, W.
white
    blood cell, w. (WBC)
    blood cells per high power field, w. (WBC/hpf)
    blood count, w. (WBC)
    cell, w. (WC)
    cell count, w. (WCC)
    clot syndrome, w.
    gangrene, w.
    matter, w.
    matter necrosis, w.
    radiation, w.
    softening, w.
Whitmore
    bacillus, W.
    disease, W.
WHO (World Health Organization)
    classification, W.
whole blood
    folate, w. (WBF)
    hematocrit, w. (WBH)
whole-body
    counter, w.

ADDITIONAL TERMS

hyperthermia, w. (WBH)
irradiation, w.
proton magnetic resonance
    imaging, w.
radiation, w. (WBR)
scan, w. (WBS)
scanner, w.
synthesis, w.
whole-brain irradiation
whole-lymphocyte fraction
whole-pelvis irradiation
whole saliva
whole-virus enzyme immunoassay
Widal
    reaction, W.
    syndrome, W.
Widal-Abrami disease
wide
    excision, w.
    -field external beam, w.
    -field radiation, w.
widespread metastases
Wilbrand prism test
wild allele
Wilder
    diet, W.
    sign, W.
wild-type
    cell, w.
    gene, w.
    virion, w.
Will Rogers phenomenon
Willebrand syndrome
Williams
    factor, W.
    sign, W.
Williamson blood test
Wills factor
Wilms
    nephroblastoma, W.
    tumor, W.
Wilson
    chamber, W.
    disease, W.
Winckel disease
window
    hypothesis, w.
    period, w.
Winston glioma
Winterbottom sign
Wintrich sign
Wintrobe
    hematocrit, W.

indices, W.
macromethod, W.
method, W.
Wintrobe and Landsberg method
Wiskott-Aldrich syndrome (WAS)
Wistar rats
Witzel gastrostomy
witzelsucht
Wobemugos
wobble hypothesis
Woldman test
Wolfe
    breast dysplasia, W.
    cheiloplasty, W.
    mammographic parenchymal
        pattern, W.
Wolff-Junghans test
Wollner system
Wolman disease
Wood light
Woodes-Fildes theory
Wookey
    neck flap, W.
    radical neck dissection, W.
Woringer-Kolopp
    disease, W.
    syndrome, W.
works (drug paraphernalia)
World Health Organization (WHO)
    classification, W.
Woronet trait
WR-2529
WR-2721 (ethiofos)
WR-2823
WR-6388
WRBC (washed red blood cells)
WRC (washed red cells)
Wright
    blood group system, W.
    stain, W.
W-shaped ileal pouch
Wu-Kabat plot
Wuchereria
    bancrofti, W.
Wymox

X

X (Kienbock unit of x-ray
    dose)
X body
X chromosome
X factor
X histiocytosis

X-linked
  agammaglobulinemia, X.
  disorders, X.
  gene, X.
  familial hypophosphatemia, X.
  hypogammaglobulinemia, X.
  infantile agammaglobulinemia,
    X.
  lymphoproliferative disease, X.
X particle
X porphyria
x radiation
xa factor
xanthelasma
xanthelasmatosis
xanthematin
xanthemia
xanthin
xanthine
  oxidase inhibitor, x.
xanthoderma
xanthoerythrodermia
  perstans, x.
xanthofibroma
  thecocellulare, x.
xanthogranuloma
  juvenile x.
xanthoma
  craniohypophyseal x.
  diabetic x.
  diabeticorum, x.
  disseminated x.
  disseminatum, x.
  eruptive x.
  eruptivum, x.
  generalized x.
  multiplex, s.
  planar x.
  plane x.
  planum, x.
  striatum palmare, x.
  tendinous x.
  tendinosum, x.
  tuberoeruptive x.
  tuberosum, x.
  tuberosum multiplex, x.
  tuberous x.
xanthoma cell
xanthomatosis
  biliary hypercholesterolemic x.
  bulbi, x.
  cerebrotendinous x.
  chronic idiopathic x.
  corneae, x.

  generalisata ossium, x.
  iridis, x.
  primary familial x.
  Wolman x.
xanthomatous
xanthopsis
xanthosarcoma
xanthosine
  monophosphate, x. (XMP)
xanthosis
Xe (xenon)
  127 radioaerosol, X.
  133, X.
  133 inhalation method, X.
  133 washout, X.
XECT (xenon-enhanced computed
  tomography)
xenembole
xenenthesis
xenoantigen
xenobiotic
xenogeneic
xenogenous
xenograft
xenon (Xe)
  127, x.
  133, x.
  arc lamp, x.
  -enhanced computer tomography,
    x.
  133 radioisotope, x.
  scan, x.
xenoplated tumor cell
Xenopus
  laevis, X.
xenotransplantation
xerocytosis
xeroderma
  pigmented x.
  pigmentosum, x. (XP)
xerodermoid
  pigmented x.
xerogram
xerography
xeromammogram
xeromammography
xeroradiograph
xeroradiography
xerosialography
xerosis
xerostomia
xerotes
xerotic
xerotomography

ADDITIONAL TERMS

XES (x-ray energy spectrometry)
Xg blood group system
Xga blood group system
XM (crossmatch)
XMG (x-ray mammogram)
XMP (xanthosine monophosphate)
XomaZyme
   -H65, X
   -791, X.
Xomed endotracheal tube
XP (xeroderma pigmentosum)
x-ray
   absorptiometry, x.
   alopecia, x.
   bath, x.
   beam, x.
   burn, x.
   contamination, x.
   crystallography, x.
   dermatitis, x.
   diffraction, x.
   dosage, x.
   emission spectrum, x.
   energy spectrometry, x. (XES)
   mammogram, x. (XMG)
   orthovoltage, x.
   photon, x.
   spectrometer, x.
   spectrum, x.
   target, x.
   template, x.
   therapy, x. (XRT)
   unit, x.
XRT (x-ray therapy)
x-strahlen
XTT reagent
Xylocaine
   jelly, X.
   spray, X.
   viscous, X.
xylose

Y y (prefix which identifies classification that was performed during or following initial multimodality therapy. Used with TNM or pTNM categories.)
Y (yttrium)
   87, Y.
   88, Y.
   90 isotope, Y.
   91, Y.

Y bodies
Y chromosome
Y-linked gene
Y protein
YAC (yeast artificial chromosome)
YAG (yttrium-aluminum-garnet)
   laser, Y.
Yakima hemoglobin
Yalow technique
Yamada-type III lesion
Yamaguchi sarcoma virus
Yates continuity correction
yaws
Ya Yan Tzu
Yb (ytterbium)
   -169 DTPA, Y.
YC8 lymphoma
yeast
   artificial chromosome, y. (YAC)
   artificial chromosome clone, y.
   eluate factor, y.
   nucleic acid, y.
yellow
   bone marrow, y.
   enzymes, y.
   jaundice, y.
   nail syndrome, y.
Yergason sign
Yersin serum
Yersinia
   enterocolitica, Y.
   pestis, Y.
   pseudotuberculosis, Y.
yersiniosis
yes oncogene
Yew
   English Y.
   Pacific Y.
y-interferon
Yo antigen
Yodoxin
yoga
yolk sac (YS)
   carcinoma, y. (YSC)
   tumor, y.
York antigen
young form
YS (yolk sac)
YSC (yolk sac carcinoma)
Yt antigen
ytterbium (Yb)
   -169 DTPA, y.
yttrium (Y)
   90 isotope, y.

ADDITIONAL TERMS

yttrium—*Continued*
    -aluminum-garnet, y. (YAG)
    hypophysectomy, y.
    pellets, y.

Zz

Z antigen
Z-bank
Z-line
Z-plasty
Z protein
Z-technique
Zacopride
Zahn lines
zalcitabine
Zanosar (streptozocin)
Zantac
Zappacosta test
Zavala lung biopsy needle
Z-DNA left-handed helix
ZDV (zidovudine)
ZDX (goserelin)
Zefazone (cefmetazole)
Zelsmyr Cytobrush
Zen macrobiotic diet
zeniplatin
Zenker
    fixative, Z.
    necrosis, Z.
zeolite
zero order kinetics
Zervas hypophysectomy kit
ZES (Zollinger-Ellison syndrome)
zeta
    potential, z.
    sedimentation rate, z. (ZSR)
    stimulation ratio, z. (ZSR)
zetacrit
Zetafuge
zidovudine (Retrovir or ZDV)
Ziehl-Neelsen
    carbolfuchsin, Z.
    stain, Z.
Zieve syndrome
ZIG (zoster immune globulin)
Zimmerman elementary particles
zinc (Zn)
    atom, z.
    -binding, z.
    chloride, z.
    chloride paste, z.
    finger, z.
    -finger motif, z.

    -finger protein, z.
    -finger structure, z.
    metalloendopeptidase, z.
    sulfate, z.
zinostatin
Zinser-Cole-Engman syndrome
zinviroxime
ZIP (zoster immune plasma)
zirconium (Zr)
    granuloma, z.
Zithromax (azithromycin)
Zixoryn
Zn (zinc)
Zofran (ondansetron)
Zoladex (goserelin)
Zollinger-Ellison
    syndrome, Z. (ZES)
    tumor, Z.
zonal
zonation pattern
zone
    electrophoresis, z.
zoning
zonostatin
zoo-agglutinin
zoografting
zooprecipitin
zootoxin
zorubicin hydrochloride
zoster
    auricularis, z.
    dermatomal z.
    herpes z.
    ophthalmic z.
    ophthalmicus, z.
zoster immune globulin (ZIG)
zoster immune plasma (ZIP)
zosteriform
zosteroid
Zostrix
Zovickian nape-of-the-neck flap
Zovirax (acyclovir)
Zr (zirconium)
ZSR (zeta sedimentation rate)
ZSR (zeta stimulation ratio)
Zurich hemoglobin
Zwanck radium pessary
zwitterion
zwitterionic
zygomycosis
zymogenic cells
zymoplastic substance
zymosan

ADDITIONAL TERMS